POSITIONING
IN
K C Clark, MBE, FSR
Volume Two
RADIOGRAPHY
NINTH EDITION

Revised by James McInnes, FSR, TE, FRPS

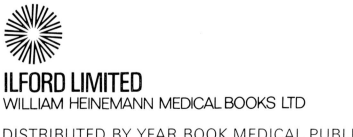

ILFORD LIMITED
WILLIAM HEINEMANN MEDICAL BOOKS LTD

DISTRIBUTED BY YEAR BOOK MEDICAL PUBLISHERS INC

First edition published in January 1939
Second edition published in January 1941
Third edition published in June 1942
Fourth edition published in April 1945
Fifth edition published in October 1949
Sixth edition published in February 1951
Seventh edition published in December 1956
Eighth edition published in July 1964
Eighth edition (revised) published in May 1967
Ninth edition (Volume 2) published 1974

ISBN 0-8151-1751-5

Library of Congress Catalog Card No. 73-90464

Distributed in Continental North, South and Central America,
Hawaii, Puerto Rico and The Phillipines by

Year Book Medical Publishers Inc
35 East Wacker Drive, Chicago

by arrangement with William Heinemann Medical Books Ltd.

Set in 10/12 pt Monotype Times New Roman, printed by letterpress
in Great Britain at The Pitman Press, Bath

INTRODUCTION

Miss K C Clark was principal of the ILFORD Department of Radiography and Medical Photography at Tavistock House, from 1935 to 1958. She had an intense interest in the teaching and development of radiographic positioning and procedure, which resulted in an invitation, by ILFORD LIMITED in 1935, to produce the publication, Positioning In Radiography, this present revised edition being the ninth edition. Her enthusiasm in all matters pertaining to this subject was so infectious and convincing, that a visit by students and radiographers to the Department was always a gratifying experience. Ably assisted by her colleagues, she was responsible for many innovations in the field of radiography, playing a notable part in the development of mass miniature radiography. Her ability and ever active endeavour to cement team-work between radiologist and radiographer gained her worldwide respect.

In 1959 she was elected an Honorary member of the Faculty of Radiologists, having been elected to Honorary Fellowship, of the British Society of Radiographers, at the conclusion of her tenure of office as President of the Society. Following this, during her visit to Australia in 1959 she was also elected to the Honorary Fellowship of the Australasian Institute of Radiography in recognition of her services to Radiography. Miss Clark died in 1968 and the Kathleen Clark Memorial Library established by the Society of Radiographers, at their premises in Upper Wimpole Street, is a fitting tribute to the respect which she commanded among radiographers and radiologists the world-over.

The continuing need for this standard work on Radiographic techniques has resulted in the publication of this, the ninth edition of Positioning In Radiography in two volumes, edited and revised by James McInnes FSR, TE, FRPS. Mr McInnes' involvement with Positioning In Radiography began in 1946 when he joined a team based at the Ilford Department of Radiography at Tavistock House in London.

Primarily concerned with teaching and investigating techniques, Mr McInnes has originated many aspects of radiography, including simultaneous contact and enlargement, multiple radiography and selective filtration, His numerous articles on tomography and associated subjects have contributed widely to radiography. In 1958 Mr McInnes became Principal of Lecture and Technical Services at Tavistock House, a position which enabled him to travel extensively throughout the world as lecturer to the X-ray Societies of Britain, Canada, America, South and West Africa.

He is a fellow of the Society of Radiographers and the Royal Photographic Society and a member of the British Institute of Radiology.

Mr McInnes' long and close association with every aspect of radiographic technique has provided an eminently suitable framework upon which to construct this up-dated authoritative work which will prove invaluable to student and established radiographer alike.

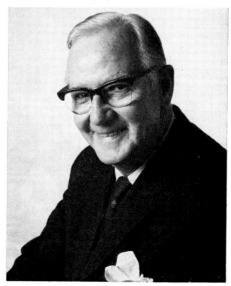

ACKNOWLEDGEMENTS

NINTH EDITION

In compiling this ninth edition of Positioning In Radiography the decision has been taken to divide the text into two volumes; part I embracing routine radiography and part II the ever growing field of specialized radiography.

In so doing, a more extensive coverage of each subject, in both volumes has been possible.

In view of the constant addition to the text in the previous eight editions, cross-reference had become excessive and a re-framing of text and illustrations has been prepared to provide a more convenient system.

The new format is in keeping with the recently published Teachers' Syllabus of the Society of Radiographers, in that the sequence of presentation consists of Basic Positioning, to indicate essential techniques for the benefit of student radiographers, supplemented by follow-up stages of *Alternative Techniques* to assist in producing the necessary diagnostic information when dealing with the less co-operative patient to "Additional" views which provide the experienced radiographer with further choice in assisting the Radiologist where, due to the discreet nature of the pathology or injury, diagnosis may be difficult.

Particular thought has been given to the inclusion of additional techniques and where these have been assessed to provide a useful practical alternative they have been added to the appropriate section, to compliment routine procedure.

Over two hundred new photographic illustrations have been incorporated in this new edition. Renewal of considerable previous illustration has taken place, to both up-date and improve the accuracy of presentation. Photographic illustration of all additional techniques has also been included.

In the production of these I am indebted to the photographic artistry and skill of Mr Michael Barrington-Martin.

I am pleased to acknowledge the considerable assistance given by GEC Medical Equipment Limited (Wembley) who, on two occasions, installed the necessary X-ray equipment in the photographic studios and to Sierex Limited and Philips Medical Systems Ltd on further occasions. The accuracy and convenience required, to present photographs of radiographic positioning technique, is largely a function of having good X-ray equipment, and on each occasion we were well served in this respect.

In connection with the above I am also indebted to Leslies Limited (Polyfoam Division) for the use of their Polyfoam positioning aids and foam table mattress, these proved a major factor in comfort, convenience and positional accuracy.

My thanks are also due to Miss H M Fowles MSR, Westminster Hospital X-ray Department for providing the facilities for photographing the tomographic positioning techniques. Thanks are also due to Miss D M Chesney, Hon FSR, TE, Coventry and Warwickshire Hospital for permission to adapt her article, "Acute Abdomen Emergency" within the format of Positioning In Radiography.

Consultation is a very necessary feature in the preparation of descriptive and accurate text, in this respect I am indebted to the following:
Miss S J Smith FSR and Mr J Causton FSR, Salford College of Technology.
Mr E Higginbottom MSR, Lodge Moor Hospital, Sheffield. Mr W J Stripp, Royal National Orthopaedic Hospital, London. Miss M England FSR, and Mr Norman Baldock FSR, Royal Northern Hospital, London.Thanks are due to Mr J Coote for making available the X-ray room facilities at Tavistock House, in order to clarify many of the problems associated with positioning technique.
Mr Kenneth Lawley and Mr Michael Smith have been responsible for the design and production of the 9th edition in the new two volume form. I am most grateful for their valued co-operation.

My thanks are due to the directors of CIBA-GEIGY Limited for making this edition possible and allowing me to be associated with this acknowledged world-wide authoritative work on radiographic positioning.

In preparing the ninth edition of Positioning In Radiography we wish to acknowledge the radiographic illustration content from the following sources:

Albert Einstein Medical Center, Philadelphia, USA
Dr J Gershon-Cohen and Miss Barbara M Curcio

Bradford Royal Infirmary, Yorkshire
Dr R J Carr

Bristol Royal Hospital, Royal Infirmary Branch
Dr J H Middlemiss

Brompton Hospital, London
Dr L G Blair and Miss V G Jones

Child Study Centre, University of London, Institute of Education and Child Health
Dr J M Tanner, group investigations

Children's Hospital Medical Center, Boston, USA
Dr E B D Neuhauser and Dr M H Wittenborg, Mr Eric Hammond

Chorley and District Hospital, Lancashire
Dr G Sullivan

Cuckfield Hospital, Sussex
Miss H E M Noller

Dublin
Dr T Garratt Hardman

Halifax, Yorkshire
Dr R I Lewis

Harefield Hospital, Middlesex
Dr L G Blair, Mr V C Snell and Mr A W Holder

Hospital for Sick Children, London
Dr L G Blair, Dr G N Weber, also Miss H Nicol and Miss M Riocreux

Hospital for Sick Children, Toronto, Canada
Dr J D Munn, Mr Richard Harmes, Mr Walter Johns, also Mr L J Cartwright

Ipswich and East Suffolk Hospital
Miss S M Stockley

Johnson and Johnson (Great Britain) Limited, Slough, Buckinghamshire

Lodge Moor Hospital, Sheffield, Yorkshire
Dr T Lodge and Mr E Higginbottom

London Hospital
Dr J J Rae and Miss F M A Vaughan

Department for Research in Industrial Medicine
Dr L J Rae, Dr A I G McLaughlin and Miss F M A Vaughan

Maidenhead Hospital, Berkshire
Dr A W Simmins, Mr David W Bain and Miss A Crofton

Manchester Royal Infirmary, Lancashire
Dr E D Gray, Dr R G Reid

Medical Arts X-ray Department, Niagara Falls, Canada
Mr Lewis Edwards

Melrose-Wakefield Hospital, Massachusetts, USA
Dr William E Davis and Mr Clarence W Coupe

Memorial Hospital, Cirencester, Gloucestershire
Dr G C Griffiths

Memorial Hospital, New York City, USA
Dr Robert S Sherman and Dr George Schwarz

Middlesex Hospital, London
Dr F Campbell Golding and Miss H J Weller, Dr M J McLoughlin and Miss Marion Frank

Mulago Hospital, Kampala, Uganda
Dr A G M Davies

National Hospital, Queen Square, London
Dr Hugh W Davies, Dr J W D Bull, Mr Harvey Jackson and Mr Peter Gortvai, Dr J Marryat, Mr A M Hastin Bennett, Mr A E Prickett, Miss A M Hamilton, Mr L S Walsh

National Heart Hospital, London
Dr Peter Kerley, CVO, CBE and Miss K M A Pritchard

New Britain Hospital, Connecticut, USA
Dr John C Larkin and Mr Nicholas R Barraco

Newcastle General Hospital, Newcastle-Upon-Tyne
Dr S Josephs

New England Center Hospital, Pratt Diagnostic Clinic, Boston, USA
Dr Alice Ettinger

Nuffield Orthopaedic Centre, Oxford (Wingfield Morris Orthopaedic Hospital)
Dr F H Kemp, Dr J L Boldero, Mr J Agerholm, Miss B Robbins

NV Optische Industrie 'De Oude Delft', Holland

Prince of Wales's General Hospital, London
Dr A Elkeles

Queen Victoria Hospital, Plastic Surgery and Jaw Injuries Centre, East Grinstead, Sussex
Dr William Campbell

Radcliffe Infirmary, Oxford
Dr F H Kemp

Robert Jones and Agnes Hunt Orthopaedic Hospital, Oswestry, Shropshire
Dr J W Foy, Mr J Rowland Hughes, Mr F B Thomas, Mr R Roaf and Mr W G Davies

Royal Cornwall Infirmary, Truro
Dr H S Bennett, Mr J G Kendall, Mrs V Wheaton

Royal Dental Hospital, London
Dr Sydney Blackman, Miss D O Gibb and Mrs D White

Royal Hospital, Sheffield, Yorkshire
Dr T Lodge and Mr G W Delahaye

Royal Marsden Hospital, London
Dr J J Stevenson, Dr J S McDonald, Dr E J Pick

Royal National Orthopaedic Hospital, London
Dr F Campbell Golding, Mr J N Wilson, Mr C W S F Manning, Mr J I P James, Mr W J Stripp

Royal National Orthopaedic Hospital, Brockley Hill, Stanmore, Middlesex
Dr F Campbell Golding, Mr J N Wilson, Mr C V S F Manning

Royal Northern Hospital, London
Dr L S Carstairs, Mr A M Hastin Bennett, and Miss M J England, Mr N Baldock

Royal Portsmouth Hospital, Hampshire
Dr R S MacHardy

St Anthony's Hospital, Cheam, Surrey
Mr Aubrey York Mason

St Mary's Hospitals for Women and Children, Manchester
Dr J Blair Hartley and Miss A Stirling Fisher

St Thomas's Hospital, London
Dr J W McLaren

St Vincent's Hospital, New York City, USA
Dr Francis F Ruzicka Jnr, and Dr M M Schechter

St Vincent's Orthopaedic Hospital, Eastcote, Pinner, Middlesex
Dr L G Blair, Mr V C Snell and Sister Francis

Salford Royal Hospital, Lancashire
Dr A H McCallum

Stuttgart, Germany
Dr Georg Thieme Verlag

Sydney, Australia
Dr Majorie Dalgarno

Temple University Hospital, Philadelphia, USA
Professor Herbert M Stauffer and Miss Margaret J McGann

The Hague, Holland
Dr V Fiorani

Universiteit Van Amsterdam, Holland
Professor Dr B G Ziedses des Plantes

University College Hospital, London
Dr David Edwards, Dr M E Grossmann, Dr M E Sidaway and Mrs S Gordon and Sister H Quirke

War Memorial Children's Hospital, London Ontario, Canada
Dr D S Rajic and Mr Bryan Fisher

Westminster Hospital, London
Dr B Strickland, Dr Roger Pyle and Dr S Holesh

Weston-Super-Mare General Hospital, Somerset
Dr H B Howell and Mr E J Quick, Mrs S S Duncan

Women's College Hospital, Toronto, Canada
Dr M E Forbes, Dr Jean Toews and Mrs Elizabeth Mills

REVIEW OF EXPOSURE TABLES

Exposure table section

It should be understood that the quoted exposures are included for guidance only, and that it is not possible to give more than relative data on each section for any particular region. These are however sufficiently compatible to the region to produce an acceptable result. The beginner, however, and those less familiar with the many variants involved, namely kilovoltage, milliampere-seconds, focus–film distance, film/screen, and grid or non-grid approach will perhaps welcome this guidance.

The output of modern X-ray apparatus has been considerably extended and in conjunction with this, the selection of exposure time from milleseconds upwards, the required film density being provided by adjustment of either milliamperage up to 1000 mA or the application of an extended kilovoltage range up to 150 kVp where applicable.

It is only by fully understanding how to balance these available factors that the radiographer is able to make such adjustment as to produce radiographs of high technical quality and diagnostic value as a matter of routine, which is the purpose of every X-ray department. This ability to make quick factor exchange calculations, is only acquired by experience of actual departmental work, and the beginner is advised to work to a recommended selection of these factors in the form of an exposure chart.

The constant study of radiographic results will then allow full appreciation of the manipulation of milliampere-seconds to control subject movement, and provide the required film density, and the choice of kilovoltage with respect to the provision of adequate penetration and the scale of subject contrast required.

There is, unfortunately, no fixed standard of contrast and density for any specified region and the radiographic quality sought is that, which should be thought best suited to the requirements of the individual radiologist. Fortunately the tolerance of the modern X-ray film in exposure latitude is such that subjective preference can be provided for.

Kilovoltage

Kilovoltage refers to the tension across the X-ray tube. Its waveform also determines the uniformity in wavelength of the X-rays emitted, most X-ray circuitry today passes virtually constant potential waveform to the target resulting in a close to homeogenity of wave-length and consequently high efficiency of the emerging X-ray beam.

The kilovoltage determines the degree of penetration of the rays and has a major influence on the contrast of the radiograph, higher kilovoltage is required as the part thickness increases to produce adequate penetration.

Initially a relative kilovoltage for each part-thickness should be formulated in the mind and eventually with experience will come the knowledge if it is necessary to diverge from this principle.

The choice of optimum kilovoltage allows the subject detail to be readily perceived in its entirety due to adequate penetration.

Where the kilovoltage is too low the image will lack detail due to under-penetration of the subject and will exhibit excessive contrast.

Correspondingly if the kilovoltage is too high, excessive penetration will reduce the radiographic contrast to too low a level to readily perceive detail.

Optimum Kilovoltage, which portrays the fact that there is a Kilovoltage value for each part which, while ensuring adequate penetration also minimizes the effect of scattered radiation and as a consequence results in maximum radiographic contrast. The application of the above is of paramount importance where the subject contrast is low, and there is a limited subject range. Where maximum radiographic contrast is desired, the system is suited to radiographic procedures, but where extenuating circumstances are present these may necessitate a variation in the choice of kilovoltage in order that further conditions may be satisfied.

Gradually we are able to appreciate the necessity for changes in these values for

(a) Variation from average thickness.
(b) Variation in individual thickness of the part.
(c) Steep changes of subject opacity within the area to be X-rayed.

In a subject with widely varying regional absorption differences the conventional kilovoltage level for part thickness would produce excessive contrast, in such an instance, an increase of 20–30 kilovolts is required to reduce the steep absorption differences, to ensure more uniform exposure throughout the subject range.

(d) Change necessary due to variation from the normal, eg. Pathology and type of Pathology.
(e) Increased subject contrast due to the introduction of contrast media.

The choice of kilovoltage to control the density of the radiograph is also becoming more prevalent than in the past.

Reason for this is primarily to minimize excessive heat loading of the target area.

This danger is present in examinations which necessitate repetitive exposures, eg. Angiography, Cineradiography, Tomography, etc.

Similarly, increasing the kilovoltage to attain the density required on the film permits a greater range of subject investigations within the rating of smaller foci and maintains greater accuracy in the focal spot dimension thereby improving definition.

The reduction in exposure time is also in keeping with adequate ellimination of subject movement.

The following provides an approximate guide as to the increased kilovoltage value required to reduce the milliamperage or millesecond exposure by half.

Range
40–60	7KVP increment
60–85	10KVP increment
85–100	15KVP increment
100–120	20KVP increment
120–150	25KVP increment

Milliampere seconds (mAs)

Is the value of the product of the high tension current in milliamperes and the duration of exposure in seconds. These two factors—milliamperes and time—are quoted in order that any recommended milliampere second value can be obtained by dividing the milliampere seconds quoted, by the milliamperage in departmental use and by so doing, the exposure in seconds is obtained. Some modern X-ray units operate within a tied system between milliamperage and kilovoltage, by so doing operating at maximum tube load. In such a procedure the mAs is set and automatically the highest mA available and subsequently the shortest exposure time is selected at that particular kilovoltage.

The milliampere second value set is the prime factor in controlling the exposure (density) on the film. Correct exposure producing with optimum kilovoltage the most suitable density and contrast that can be obtained.

Under exposure will result in lack of density and lack of contrast.

Over exposure resulting in excessive density and low contrast.

While most films exhibit considerable tolerance to errors in exposure (milliampere seconds) correct exposure becomes more critical and necessary where high kilovoltage technique is employed, in order that maximum contrast is obtained to amplify the low radiographic subject contrast.

Where exposure time is critical due to subject movement selection of the highest milliamperage will allow the use of suitable short exposure time. Where, however, time of exposure is not so exacting, selection of lower mA values may be more practical in order to extend tube life.

As a consequence of this the following milliamperages are suggested:–

Limbs—With or without intensifying screens—100–200 milliamperes.

Skull, Vertebral Column, Pelvis—highest mA within rating of smallest foci.

Heart and Lungs —500–800 milliamperes.
Alimentary Tract—500 milliamperes.
Gall-bladder   —500 milliamperes.
Urinary Tract   —500 milliamperes.

Dental—8–10 milliamperes according to dental unit output. Screening conventional—3 milliamperes at 70–80 kilovolts with image intensifier—0·3 milliamperes.

It is particularly useful to have a free control adjustment of the 100 milliampere setting in order that low values of mA can be obtained applicable to the requirements of long exposure breathing techniques, and also milliamperage values in keeping with the excursion time required for tomographic movement.

Distance

Indicates the focus–film distance employed, where grid technique is in use the FFD is usually dictated by the radial–focus distance of the grid in order to obtain uniformity of exposure over the entire subject (for example—AP pelvis). Generally this is either 36–40 inches (90–100 cm). In instances, however, where the subject is centralized to the grid (lateral spine) the focus–film distance may be increased to 120 cms to improve the focus-object to object-film ratio to reduce the unsharpness of the image due to subject film displacement.

In techniques where true size is imperative (for example—chest and heart radiography) extended FFD are employed 5 to 6 feet (150–180 cm).

The advent of small focal spot sizes in the order of ·3 and ·6 mm however, has reduced the necessity for any alteration in FFD in general Bucky radiography, the advantage of improved sharpness being directly proportional to the focal spot size whereas with extended focus–film distances the improvement in sharpness is only inversely proportional, added to this, the further possibility of subject movement at the longer exposure required for the extended distance.

Change in exposure with increased FFD can be calculated by applying the formula—

$$\frac{\text{New distance squared}}{\text{Original distance squared}} \times \text{Original exposure} =$$
$$= \text{New Exposure}$$

Collimation of the beam is important; the use of a cone or diaphragm or both of minimum aperture conforming to the size and shape of the area to be covered is imperative, to improve definition and provide patient protection.

To reduce further radiation dosage to the patient each X-ray tube is fitted with a conventional 2 mm aluminimum filter placed at the tube aperture. It should be understood that heavier filtration will effect both contrast and exposure.

Radiographic Grids. This includes both moving and stationary grids, the moving type grid requiring a ×4 increase in exposure relative to a non-grid exposure and the stationary grid a ×3 increase.

Grid efficiency is dependent on two factors and can be judged on two essential features namely Primary Transmission and Secondary Elimination, these features are determined by the composition of the grid and its grid ratio.

Satisfactory and matched performance in both respects can be obtained with a 7-1 metal grid and a 10-1 plastic type with kilovoltage up to 100 kVP.

Grid ratios of 12-1 metal; 16-1 plastic are available to give improved performance at kilovoltages above 100 kVP, but the advantage compared with their high primary absorption, particularly where short exposure does not coincide over a uniform de-centralized grid excursion is problematical.

In such an instance conventional grids complimented by selective filtration behind the grid would appear to be more favourable.

Fineline Grids (Stationary). These grids are of such fineline construction that the lead strips are virtually indiscernible, their major advantage is that they obviate the problem of grid movement suited to ultra short exposures, and have an efficiency comparable to 7-1 ratio moving grid.

Filtration. Adequate filtration should always be present in the portal aspect of the tube to ensure that longer X-ray wavelengths which would be absorbed within the patient; and as a consequence do not contribute to useful film density are eliminated prior to entry. This takes the form of a recommended 2 mm aluminium thickness in the 60–100 kilovoltage range.

Filtration can also be used to ensure that high absorption differences within an area of the body are reproduced with a more uniform scale of contrast. Depending on the shape of the part this can either take the form of a wedge-type filter placed in the portal aspect of the tube so that its thickest dimension is over the area of least absorption, or alternatively by increasing the thickness of the conventional tube filter or replacing this with an appropriate thickness of copper.

A comparison of tube position with filtration of this type and selective filtration with sheet tin on the under surface of the grid will lead however to a recommendation for the under-grid filtration position in that the former does not eliminate a high degree of often unsuspected grid scatter from reaching the film.

Films

To-day the type of X-ray film chosen is virtually dictated by the speed of processing requirements, this ranges through automatic dry to dry cycles of 7 minutes, $3\frac{1}{2}$ minutes and 90 seconds, the latter now predominating. The films characteristics have therefore to be suited to both this rapid transport and high activity in developing, fixing and drying. This has innovated what can be regarded as a universal type film which suited to the extreme 90 second processing produces a standard result in all forms of processing. Its general use is in conjunction with intensifying screens but for extremity work where 90 second processing only, is in vogue it satisfies the requirements of non-screen procedure, alternatively where increased contrast is desired reduced dosage and exposure time can be obtained by using it in conjunction with slower speed high definition screens.

Choice of film and screens

The optimum choice of film and screen speed to be used can only be adjudged when the total speed of the system namely output complimented by film and screen speed provides for the elimination of movement and a low geometrical unsharpness value, the choice of screen should then be that, which provides a physical unsharpness in line with the prevailing unsharpness.

It is advisable that departments use screens of one manufacture as quoted high definition, standard (universal) and fast screens do not necessarily mean that these are matched in speed to similarly quoted screens from other sources.

Intensifying screens

The following calcium tungstate screens are available—Fast Tungstate, Standard and High Definition.

The Standard Screen is a general purpose screen of high quality and efficiency. Fast Tungstate screens require only half of the exposure needed for standard screens with scarcely any perceptible loss of definition. The High Definition screen requires 50% more exposure than the standard screen but where exposure conditions permit, the reduction in speed is well compensated by the improved definition.

Subject. The patient is the most variable factor of all and exposure must be related to the individual, the region of examination, age (child, adult, old person), thickness and condition of tissues (muscular, non-muscular, pathological), and the presence of plaster or other splints and of dressings.

The suggested techniques are based on a subject of average physique, for smaller or larger subjects, the exposure could be increased or decreased respectively by from 25 to 50 per cent in mAS or relatively by 5 to 10 kilovolts.

X-Ray film quality

Maximum sharpness is obtained when there is a uniformity in the unsharpness associated with movement; geometrical projection, the physical screen unsharpness, and when each is at a minimum value in respect to the conditions pervading during the examination.

Subject movement unsharpness

Although of major importance the effect on radiographic unsharpness tends to be least appreciated, bearing in mind that however we improve projection and screen unsharpness this will not offset the result of permitted movement in the radiograph. The reason would appear to be that we are not sufficiently enlightened as to the rate of movement entailed in subject areas influenced by involuntary movement under normal and abnormal conditions and circulatory flow when envisaged with the introduction of opaque media in solution.

Where subject movement can be controlled by the joint effort of the patient and the radiographer's approach to the patient no great problem exists, however, in areas associated with involuntary movement; both, how brief the exposure should be, and how it should be obtained can present a problem.

The advent of what is virtually constant potential wave-form with its greater efficiency in output permits the selection of exposure times in the millesecond range either (a) with high milliamperage or (b) with high kilovoltage, to the extent that the insidious presence of movement in the radiograph need no longer be tolerated.

Geometrical unsharpness

Two features should be borne in mind (when choosing the most appropriate focal spot dimension). (a) Geometrical unsharpness is directly proportional to the focal spot dimension. (b) The rating of the focal spot with respect to the energy required for the examination.

If we consider a typical lumbar-spine examination in the lateral position, in such an examination the subject–film displacement is in the region of 25 cm. With a conventional 100 cm FFD and 2 mm focal spot; the geometrical unsharpness value is 0·6 mm. In such an instance the effect on definition would be dominated by the unacceptable geometrical unsharpness, a 1 mm focus would reduce this to 0·3 mm in keeping with the physical unsharpness of standard type screens. An 0·5 mm foci would reduce this to 0·15 mm whereupon the full benefit of high definition screens could be fully appreciated relative to the improved sharpness.

Contrast
This is a function of

(a) The X-ray film contrast in conjunction with its processing procedure, combined with the joint result in reduction of the amount of secondary radiation reaching the film by the following procedures.
(b) The limitation of the area in which scattered radiation can be produced by confining the beam to the required area only.
(c) Using compression of the part where practicable, permitting lower kilovoltage to be used.
(d) Adequate removal of scattered radiation emanating from the patient by using efficient types of grids.
(e) The prevention of backscatter where there is a steep change between subject filtration and surround.

Sharpness

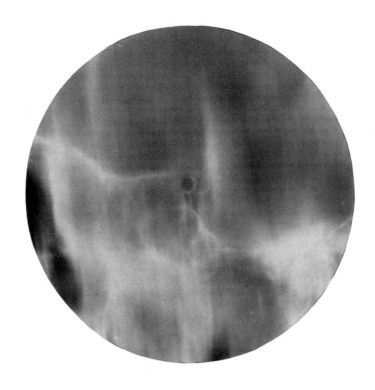

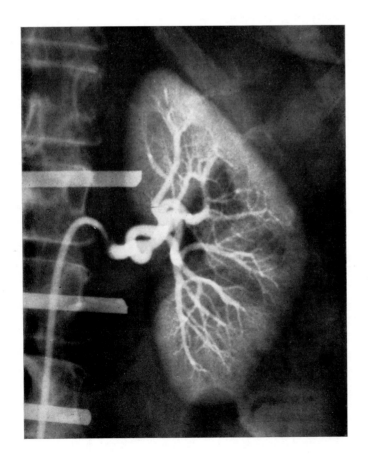

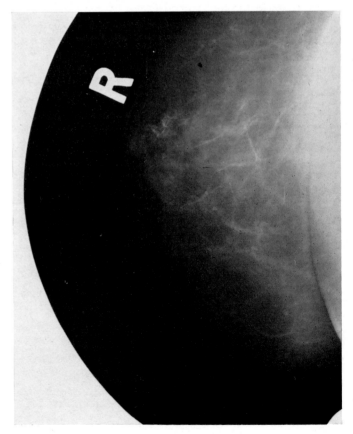

Contrast

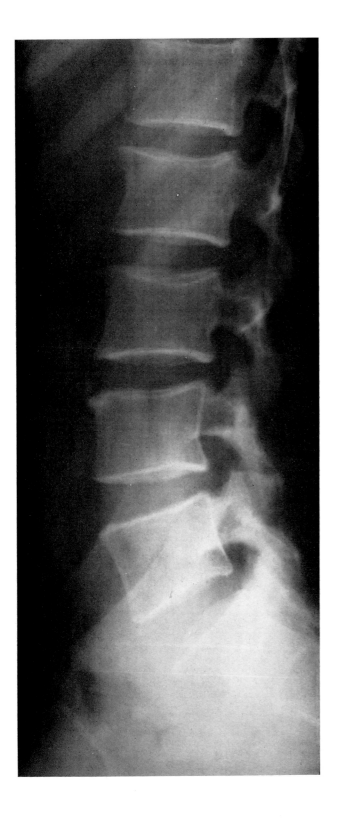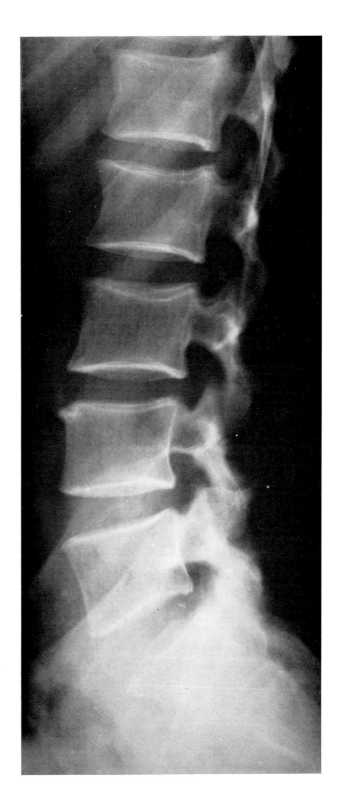

CONTENTS
VOLUME TWO

SECTION 19
Dental
Anatomical features. Examining mouth, dental request formula, planes and angles. Radiation protection. Equipment. Film-holders. Identification. Mounting. Intra-oral, extra-oral, occlusal, crowns, edentulous, localization.

Panagraphy (Pan-Oral)
Panoramic survey upper and lower jaws. Intra-oral X-ray tube.

Rotography
Roto-tomography. Facio-maxillary investigation.

SECTION 20
Salivary Glands
Anatomical features. Parotid. Submandibular. Sublingual. Sialography, opaque medium.

Lacrimal System
Anatomical features. Opaque injection, timing exposures. Macroradiography.

SECTION 21
Temporal Bones
Anatomical features. Mastoid, petrous. Comparative positional radiographs with annotated tracing diagrams. Conventional and skull table technique, macroradiography, middle ear. Multisection, auditory ossicles.

Optic Foramina
Conventional Couch, and skull table technique. Tomography.

Additional Skull Procedure
Reversed optic foramen. Reversed Towne's position, alternative skull procedures.

SECTION 22
Ventriculography and Encephalography
Anatomical features, planes, lines and landmarks. Comparative series of radiographs with annotated tracing diagrams. Contrast media, general- air injection, opaque medium for aqueduct and fourth ventricle. Details of skull table. Auto-tomography for third and fourth ventricles.

Stereotaxis
Cerebral localization. Equipment. Two methods.

Ultrasound Investigation Gamma Ray Scanning
Principle. Cerebral application, oscillographs.

SECTION 23
Myelography
Spinal cord, anatomical features. Sub-arachnoid space, injection of opaque medium, or air. Tilting couch, biplane localization, spot filming. Intervertebral discs.

SECTION 24
Angiography
Film changers, manual, automatic, biplane. Films. Large, miniature cine. Opaque media, injection procedures. Cerebral, Cardiac angiography, Sub-traction technique, Abdominal aorto-graphy, general renal, selective renal. Tomography macroradiography.

SECTION 25
Soft Tissue
Mammary glands, positioning and ex-posure technique. Investigations for pathology. Limbs, vessels, trunk, adenoids, auditory tubes.

SECTION 26
Macroradiography
Principles of, Tube foci Applications, Elbow, wrist, Petrous, Chest, Lacrimal system.

SECTION 27
Multiple Radiography
Steep subject range application (examples) Duplication Technique (examples) Simultaneous Contact and Enlargement technique.

SECTION 28
Tomography
Principles of, apparatus essentials. Linear movements, Testing accuracy, Section intervals, efficient blurring Symmetrical-Unsymmetrical movement Zonography, Circular, Hypocycloidal movements. Localization procedure, Angle of Move-ment related to Respiratory Tract Verte-bral Column, etc. Multisection, Tomo-graphy Chart; guide to levels. Axial Transverse Tomography.

SECTION 29
Stereography
Procedure-presentation for viewing, stereoscopes, stereometry.

SECTION 30
Female Reproductive System
Anatomical features. Radiation restriction. Compression technique as approved. Hysterosalpingography, premedication. Opaque melium. Gynacoography pre-medication. Air insufflation. Pregnancy; early; advanced; multiple Placentography, Placenta praevia. Urography, Amniography. Stillborn foetus. Pelvimetry. Pelvic in-clination. Foetal head mensuration.

SECTION 31
High Kilovoltage
Application of High Kilovoltage. Exposure Time, Focal spot sizes Subject contrast, repetitive exposure.

Selective Filtration
Reduction in the effect of scatter using metals, with or without grid technique.

SECTION 32
Foreign Bodies
Foreign body types, opaque and non-opaque, surgical swab. Initial confirmation. Anatomical location-limbs, head, trunk, respiratory system, alimentary tract. Localization, equipment, experiments with phantoms. Methods-by screening, by triangulation, by parallax. Orbital cavity, related to centre of eye, related to anterior corneal margins.

SECTION 33
Miniature Radiography
Mobile equipment, protection, optics, fluorescent screens. Film-types, sizes, processing. Exposure and uniformity, mass surveys-chest. Viewing. Confirmation by large film, by tomography.

SECTION 34
Cineradiography
Equipment. Image intensifier range of units. X-ray tube, focus, rating, Cine camera, camera speeds. Cine film-types, sizes, processing. Television viewing, direct, remote, monitoring. Recording on magnetic tape, remote control. Image retaining panel. Examples-cerebral and cardiac angiography, pyelography, micturition, oesophagus, stomach. Cine projection, projectors. Editing table. Copying. Enlarging selected frames. Spot filming, fullsize, 70 millimetre, 100 millimetre.

SUPPLEMENT ONE
Contrast and Opaque Media

SUPPLEMENT TWO
The Effects of Radiation, and Protection
Methods in Diagnostic Radiology

SUPPLEMENT THREE
Working Metric Equivalents of Dimensions and
Quantities

The Ninth Edition of
Positioning in Radiography
has been produced in two volumes.
An outline of the contents
of volume one is shown below:

CONTENTS
VOLUME ONE

SECTION 1
Upper Limb

SECTION 2
Humerus and Shoulder Girdle

SECTION 3
Lower Limb

SECTION 4
Hip Joint and Upper third of Femur

SECTION 5
Pelvic Girdle

SECTION 6
Vertebral Column

SECTION 7
Vertebral Column

SECTION 8
Bones of Thorax

SECTION 9
Skull

SECTION 10
Mandible

SECTION 11
Paranasal Sinuses

SECTION 12
Subject types

SECTION 13
Heart and Aorta

SECTION 14
Respiratory System

SECTION 15
Alimentary Tract

SECTION 16
Abdomen

SECTION 17
Biliary Tract

SECTION 18
Urinary Tract

19

DENTAL
PANAGRAPHY
ROTOGRAPHY

19 SECTION 19

DENTAL

The terminology for the mouth differs from that of other regions particularly in the absence of such general terms as antero-posterior and lateral.

The Dental arches

On examining the mouth the upper and lower dental arches appear as in radiographs (1641) of the upper teeth lodged in the maxilla above, and (1642) of the lower teeth lodged in the mandible below. The term mesial applies to the anterior part of the arches toward the canine region, and distal to the posterior part toward the molar teeth. The terms labial or buccal refer to the outer aspect or cheek side of the jaw and lingual or palatal to the inner side of the jaw within the mouth cavity, and as would be described in other regions of the body as external and internal.

Dentitions

The human being develops two sets of teeth, referred to as dentitions. These are the temporary or deciduous set, also referred to as the milk teeth, numbering twenty (1652), which appear between the ages of six months and two years. The deciduous set gives place to the permanent teeth, thirty-two in number (1653), which erupt from the sixth year onward, the last four molars, or wisdom teeth, appearing normally during the eighteenth year. The wisdom teeth may not erupt, however, until as late as the twenty-sixth year, and may occasionally remain embedded in the jaw, for which reason, even if no wisdom tooth is visible in the mouth, this area should always be included in the complete examination (1655). On the other hand, it is possible for the wisdom teeth to be absent entirely.

In extra-oral films of a child aged eight years (1643,1644), both temporary and permanent teeth are present.

Panoramic projections of the adult dentitions serve for guidance in showing the arrangement of the permanent teeth (1649).

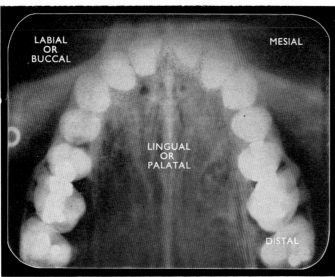

1641

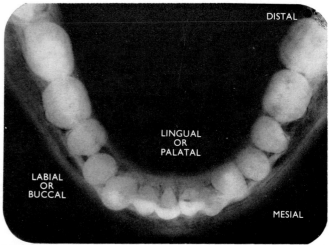

1642

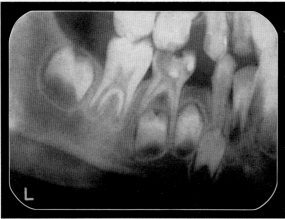

1643

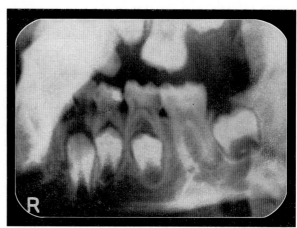

1644

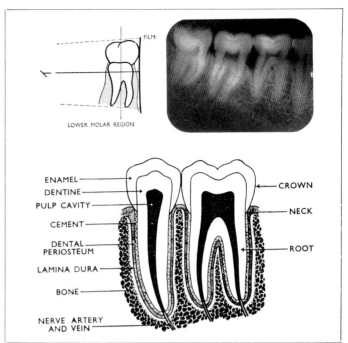

1646/1647

Anatomy

Each tooth, consisting briefly of crown, neck and root or roots —each root terminating in an apex—is set in the jaw with, normally, only the crown visible, the remainder of the structure being embedded in the alveolar part of the jaw. The alveoli are covered with the soft tissue forming the gum (1645).

A film, therefore, placed in the mouth in contact with the crown of a tooth and with the gum is somewhat removed from the root of the tooth, the angle between tooth and film varying from patient to patient and according to the region of the mouth: it is greatest in the upper incisor area (1645) while in the lower molar region it is negligible, it being possible, in fact, to work here with the film parallel to the tooth (1646).

The anatomical structure of the individual tooth and its relationship within the tooth socket is shown in (1647) with its relative radiographic interpretation in (1648). In addition to the crown, neck and root, the differential substances of the pulp cavity, dentine and enamel are clearly defined in the radiograph, also the finer details such as the periodontal membrane, the lamina dura, the apex of the root and the inter-dental table (1647,1648).

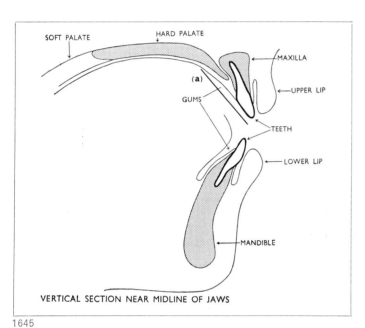

1645

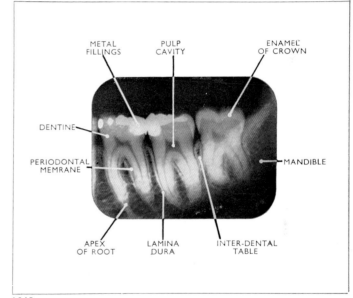

1648

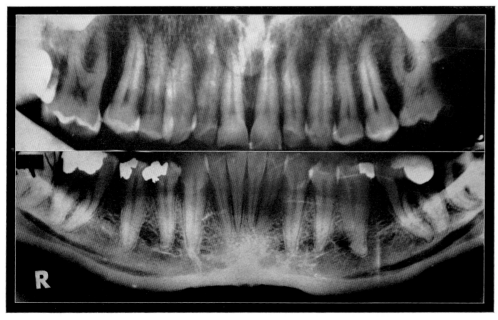

1649

471

Dental request formula

Requests for dental X-ray examination are made in accordance with the dental formula (1650,1651), the number of teeth to be examined being specified. Similar indication may be given in the case of the toothless, or edentulous, subject to be examined for the location of buried roots or abnormal condition of the alveolar margin. The examination of children may be required when teeth of both dentitions are present.

The deciduous teeth are referred to by serial letters from 'a' to 'e' on passing from central incisor distally to second milk molar (1650,1652).

Films

Dental films are made in two types, Standard and Fast, the exposure for the Fast film being reduced to half of that required for the Standard film. They may be used according to the technique preferred, and are packed singly or in pairs, use of the latter pack enabling one complete set of films to be retained for

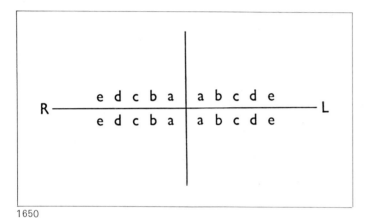

1650

The permanent teeth are referred to by serial numbers from '1' to '8' on passing distally from central incisor to third molar (1651a).

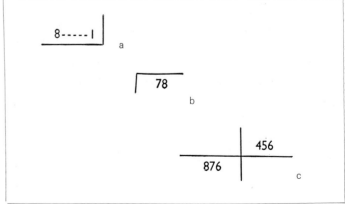

1651a

Requests for selected teeth or for individual groups of teeth would be given as follows (1651b):
(a) Upper right, 1 to 8.
(b) Lower left, 7 and 8.
(c) Upper left, 4, 5, 6, and lower right, 6, 7, 8.

record purposes. The film-pack contains a lead foil between film and label to absorb secondary X radiation, definition being thus enhanced. An emboss on each film enables identification to be made of the individual exposures. The film-packs are damp-proof.

Intra-oral films are made in standard and sub-standard sizes, the former being $1\frac{1}{4} \times 1\frac{5}{8}$ inches and the latter $1 \times 1\frac{1}{4}$ inches. The smaller films are convenient when examining the incisor and canine regions in narrow and shallow mouths, and they are also particularly suitable for children.

A larger film, termed 'occlusal', $2\frac{1}{4} \times 3$ inches in size, is so named from its position—in the occlusal plane between the jaws—during exposure. This is supplied in packs similar in type to those of the smaller intra-oral films.

Other sizes of film used for investigation of mouth and jaws are the whole-plate and half-plate, which are employed for extra-oral examination.

Equipment

Patients are usually examined in the sitting position but as a request for the examination of the teeth of a sick patient sometimes involves the horizontal position, the general purpose radiographer should be able to use either. This should present no difficulty once the angulation for dental technique is understood.

As dental units are shock-free, the special dental cone is used in contact with the skin, thus, the focus–film distance and the technique employed may be governed by the type of unit and length of cone supplied. These units move freely and the patient may, therefore, remain seated in the dental chair, or in a chair fitted with a modified head support, while the tube is moved round the head to the various positions. In using the general purpose unit however, the patient is usually supine and the head is moved to the various necessary positions in relation to the X-ray tube. A focus–film distance of from 20 to 24 inches (50 to 72 cm) is employed, again using the small localizing cone with its restricted diaphragm aperture to cover only a small margin beyond the size of the dental film for intra–oral work.

1651b

DECIDUOUS TEETH

UPPER JAW

CANINE (2)

INCISOR (4)

MOLAR (4)

e d c b a a b c d e

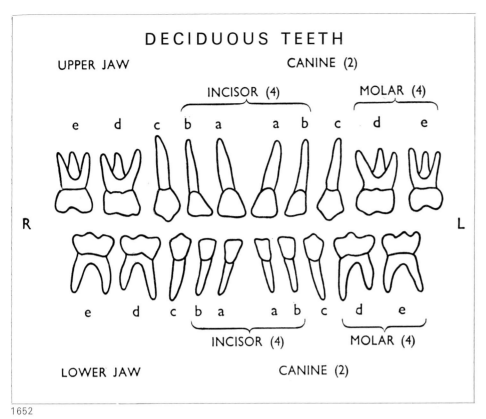

R

L

e d c b a a b c d e

INCISOR (4)

MOLAR (4)

LOWER JAW

CANINE (2)

1652

PERMANENT TEETH

UPPER JAW

CANINE (2)

INCISOR (4)

PREMOLAR (4)

MOLAR (6)

8 7 6 5 4 3 2 1 1 2 3 4 5 6 7 8

R

L

8 7 6 5 4 3 2 1 1 2 3 4 5 6 7 8

INCISOR (4)

PREMOLAR (4)

MOLAR (6)

LOWER JAW

CANINE (2)

1653

Film-holders
Placing the film in position

Dental film holders should support the films, but in their absence, the patient should hold each film in position after it has been placed correctly behind the appropriate teeth, using the thumb for the incisor region, the fingers being extended out of the way or used as a support against the face. For the remainder of the teeth, use is made of the index finger of the hand opposite to that of the side of the jaw being radiographed; that is to say, the first finger of the patient's left hand will be placed behind the films for teeth on the right side of the mouth, and vice versa.

In no circumstances should the operator's own hands be used to hold the film, as this practice may lead to injury to the fingers through frequent exposure to the direct X-ray beam.

To obviate the risk of displaced films through inadequate co-operation from the patient, film holders should always be used when possible.

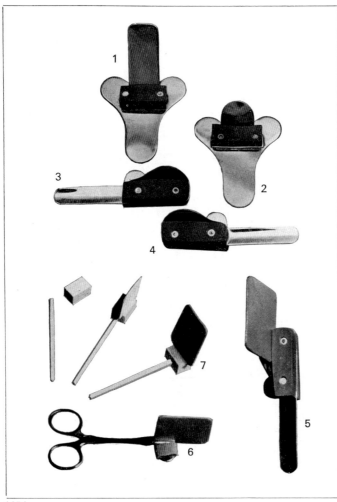

1654

Whenever holders of any kind are employed there must, of course, be a sufficient number of teeth in the jaw to hold them firmly, although, if necessary, a dental plate can be left in the jaw which is not being examined. Some of the various types of dental film holders are described below.

Colyers's dental film holders. These consist of a group of four stainless-steel holders each carrying, on a suitable handle, a metal film support and hard-rubber bite block.

No. 1 holder is designed to carry the film, placed long edge vertically, for the upper incisor and canine region.

No. 2 holder is shaped to suspend the film downwards in the central curve of the lower arch, for the lower incisor teeth.

No 3 holds the films for both the upper left premolar and molar teeth, and the lower right premolar and molar teeth.

No 4 caters for the upper right and lower left corresponding teeth.

Since these last two holders are fairly large and cannot be tolerated far back in the mouth, the film for the molars can be placed to extend beyond the bite block (5).

Forceps holders. The forceps are so constructed that the film edge is retained by a locking device and a small rubber-covered bite block is included. The forceps are light in weight, and are easy to manipulate and adjust to the various positions. It is important that the operator should not continue to hold the forceps while the exposure is being made (6).

Balsa-wood bite blocks. Balsa wood is silky to the touch and very light in weight, and the bite blocks are easily introduced into the mouth. They can be shaped with a slot for the film, and an adaptable handle simplifies adjustment in the mouth.

Such blocks are inexpensive and can be thrown away after use, which saves the work of re-sterilization; they should, however, be made of the harder varieties of balsa wood (7).

No matter what kind of film holder is used, it should always be loaded with the tube-facing surface of the film turned towards the bite block.

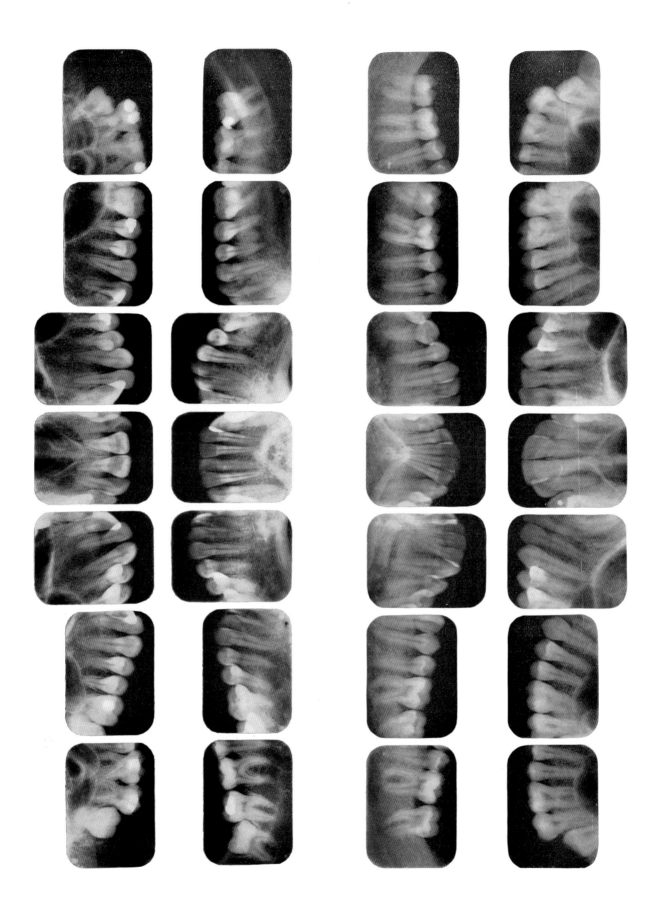

Technique

To show a complete set of teeth, the size and number of films used depend upon the shape of the mouth. For certain subjects ten films may suffice; in others fourteen or even more may be necessary. Centring is therefore shown in this section for both a ten-film and a fourteen-film series.

For vertical technique the patient, usually sitting in a dental chair, is placed, for both upper and lower jaw examinations, with the head supported and immobilized against the neck-rest with the median-saggittal plane vertical, and the occlusal plane horizontal, for each jaw in turn. It should be possible to maintain the appropriate position throughout the examination; with the patient in the horizontal position, however, a certain movement of head and tube is necessary. Two diagrams show, with the mouth open, the horizontal adjustment of the upper occlusal plane (1656) and the lower occlusal plane (1657).

The positioning line extending from the tragus of the ear to the ala of the nose, about which radiographic centring points are commonly negotiated for the upper teeth, is 1½ inches above the occlusal plane (1656).

As an aid to assessing the level of the lower occlusal plane with the mouth open in variable degree, a positioning line extending between the tragus of the ear and the angle of the mouth is three-quarters of an inch above the lower occlusal plane (1657). Centring for the lower teeth is in relation to just above the level of the lower border of the mandible and spacing is in relation to the centring for the upper teeth, hence in the illustration (1659) the perpendicular lines extending between the approximate centring points for upper and lower teeth from mesial to distal aspects.

The range of angulation normally employed in relation to the occlusal plane is seen in profile (1658) and en face in (1659). These angles will, of course, vary slightly for the individual subject according to the possible variations in the angle of the embedded teeth, but they do serve for guidance until experience is gained in observing the lie of the teeth.

Full adult dentition is shown on page 475 with grouping which may be needed for the incisor, canine premolars and molar region.

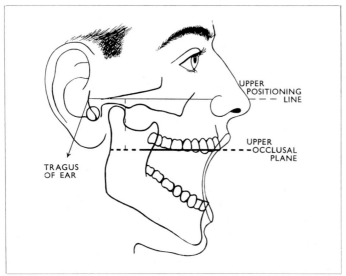

1656

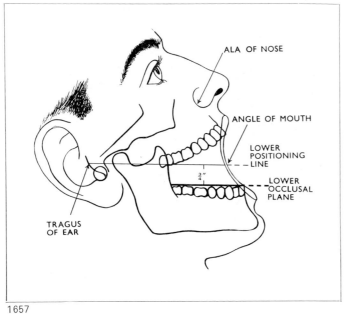

476

1657

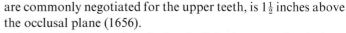

1658

Correct projection

At the short focus–film distance used for dental radiography, the importance of the correct projection of the teeth should be fully appreciated.

The aim in projection should be to direct the beam at right angles to the line bisecting the angle between tooth and film, as this gives the nearest approach to the normal shadow length of the tooth (1660). Projection toward the crown gives rise to foreshortening (1661), that toward the apex resulting in elongation of the tooth shadow (1662), and while some degree of foreshortening is permissible, elongation is to be avoided. The central ray should be directed toward the apical half-section of the tooth. The diagrams show varying tube angulation applied to the incisor region, and the accompanying radiographs show the result of such tube angulation (1660,1661,1662).

Lateral distortion—which varies the breadth and, therefore, allows overlapping of the tooth shadows—is also to be guarded against (1663a). While it is sometimes unavoidable, owing to the manner of growth of the teeth or to the shape of the mouth, careful centring and additional exposures will do much to minimize its effect (1663b). The shape of the mouth and direc-

tion of the teeth should be noted before commencing the examination: the broad mouth showing a good, regular, anterior curve is easily negotiated, but the very narrow mouth can sometimes only be demonstrated satisfactorily by using small substandard films and by centring for each of the front teeth in turn. A shallow palate also requires greater tube angulation that that necessary for a high palate.

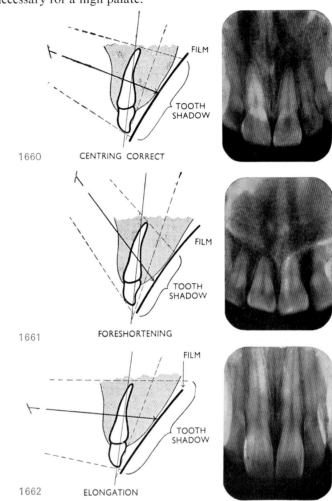

1660 CENTRING CORRECT

1661 FORESHORTENING

1662 ELONGATION

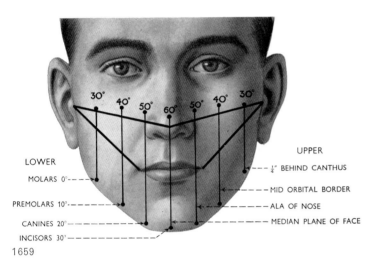

LOWER
MOLARS 0°
PREMOLARS 10°
CANINES 20°
INCISORS 30°

UPPER
¼″ BEHIND CANTHUS
MID ORBITAL BORDER
ALA OF NOSE
MEDIAN PLANE OF FACE

1659

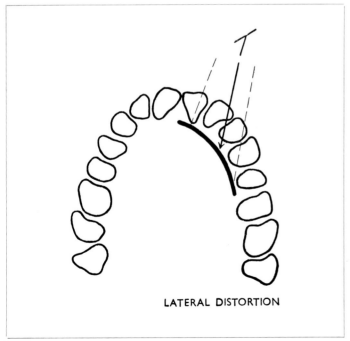

LATERAL DISTORTION

1663a

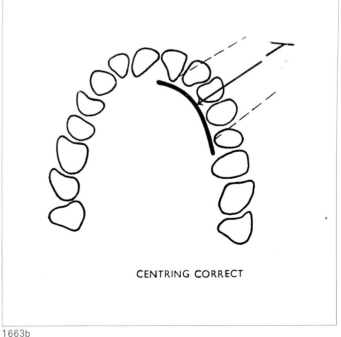

CENTRING CORRECT

1663b

Radiation protection

Protection from radiation for both patient and operator is important in dental radiography, particularly in view of the short-distance technique employed and the number of overlap exposures necessary to include a complete dentition.

A 2-millimetre aluminium filter at the tube aperture, usually incorporated in the unit by the manufacturer, is imperative for the suppression of unwanted soft radiation. Protective lead–rubber aprons extending from beneath the chin to the lap (1664a) to protect the patient are available in suitable sizes for children and adults.

On using the special dental localizing cone with its small angled aperture (1664b) limited to little more than the actual size of the dental films employed for intra-oral work, there is only a small margin overlap beyond the three or four teeth involved.

Limitation in the number of essential exposures with accurate positioning and centring to avoid repeat exposures is imperative.

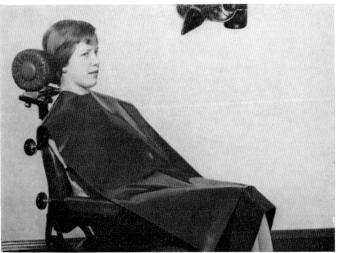

1664a

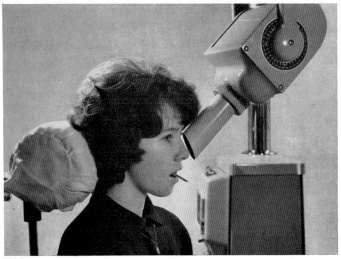

1664b

Furthermore, the use of the fast dental film reduces exposure to a minimum.

Finally, the operator should never hold the films in position in the patient's mouth during exposure. Film-holders are available for this purpose and as will be seen later the patient may be able to hold the film in position; each film-pack incorporates a backing of protective lead foil. Also, for the operator the maximum working distance from the X-ray unit is an essential protective factor.

Exposure conditions

Dental radiography tends to become the specialized work of the dental surgeon, but as a certain amount of investigation of the teeth continues to be carried out in the general X-ray department, apparatus varies accordingly from the small, specially designed dental unit to the large, general purpose unit.

Although the output required for dental radiography ranges from 55 to 65 kilovolts, units are available which carry a lower or a higher rating, or both, from 45 to 70 kV.

The smaller units generally have a fixed rating of between 45 and 60 kilovolts, and a fixed current of 8 or 10 milliamperes. There is, however, one very small unit rated at 45 kilovolts and 5 milliamperes which is used at the very short focus–film distance of 4 inches. All units are fitted permanently with a 2-millimetre aluminium filter.

Another unit has a long cone for 16-inch distance technique, accompanied by a special film-holder to enable the film pack to be held vertically in the mouth, thus requiring less tube angulation. Otherwise, special dental cones are fitted to the units to allow for set distances which range from $5\frac{1}{2}$ to 9 inches. As stated previously, these dental cones have a very small aperture which at a known distance covers little more area than the intra-oral dental film.

The usual exposure timers of the clockwork type need to be checked for accuracy from time to time. The more recent units allow for timing from 0·1 second to 10 seconds.

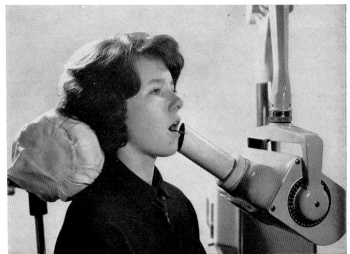

1664c

Exposure table for standard and fast dental films

The correct exposure for each region varies with type of subject, output of the X-ray tube, focus–film distance and processing.

The table below gives the exposure recommended for an adult, using a unit with 9 inches focus–film distance, giving 10 milliamperes at 60 kVp, with 2 mm aluminium filtration as recommended by the Code of Practice.

Region	Exposure time	
	Standard	Fast
Upper Incisors	1 sec	$\frac{1}{2}$ sec
Upper Canines	1 sec	$\frac{1}{2}$ sec
Upper Premolars	1 sec	$\frac{1}{2}$ sec
Upper Molars	$1\frac{1}{2}$ sec	$\frac{3}{4}$ sec
Lower Incisors	$\frac{1}{2}$ sec	$\frac{1}{4}$ sec
Lower Canines	1 sec	$\frac{1}{2}$ sec
Lower Premolars	1 sec	$\frac{1}{2}$ sec
Lower Molars	1 sec	$\frac{1}{2}$ sec
Upper Occlusal	$2\frac{1}{2}$ sec	$1\frac{1}{4}$ sec at 12 in FFD
Lower Occlusal	$1\frac{1}{2}$ sec	$\frac{3}{4}$ sec at 10 in FFD

These exposure times apply to an adult subject of average physique. For the general purpose unit, the focus–film distance should be doubled and the milliampere seconds adjusted accordingly.

Processing

Processing may be carried out in the general X-ray developing tanks, but it is advisable to use the special set of dental tanks so that these small films can be kept away from the bulk of large films passing through the dark-room. The specialist worker will certainly use the small dental processing unit. To obtain satisfactory dental radiographs, processing must be meticulous, especially as regards time and temperature, usually four minutes at 68°F, and the periodic renewal of the developing solution.

The developing hanger makes possible the processing of a complete set of films in the position in which they will be finally mounted, the patient's identification number or name being noted on the small celluloid tab fitted for the purpose (1665, 1666).

Identification

Individual films should on no account be pencil marked before being processed. Identification of position is facilitated by the provision, near one corner of each film, of a small embossed 'pip' corresponding in position with a similar embossment on the front pink paper-covered surface of the pack. When inserting the pack in the mouth the pink surface is placed facing the tube, thus ensuring that the raised side of the embossment on the enclosed film is toward the teeth to be examined. At the same time, the film should be placed in such a way that the embossment lies nearest the crowns, thus avoiding any possibility of obscuring the more important apices (1665).

Films should be mounted to appear as the mouth is seen by the surgeon from the labial aspect, that is, with the patient's right to the left of the mount and with the embossed convexity toward the observer. It is appreciated, however, that certain workers prefer to view dental radiographs as the teeth would be seen from the lingual aspect, in which case the mounting of the films is reversed, the right and left sides of the mouth being placed to right and left sides of the mount, and therefore with the embossed concavity towards the observer. In handling dental radiographs, great care should be taken to avoid finger marks, and workers who find this a problem should handle the film between tissue paper or should use, as recommended, the celluloid dental film loaders supplied for the cardboard mounts.

Viewing

In a complete series, the films should be so arranged that each tooth appears free from all distortion in at least one film (1655), page 473. On completing such a series of exposures, the films should be developed and checked, if possible, before the patient leaves, in order that any fault may be rectified or that any unusual variation from the normal may be further investigated.

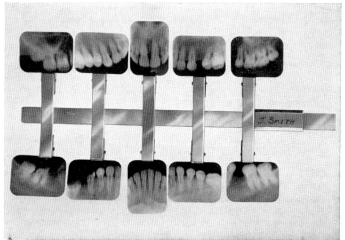

1665

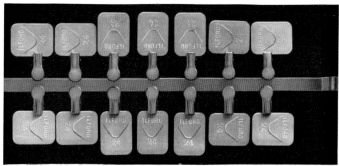

1666

Upper jaw

Angulation of the tube for the teeth of the upper jaw

Incisors; tube-occlusal plane angle 60°
Canines; tube-occlusal plane angle 50°
Premolars; tube-occlusal plane angle 40°
Molars; tube-occlusal plane angle 30°

For the shallow dish-shaped mouth with prominent incisors, the tube occlusal plane angle needs to be increased, possibly to 70°, and for subjects with receding teeth or high palate, the angle should be decreased.

Centring the tube for the upper teeth

Incisors. With the film placed long edge upright in the mouth the tube, angled at 60° to the occlusal line, is centred in the mid-line of the face, where the occlusal line would be were it produced toward the face. For the average patient this is usually the tip of the nose, but may be above or below the tip, according to its shape and the height of the palate. This should give a radiograph of the central and lateral incisors, (1668,1669, 1670a,1670b).

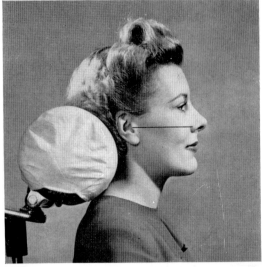

1667

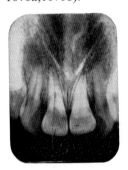

1670a

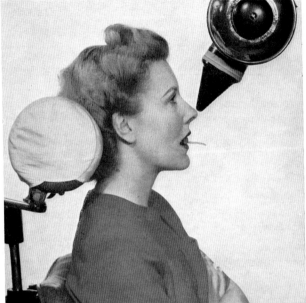

1668

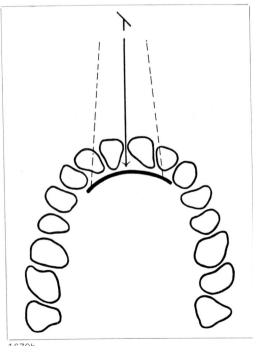

1670b

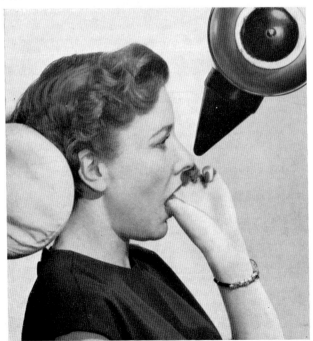

1669

Canines. The film can be inserted in the mouth with the long edge upright and the tube centre above the ala of the nose at an angle of 50° to the occlusal plane. It is as well to lift the lip to see the position of the canine tooth, as it may be slightly lateral to the ala and the tube should then be centred further back.

If the mouth is narrow, difficulty may be experienced in placing the film owing to the position of these teeth at the turn of the arch and to the shape of the palate. It may be better to use a small film (1 × 1¼ in.) in preference to the standard-size film, concentrating on getting a good view of the one tooth. This film will be large enough to include the long root of the canine tooth if used vertically in the mouth, and probably a second view of the lateral incisor will be obtained. On the other hand, in the wide-mouth type of patient, placing the film is so much easier that it may be possible to use the standard-size film long edge horizontally, with the short edge placed at the median line between the central incisors. In this instance the tube should be directed between the lateral incisor and the canine. This will give a good view of both these teeth, proving especially useful in cases where the width of the mouth has made it impossible to include the lateral incisor on the first film taken for the incisors.

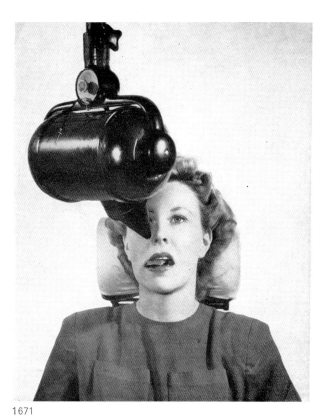

1671

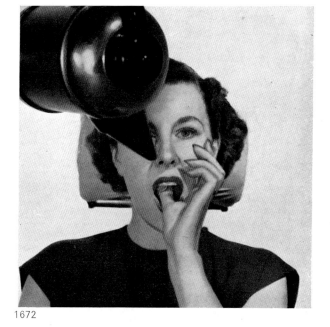

1672

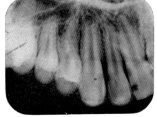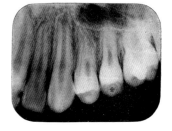

1673

Premolars. Using the ordinary size film long edge transversely, and with the tube angled at 40° to the occlusal plane, drop an imaginary line from a point mid-way between the inner and outer canthus of the eye, and swinging the tube around the curve of the cheek, centre above the occlusal line on this perpendicular.

The film should show the two premolars evenly spaced (1675 and 1677). Due to its distance from the film and the angle of the tube, the image of the buccal cusp is projected below that of the palatal one. (1674, 1675, 1676, 1677)

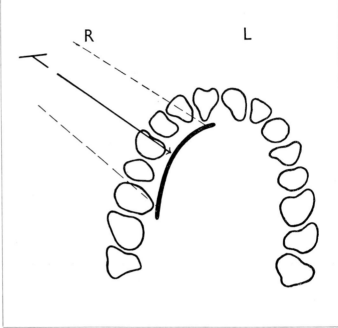

1677

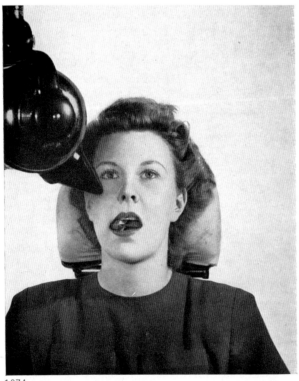

1674

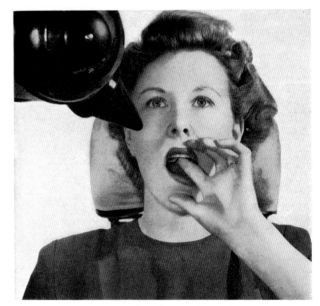

1675

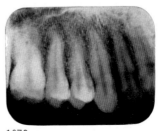
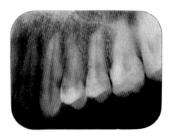

1676

Molars. The difficulty in this region is to get the patient to tolerate the film placed so far back in the mouth, and then to avoid obscuring the image of the molars by projecting the shadow of the zygomatic bone over their roots. The film position can be eased if the upper corner of the pack is bent slightly over the finger, to prevent it coming too harshly into contact with the soft palate. To avoid the zygomatic bone, drop an imaginary line down the cheek from a point ¼ in. behind the outer canthus of the eye, and centre the tube on this perpendicular at the level of or below the occlusal line. Placing the finger on the zygomatic bone to locate it, try to avoid projecting its shadow on to the film by directing the tube cone just under its lower border (1678,1679.)

(1680a) is a diagram of the lateral view of the zygomatic bone and (1680b) a diagram from the anterior showing the X-ray beam directed at 30° under the bone to avoid its shadow. In 1680c an alternative method is suggested, provided a film holder having a wide bite block is available. A dental roll is placed between tooth and film to bring the film parallel to the general line of the tooth so that the X-ray beam can be projected horizontally. If this method is employed, the focus–film distance should be increased to compensate for the increased subject–film distance and the exposure time adjusted accordingly.

All three molars should be shown on this film, probably with the floor of the maxillary sinus dipping down between the roots. (1681a) shows the teeth clearly but in (1681b) the roots are obscured by the shadow of the zygomatic bone due to faulty projection.

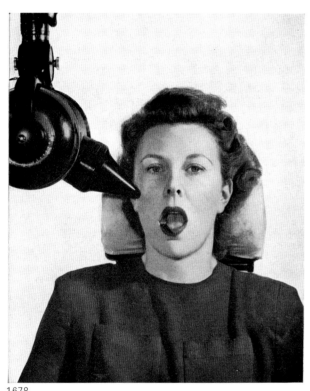

1678

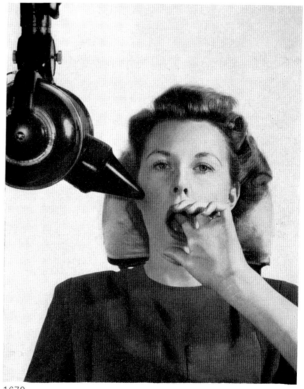

1679

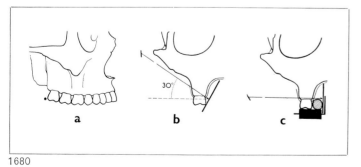

1680

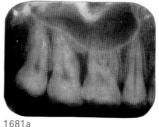

1681a

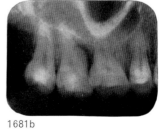

1681b

Lower jaw

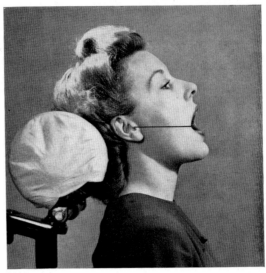

1682

Centring the tube for the lower teeth

Incisors. As a general rule, the film when used long edge transversely needs bending before it can be coaxed into place at the apex of the arch of the jaw. It can, of course, be used with the long edge vertically but it may be easier to use one of the smaller films, especially if there is painful inflammation present in the mucous membrane of the floor of the mouth. This small film will demonstrate the same area, and as it can be inserted without bending, pressure marks and distortion of the image of the roots of the teeth are avoided.

With the head tilted back to bring the lower occlusal line horizontal, the tube is centred upward to the symphysis menti at an angle of 25° to 30° to the occlusal plane (1683,1684.)

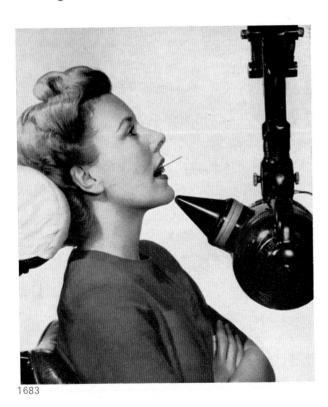

1683

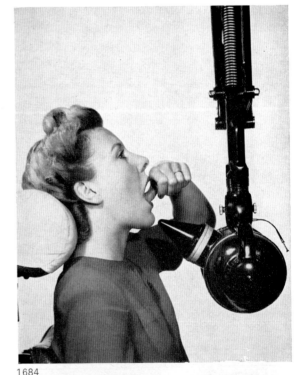

1684

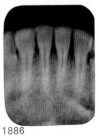

1685   1886

Canines. The standard-size film may be used long edge horizontally or vertically, or again it may be more expedient to use the smaller film, concentrating on getting a good radiograph of the canine only. The tube position is ascertained by dropping an imaginary line from the outer edge of the ala of the nose, and centring at the point where this line reaches the lower border of the mandible; the tube is angled at 20° to the occlusal plane.

If the standard size film is used horizontally, it may be possible to include the view of the premolars (1689), and so complete the examination of the lower jaw with five films instead of seven (1687, 1688, 1689).

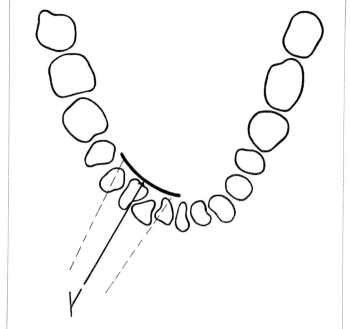

1690

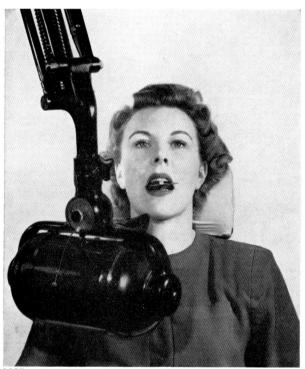

1687

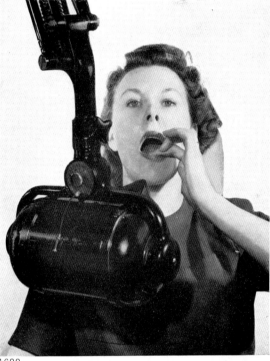

1688

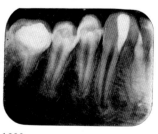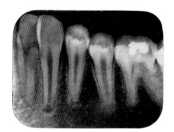

1689

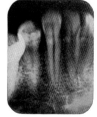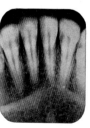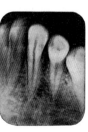

1691

Premolars. A standard-size film is used transversely with the tube swung round to direct the beam squarely to the film plane from the lateral angle. The tube position is found by referring again to the mid-point between the inner and outer canthus of the eye, from which an imaginary line is dropped until it reaches the lower mandibular edge. Centre at this point with the tube angled at 10° to the occlusal plane (1692,1693,1694).

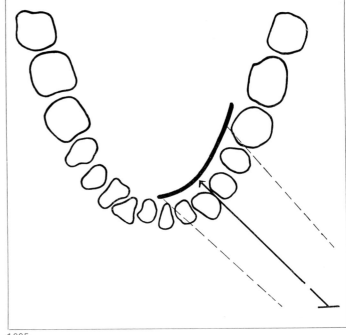

1695

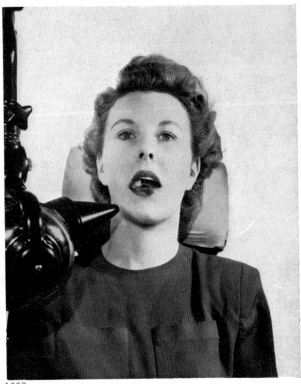

1692

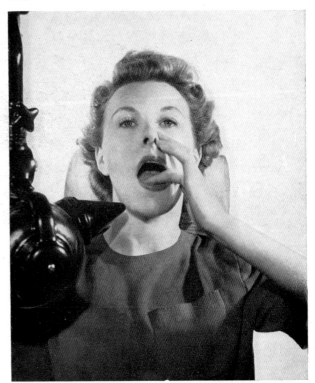

1693

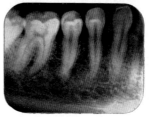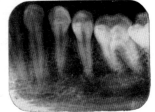

1694

Molars. The standard-size film is again used and the centring point found by producing the line, drawn from a quarter of an inch behind the outer canthus of the eye, as used for the upper molars. As the tube is at 0° to the occlusal plane, ie, horizontal, the film lying parallel to the molar teeth, the centring point will be a little higher than for the other teeth in the lower jaw, namely, above the lower border of the mandible, (1696,1697, 1698) shows the third molar fully developed and (1699) an unerupted third molar.

The angle of the mandible will serve as a guide in locating the molar group since all these teeth are well in front of this position.

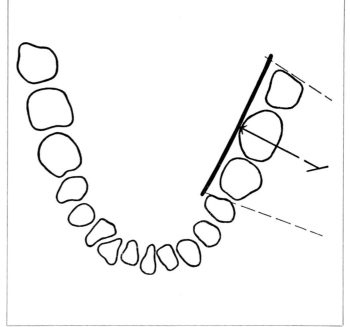

1700

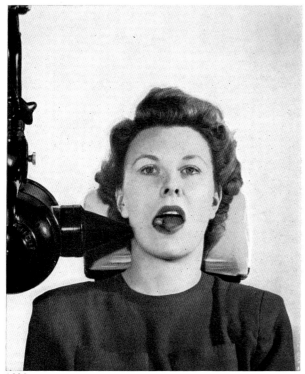

1696

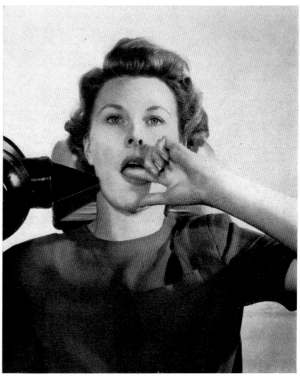

1697

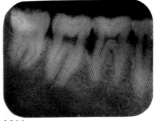

1698

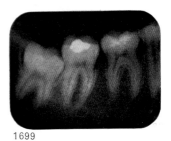

1699

Edentulous subjects

When the edentulous patient is to be examined, the date of extraction of the teeth will need to be considered. Recent extractions leave the alveolar margin intact with the sockets still showing the white line of the lamina dura in the radiograph (1701), but in toothless jaws of long standing, the alveolar margin will have been absorbed and the dental film will lean backward or forward according to the position in the mouth. For this reason it is desirable to increase the angulation of the tube, unless a dental film holder with a dental roll can be used to keep the film more upright. Replacement of a denture in the jaw not being examined will help to grip the film holder while the exposure is being made. Good definition is essential to show the condition of the bone; as a guide to the required quality of film, it should be such that the dental canals are clearly demonstrated (1702).

The X-ray exposure time should be reduced as the teeth are not present.

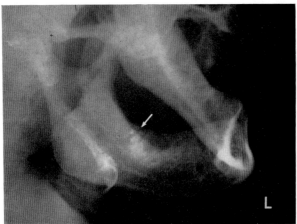

1703

If any difficulty is experienced in localizing the position of a buried root, the taking of a general extra-oral or occlusal film is advisable. (1703).

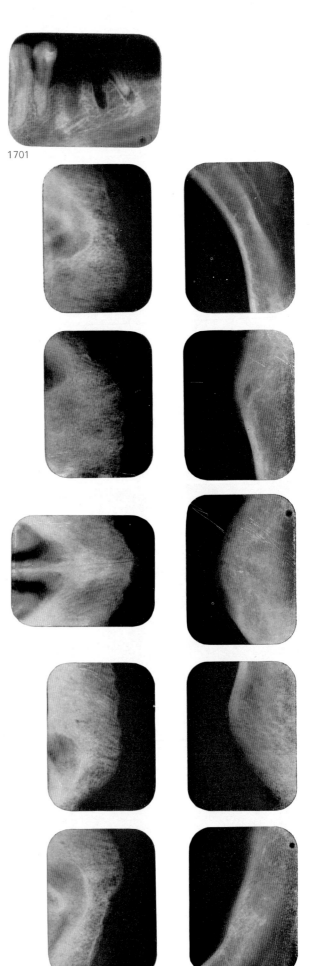

1701

1702

Investigation of crowns

The examination of the crowns can usually be completed with four or five films, each radiograph showing a group of both upper and lower teeth. Special holders have been designed to support the film mid-way between the jaws by a central bite-block, and in the drawings in (1704) alternative designs for the holders are suggested. Film holders are also made of tasteless tubular plastics material supplied in lengths of about 1 ft from which a piece of appropriate size can be cut for holding the film (1705); this material, being inexpensive, can be discarded after use. Illustration (1705) shows how the film is inserted after folding the plastics holder into a T-shape to bring the bite-block into a central position in relation to the film. With the tube-side facing the support, the film is introduced into the mouth, the teeth closing over the bite-block to maintain the position. The tube is centred at right-angles to the film (1706), with the central ray parallel to the plane of occlusion, which in the molar area usually means an angulation of the tube 5° downward. The radiographs show the upper and lower crowns with the density of the bite-block, if metal, appearing as a thin white strip between them (1707). In the case of the incisors this examination is often omitted as they can more easily be examined visually.

If special film holders are not available, a small tab of adhesive tape can be attached to the middle of the front surface of the film, on which the patient is instructed to bite so that again the film is held in place against the crowns. It is advisable to test the transradiancy of the tape as many adhesives are radio-opaque (1708).

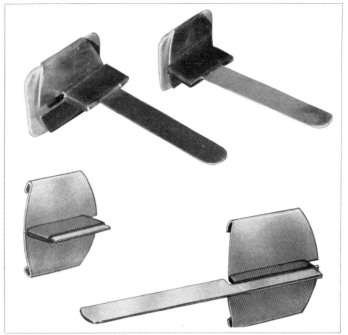

1704

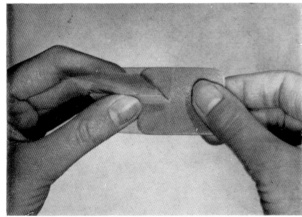

1705

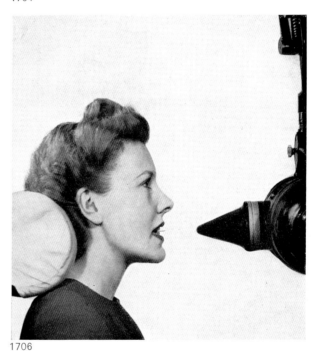

1706

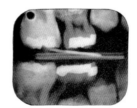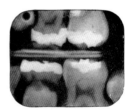

1707

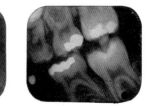

1708

Occlusal

Occlusal view of the upper incisor region

A No 3 occlusal film is inserted in the mouth by its narrow edge and the tube is centred, as for the ordinary dental film view of the incisors, just above the level of the produced occlusal line (1709). The tube-occlusal plane angle must be increased to 70° because the horizontal position of the film increased the tooth-film angle. The pink side of the wrapped film should, of course, face the tube. This radiograph, besides showing the incisor teeth, will show the incisive fossa and possibly the canals, together with the central area of the palate and, above them, the trans-radiant air-filled nasal cavity (1710).

Oblique Occlusal views of the upper jaw

Using the same type of film but placing it, if possible, long edge transversely, the tube is angled at 65° to the occlusal plane (1711). The increase in the angulation is again necessary owing to the horizontal position of the film. Centre halfway along the orbital border for the lateral incisor and canine teeth, or just below the outer canthus of the eye for the premolar and molar region (1711,1712).

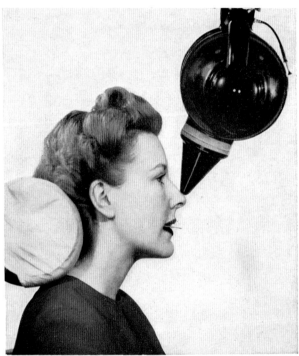

1709

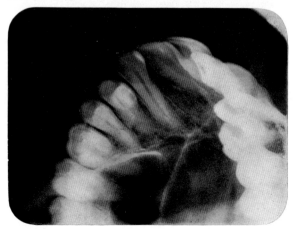

1711

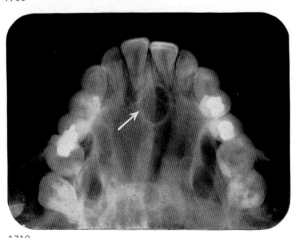

1710

1712

Occlusal view of the lower incisor region

The patient's head is tilted to bring the lower occlusal plane horizontal and, using a No 3 occlusal film, the tube is centred to the lower border of the mandible at the symphysis menti in the same way as for the intra-oral radiograph of the incisors. The tube is angled at 35°–40° to the lower occlusal plane, the increased angle being required because of the horizontal position of the film (1713).

Because the larger film is used, a radiograph of the whole area of the symphysis menti is obtained right down to the lower border of the mandible (1714).

Occlusal plan view of the lower jaw

For this radiograph the film is placed between the jaws as for the previous view, the head being bent well back to enable the tube to be centred at the neck, mid-way between the angles of the mandible and perpendicular to the plane of the film (1715). To accomplish this it must be possible to tilt the head far enough back to allow the tube to be placed well down and almost on to the patient's chest. It may be found that a prominent thyroid cartilage (Adam's apple), particularly in the male subject, makes

it impossible to centre as far back as suggested, but the backward tilt of the head, if well maintained, helps to provide the necessary clearance.

This gives a plan view of the lower dental arch, and is useful to demonstrate fracture displacements (1716), the position of unerupted teeth, or direction of roots of displaced teeth (1715), 1717).

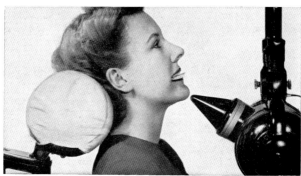

1713

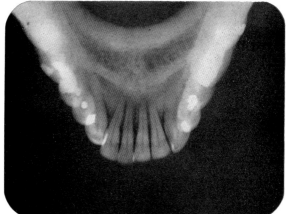

1714

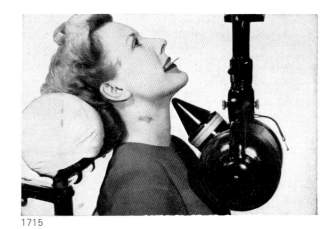

1715

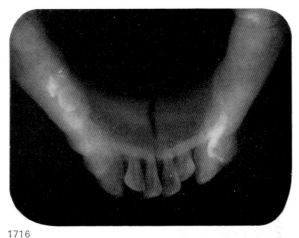

1716

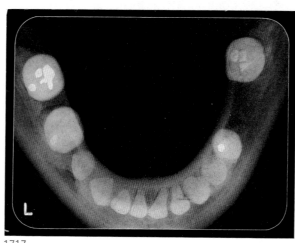

1717

Extra-Oral

The Mandible to show the ramus

For this view, a half-plate or whole-plate cassette is needed and is loaded in the darkroom with Rapid R film placed between intensifying screens.

The radiographs can be taken with the patient standing with the head bent over an angle board (1718), or alternatively seated in the dental chair (1719) or seated at a table (1720), in each the subject is positioned to bring the median line of the face parallel to the film and the interorbital line at right-angles, the tube being directed at 110°–120° to the film. The submental triangle of the patient's neck should be observed if looked at from the position of the X-ray tube (1721,1722).

The Mandible to show the body

The angle board, set at 25°, can be used for this film also, the patient's head being turned toward the cassette to place the body of the jaw on the film. Centre the tube 2 inch below the angle of the jaw remote from the film as before (1723,1724,1725).

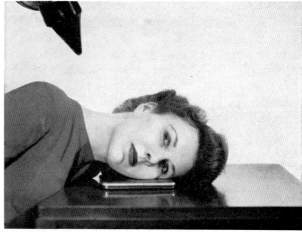
1720

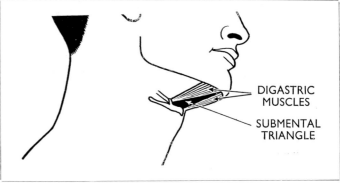

DIGASTRIC MUSCLES

SUBMENTAL TRIANGLE

1721

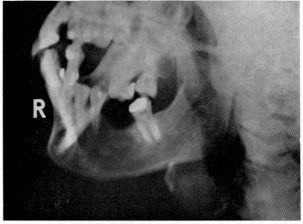
1722

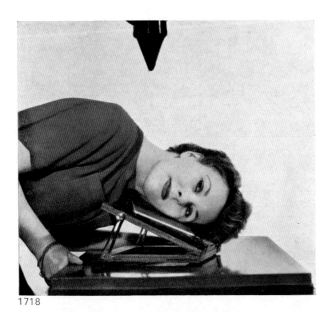
1718

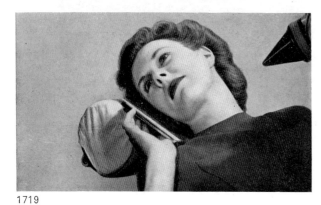
1719

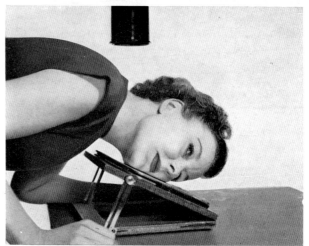
1723

Superior-inferior, collar radiography

Referring to the axial projection of the mandible, page 491, the technique may well be modified for the injured subject. A specially designed cassette enables the film to be placed immediately below the mandible from right to left temporo-mandibular joints.

The cassette, which can be used on any conventional table, here demonstrated with the skull table, serves to produce a satisfactory plan projection of the mandible including the condyles.

Centre to the median-sagittal plane with the tube angled approximately 15 degrees forward toward the mandible molar regions (1726,1727,1728).

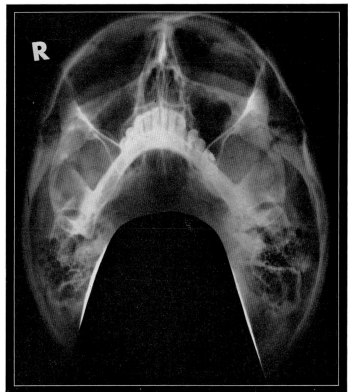

1727

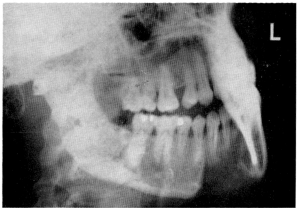

1724

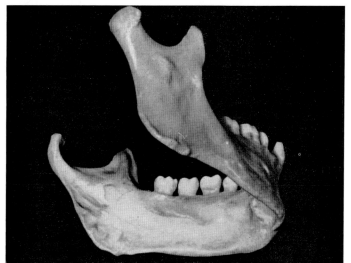

1725

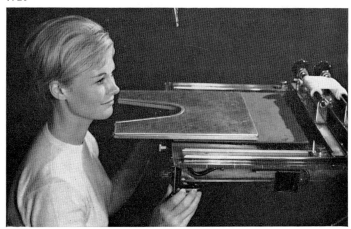

1726

1728

Panagraphy

Panagraphy—pan-oral radiography—is the examination of the upper and lower dental arches by means of an X-ray source operating within the oral cavity with the film placed exteriorly.

Pan-oral radiography has become practicable through the introduction of a special X-ray tube (1730). The bulk of this oil-immersed tube containing the filament and magnetic focusing of the cathode stream is outside the mouth, while the anode at the end of a narrow metal sheath is within the mouth. The tube has a low rating of 0·1 second at 0·5 milliampere and 60 kilovolts, and exposures are thus limited to one per second. As the anode is earthed there is no danger of electrical shock. Lead protection of the anode stem with 2 mm aluminium filtration of the target area reduces radiation to a minimum for the two exposures required for the complete examination of the upper and lower jaws, as against the ten to fourteen exposures by conventional methods.

The focal point 1/250 inch in diameter or 0·1 millimetre is at the tip of the pyramidal shaped anode. This pin-point focus ensures maximum definition and with good contrast, and also with the benefit diagnostically of a magnification of ×2 due to the short focus–object distance and the distance between the teeth and the externally placed film. The electrical capacity is low on account of the minute focal point, but it is ample at the short focus–film distance of about 4 centimetres. Constant potential ensures the maximum of effective radiation for a given input.

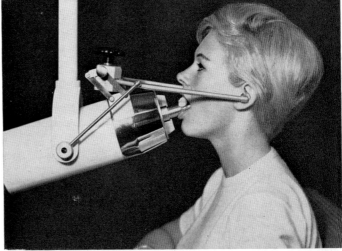

1730

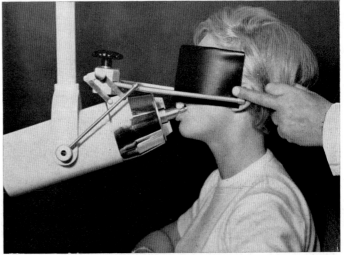

1731

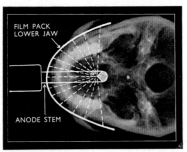

FILM PACK
LOWER JAW

ANODE STEM

1729

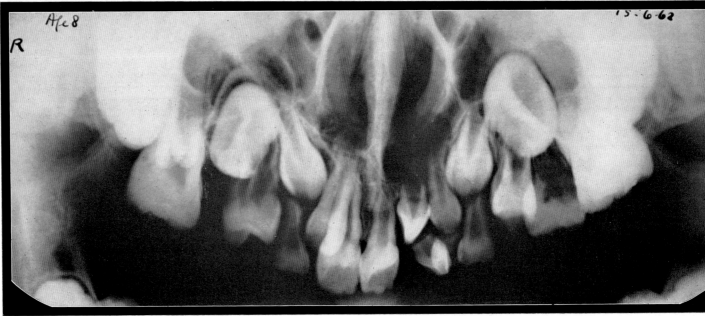

1732

Rapid R film is used in a 4 × 10 inch flexible cassette which is lined with a layer of calcium tungstate to serve in lieu of normal intensifying screens. The outer side of the cassette is lead-backed for absorption of scattered radiation and for protection when it is necessary for the patient to hold the cassette in position.

Within the oral cavity the pin-point focus becomes the axis for the arc of the curve of the teeth toward which the radiation emanates over the wide angle of 270 degrees in two planes, on its passage to the film (1729). The film-cassette is wrapped around the patient's cheeks from ear to ear and positioned appropriately in turn for the upper and lower teeth (1731, 1734).

Adjustable sleeves for the anode are provided, 1 inch in diameter for adults and $\frac{3}{4}$ of an inch for children. Each sleeve has a bite ridge for the incisor teeth to enable the insertion of the anode stem into the mouth to be adjusted in depth to about 2 inches for adults and $1\frac{1}{2}$ inches for children. A sterile polythene cover is renewable for each patient.

The flexible film-pack, approximately 4 × 10 inches, is placed around the face to extend from ear lobe to ear lobe with its lower edge just above the anode stem as it enters the mouth, and generally a little below the level of the occlusal plane. A nylon band or a special chair attachment may be used to maintain the film-cassette in position but the patient is usually sufficiently co-operative to hold the cassette. To avoid obscuring the positions for these demonstration photographs (1731, 1734) the film-cassette is being held in place by a second person (1730, 1731, 1732, 1735).

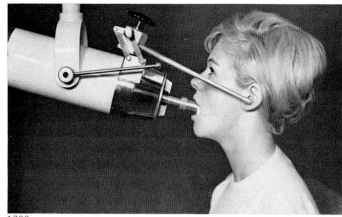

1733

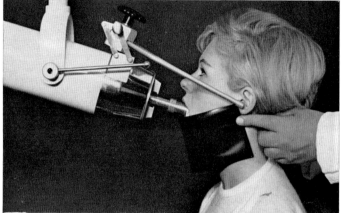

1734

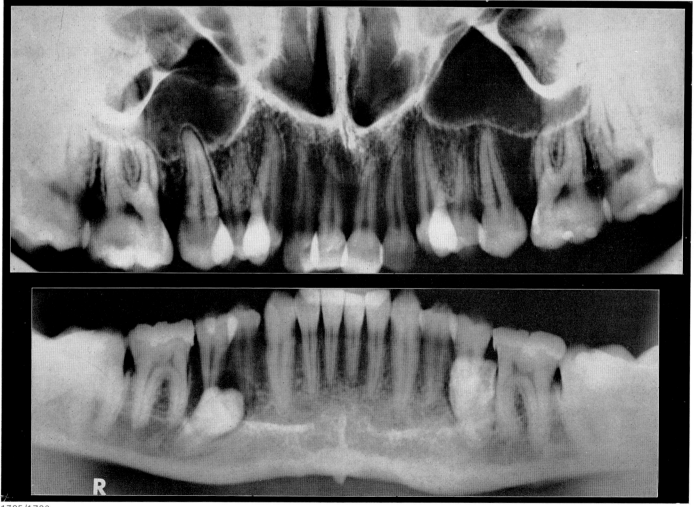

1735/1736

Upper jaw

The seated patient, immobilized against a back and neck support, is placed with the median-sagittal plane vertical and the upper occlusal plane horizontal. An attachment to the tube which can be reversed for upper or lower teeth is adjusted to the angle required for the upper occlusal plane and with the earplugs introduced enables the position of the head to be finally checked before the exposure is made. The tube is angled 30 degrees upward, and having adjusted the bite position to 2 inches for an adult, the anode head is gently introduced into the mouth and the patient is instructed to close the teeth on to the padded bite ring. There is no complaint of discomfort.

Lower jaw

Again, with the median-sagittal plane vertical and the lower occlusal plane horizontal, the earplugs are adjusted and the tube is angled 20 degrees downward. The tube anode is introduced into the mouth and the film-cassette is held in position with its upper border just below the lower tube-anode position and extending with an upward curve to the level of the tragus of the ear from right to left sides (1733, 1734, 1736).

Rotography

Rotography, roto-tomography, is a method for producing radiographs of curved objects such as the mandible, or sections of the skull. In principle the system is a combination of tomography and slit scanography, involving synchronous rotary movements of the patient and film (1737).

In operation, the patient and the curved film rotate in opposite directions, while a stationary X-ray tube projects the image horizontally. By the patient and the film rotating at the same speed, the image of one 'plane' moves with the film and is therefore recorded more sharply than the images of other 'planes' which move at different speeds. To ensure that the section recorded has a suitable thickness and to avoid too many film curvatures, provision is made for a narrow X-ray beam by employing a vertical slit diaphragm 1/32 inch (0·8 millimetre) wide at the tube aperture; there is also a correspondingly proportional vertical slit diaphragm between the patient and the cassette to shield the film from scattered radiation.

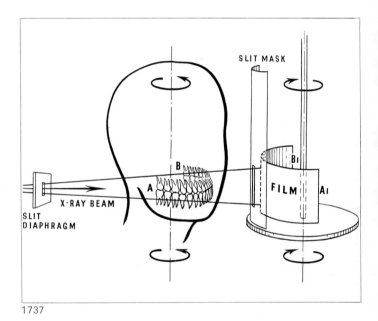

1737

The apparatus for immobilizing the patient's head in the correct position, a modified craniostat attached to the patient's chair, consists of a head-clamp with adjustable pads, plastic earplugs and a chin-rest with adjacent centring device. The special 4 × 10 inch X-ray flexible film-cassette is clamped to a turntable which is interlocked to rotate correctly with the patient's chair. The cassette is made to conform to a shape corresponding to that of the patient's jaw. For guidance an outline of the individual jaw can be checked from a bite made in wax. The holder shown in (1739) is hinged to provide a certain amount of adjustment. More than one type of holder may be provided.

The craniostat can be adjusted in respect of the axis of rotation forward or backward, to include for instance the whole of the mandible and temporo-mandibular joints, or on making a forward sagittal movement of the axis to confine the examination to the teeth. The film turntable is scaled to correspond with the scale on the headclamp for synchronous adjustment. Locating pins on the curved cassette-holder and on the chin-rest ensure the correct relationship between film and skull.

For these facio-maxillary examinations, although the apparatus rotates to a full circle, electrical contacts ensure that the exposure is made only during 180 degrees, beginning and ending in the precise pre-estimated position of the head. In (1739) the exposure is beginning, and in (1740) is approaching half-way. Two density wedges serve to produce uniformity in the molar region as compared with that of the incisor region where X-ray projection is through the cervical vertebrae. A mechanical practice rotation with the patient in position promotes confidence followed by ready co-operation during the actual exposure. Usually there is no discomfort to the patient.

Using Rapid R film and fast intensifying screens an average exposure is 300 milliampere-seconds at 80 kilovolts, the time being 10 seconds, tube current 30 milliamperes, at the incorporated focus–film distance and with the slit diaphragm of 1/32 inch wide (0·8 millimetre). The axis of rotation is irradiated throughout the whole of this exposure, but the skin surface and teeth are irradiated for only a fraction of the exposure. To avoid the pituitary fossa being on the axis of radiation the vertical dimension of the slit diaphragm is adjusted in height or moved forward in the sagittal plane to exclude exposure to the pituitary body.

Using a 3 millimetre aluminium filter and with the narrow diaphragm, radiation exposure is at a minimum.

Rotographs record the following conditions:
(1741a) a fracture at the angle of the mandible.
(1741b) showing the condylar heads with the mouth open.
(1742) a child of four years showing both dentitions with fracture dislocation of the right condyle.

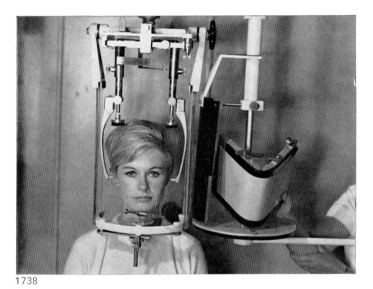
1738

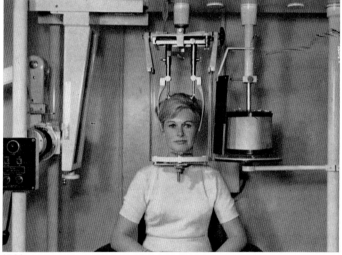
1739

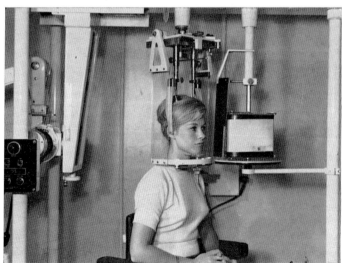
1740

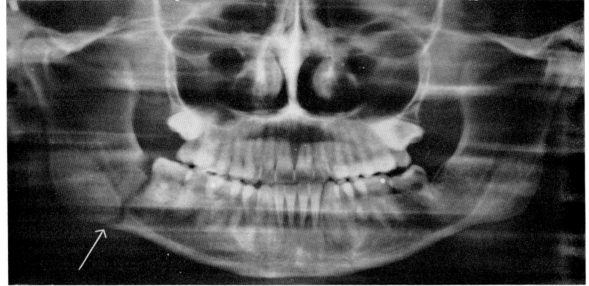

1741a

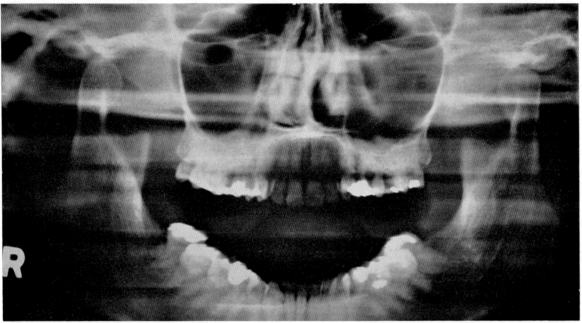

1741b

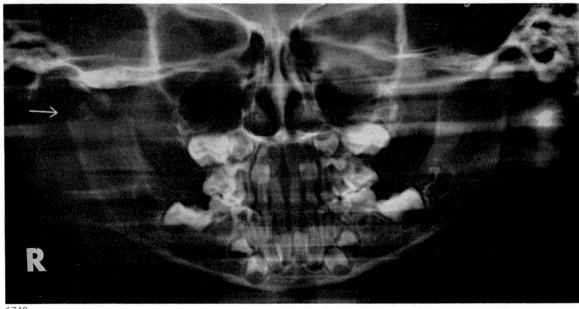

1742

20

SALIVARY GLANDS
LACRIMAL SYSTEM

SALIVARY GLANDS

These glands, consisting of three pairs—parotid, sub-mandibular and sublingual—are situated adjacent to right and left sides and floor of the buccal cavity (1743). They secrete the saliva which passes, via the respective ducts, into the mouth.

The saliva flow may be interrupted by the blocking of the ducts by solid accretions, or calculi, some of which are radio-opaque and can thus be shown in a radiograph.

The examination of the glands and ducts following the injection of opaque medium is termed sialography. The opaque medium is in the form of iodized oil fluid available under various proprietary names which are listed in Supplement 1.

Parotid

The parotid glands, the largest of the three pairs, are situated on the right and left sides of the face and slightly in front of, and below, the ears. The parotid duct leads from the gland, through the tissues of the cheek, to open in the mouth on a papilla opposite the second upper molar tooth. The duct bends inward at the anterior border of the masseter muscle.

The presence of a calculus in the parotid duct can sometimes be demonstrated by placing a dental film in the mouth in front of the upper molars and against the cheek. A short X-ray exposure is sufficient as the calculus may very easily be obliterated by over-exposure. Radiographs (1744) and (1745) are an example of this method, the intra-oral film confirming the presence of the calculus which was only suggested in the occipito-frontal film of the same subject.

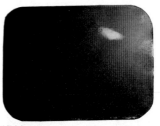

1744

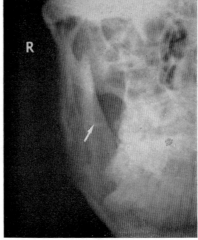

1745

![Diagram of the salivary glands](labelled: PAROTID DUCT, PAROTID GLAND, SUBMANDIBULAR GLAND, SUBMANDIBULAR DUCT, SUBLINGUAL GLAND)

1743

The glands are usually radiographed singly following an injection of iodized oil fluid which is injected through the parotid duct, a very fine catheter being used. The catheter is usually left in the duct during the X-ray examination: only one side is injected at a time. As it is not essential for the injection to be made immediately preceding the exposure, the operation may be carried out in another room or department, delay in the X-ray room being thus avoided. The resulting radiographs show the duct and the fine ramifications within the gland substance.

Lateral oblique

Positioning is similar to that used for the mandible, and either of the methods described in this section may be applied. Illustration (1746) shows the head straight with the tube angled: the shadows of the two sides, right and left, are separated, thus showing the greatest possible detail in the parotid region.

The head is placed in the lateral position with the base line at right angles to the tube direction.

■ Centre below and behind the angle of the jaw with the tube tilted 25 degrees toward the head (1746,1747)

Lateral

As an alternative, with the head lateral and the tube straight, the jaws overshadow from right to left sides. The neck is slightly extended to give the maximum clearance for the parotid gland to be shown in the space between the mandible and the cervical vertebrae.

■ Centre with the tube straight, over the angle of the jaw (1748,1749)

kVP	mAS	FFD	Film ILFORD	Screens ILFORD	Grid
60	5	36″(90cm)	RAPID R	FT	—

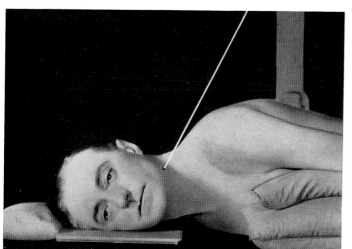

1746

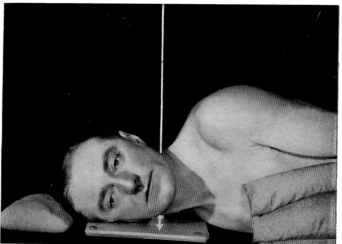

1748

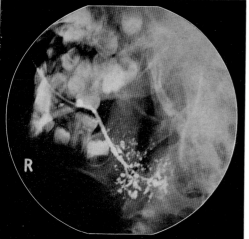

1747

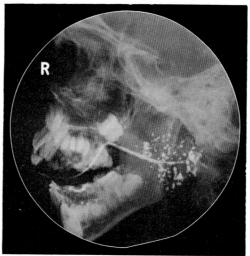

1749

Profile

A further projection of the parotid gland is obtained from either postero-anterior or antero-posterior aspects of the head, either projection being suitable, since the parotid gland is approximately mid-way between the anterior and posterior aspects.

Antero-posterior

With the patient supine, the head is raised on a small non-opaque pad and the chin lowered toward the chest to bring the base line and median plane at right angles to the film.

■ Centre in the mid-line, immediately below the mouth (1750,1751,1752)

kVp	mAS	FFD	Film ILFORD	Screens ILFORD	Grid
65	15	36″(90cm)	RAPID R	FT	Grid

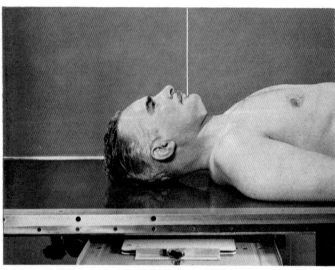

1750

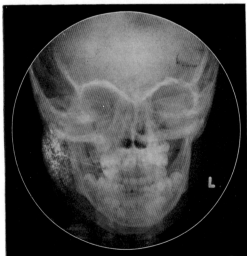

1751

When only one side is to be included it is still necessary to centre to the mid-line, as the parotid gland is mainly superficial to the bone structures and the oblique ray serves to project the soft structures clear of the bone. It is most important to remember that soft structures are being radiographed, and that for these projections films of sufficient density to show good bone detail are not suitable to demonstrate the parotid glands and ducts.

In the sialogram (1751) the parotid gland is clearly demonstrated, with the duct leading to the second upper molar region.

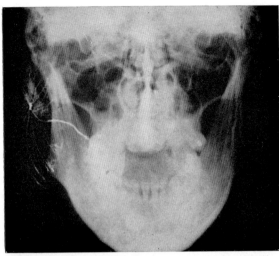

1752

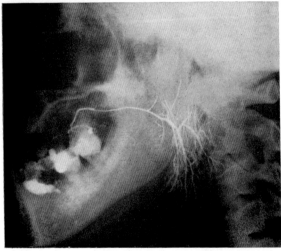

1753

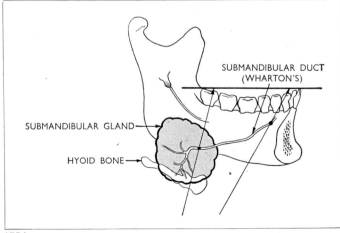

SUBMANDIBULAR DUCT (WHARTON'S)

SUBMANDIBULAR GLAND

HYOID BONE

1754

Salivary glands

Submandibular (Submaxillary)

The submandibular glands are situated on either side of the neck, being internal to, and below, the body of the mandible, the saliva passing via the submandibular duct, which runs backward, upward and then forward along the floor of the mouth to open on a small papilla at the side of the frenulum of the tongue. Two or three projections are made, infero-superior and lateral.

Infero-superior (occlusal) (1)

The patient is seated with the head well back over a suitable support. An occlusal film is placed between the jaws, well over toward the side being examined to include the whole of the gland, and is held in position between the lightly closed teeth.
■ Centre from beneath the jaw, with the axial ray at right angles to the film (1755)

Infero-superior (2)

It is possible that a small opacity may still be hidden behind the tooth shadow at the posterior angle of the duct which may be disclosed on using the following technique.

With the chin raised and the head turned away from the affected side, the occlusal film is inserted into the mouth, and placed diagonally with the greatest dimension along the jaw of the affected side and held lightly in position between the teeth. In this way the film can be placed well back along the jaw.
■ Centre beyond the angle of the jaw at right angles to the film (1756, 1757)

Note—The value of this technique is seen by comparing radiographs taken of the one subject (1758) showing two opacities, with (1757) showing only one opacity.

kVp	mAS	FFD	FILM	Screens ILFORD	Grid
60	20	30″(75cm)	FAST	OCCLUSAL	—

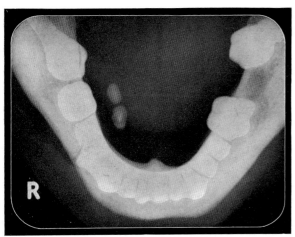

1755

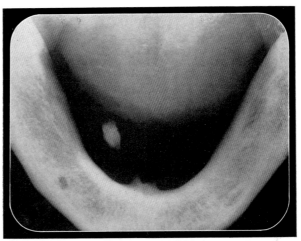

1757

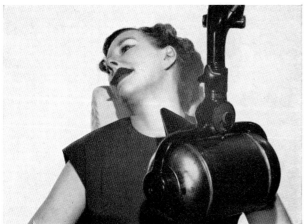

1756

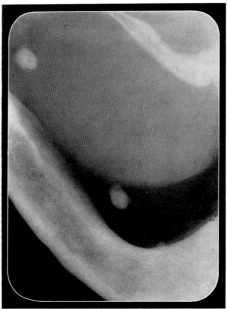

1758

Lateral

Either of the lateral projections used for the parotid gland may be applied. Of these the true lateral is the more suitable, the result of such positioning being shown in (1759).

In making these projections the presence of a calculus not sufficiently opaque to show through the bone may be confirmed by depressing the floor of the mouth with a cotton-wool pad under the tongue on the affected side. This will press the opacity beyond the shadow of the mandible (1759).

The calculus is often at the bend of the duct, somewhat medial to the roots of the third molar.

Sialograms of the submandibular glands show in (1760,1761) the normal passage of the iodized oil fluid along the submandibular duct to the gland just below the mandible.

It should be noted that (1760) was taken with pressure maintained on the syringe, and (1761) after the syringe had been removed.

Sublingual

These glands are situated in the floor of the mouth and beneath the tongue; several ducts end by small openings on the sublingual fold on either side of the frenulum and some may open into the submandibular duct.

The same projection may be taken as for the submandibular glands, but of these the occlusal projection is the more important, and is frequently the only exposure made. As the glands are more anterior than the submandibular it is not necessary to press the occlusal film so far back in the mouth (1762).

kVP	mAS	FFD	Film IILFORD	Screens ILFORD	Grid
60	5	36"(90cm)	RAPID R	FT	—

kVp	mAS	FFD	Film FILM	Screens ILFORD	Grid
60	20	36"(90cm)	FAST OCCLUSAL	—	—

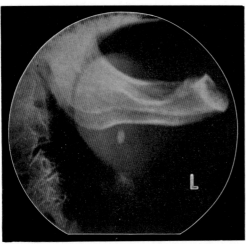

1759

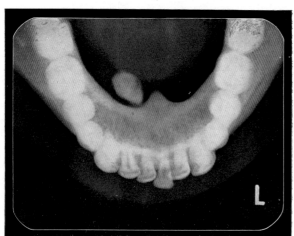

1762

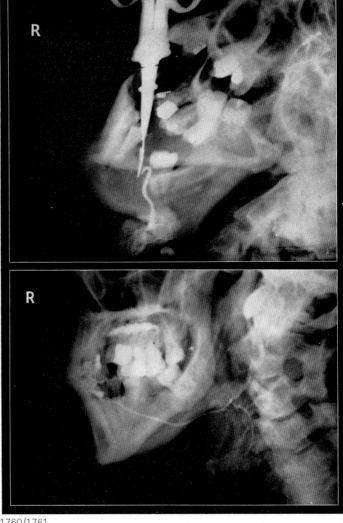

1760/1761

Lacrimal system

The lacrimal apparatus of each eye consists of the lacrimal gland, which secretes the tears, and the lacrimal passages, through which the tears pass from the eye to the nose (1763).

The lacrimal gland is in the upper and outer part of the orbital cavity, and the lacrimal passages commence near the inner canthus of the eye. These passages are made up of the canaliculi, one in each lid. They commence in orifices called puncta lacrimalia, which lie on the lid margin in apposition with the eyeball, and they cannot be seen until the lids are everted. The tears enter the canaliculi through the puncta and flow first in a vertical direction for 2 millimetres and then horizontally for 7 millimetres to the point where the canaliculi fuse to enter the lacrimal sac. The lacrimal sac continues into the naso-lacrimal duct and is defined from it by a narrowing of this part of the drainage system, approximately 1 centimetre from the point of entry of the canaliculi, into its apex. The sac and naso-lacrimal duct form a passageway 3 centimetres long, which ends below the inferior concha, well back in the nose. The bony naso-lacrimal canal is approximately 1 centimetre long. The lacrimal sac lies on the lateral aspect of the nose in the lacrimal fossa of the orbit.

The lacrimal passages are examined radiographically by the injection of an iodized oil of low viscosity, such as Neo-Hydriol fluid (see Supplement 1). The examination is carried out primarily to determine the cause of imperfect flow of the tears when the eye is watering.

With the patient lying on the X-ray couch, two or three drops of a local anaesthetic (Ophthaine) are put into the lacrimal lake. The lower lid is everted and with a blunt dilator, placed first in a vertical direction and then horizontally, the punctum is dilated sufficiently to accept a silver lacrimal cannula. The lacrimal cannula is fitted to a 2 millilitre syringe loaded with the opaque medium.

The injection is continued until the patient tastes the fluid or until it regurgitates from the upper or lower punctum. On turning the patient over to face the couch radiographs are taken in the occipito-mental and lateral positions (1764, 1765); the naso-pharynx must be included. The procedure is repeated for the other eye.

In normal subjects the ducts empty in fifteen to thirty seconds, and the medium is seen on the floor of the nose. In those with watering of the eye, an obstruction in the passages is shown by retention of the medium in the passage above the obstruction, often with gross dilation of the sac.

In positioning the patient it should be remembered that the naso-lacrimal duct is inclined backward, and in order to have it parallel with the film, and thus projected without distortion, the orbito-meatal angle should be reduced from 45 to 40 degrees.

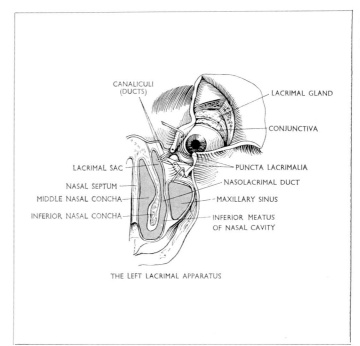

CANALICULI (DUCTS)

LACRIMAL GLAND

CONJUNCTIVA

LACRIMAL SAC

PUNCTA LACRIMALIA

NASAL SEPTUM

NASOLACRIMAL DUCT

MIDDLE NASAL CONCHA

MAXILLARY SINUS

INFERIOR NASAL CONCHA

INFERIOR MEATUS OF NASAL CAVITY

THE LEFT LACRIMAL APPARATUS

1763

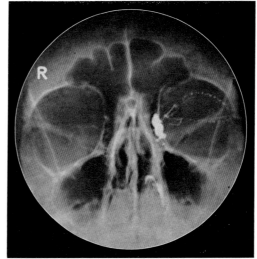

1764

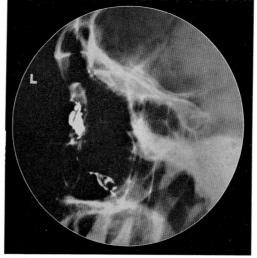

1765

21

TEMPORAL BONES
OPTIC FORAMINA

ADDITIONAL
SKULL PROCEDURES

TEMPORAL BONES

Anatomical position and structure

The temporal bones form part of the lateral aspects and floor of the cranium. Each consists of squamous, mastoid, petrous and tympanic portions and styloid process. Of these, this section deals chiefly with the mastoid and petrous portions, and only brief reference is made to the remainder of the temporal bone.

The squamous portion is a flat area of thin bone situated above, in front of, and behind the ear (1771a).

The tympanic portion forms the antero-inferior part of the external auditory meatus and enters into the mandibular fossa (1771a).

The styloid process is long and slender, and projects downward toward the angle of the jaw (1768).

The mastoid portion, behind the ear, contains the mastoid (or tympanic) antrum and the mastoid air cells, which vary in shape, number and size from subject to subject (1766,1771a).

The petrous portion, or pyramid, is the most complex part of the temporal bone, being wedged between the sphenoid and occipital bones in the base of the cranium, and containing the essential parts of the organ of hearing and equilibrium (1767, 1771c).

The organ of hearing and equilibrium consists of three parts, the external ear, the middle ear or tympanic cavity, and the internal ear or labyrinth (1767).

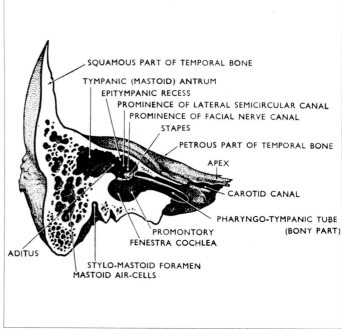

1766

The external ear consists of the auricle (the expanded portion), and the external auditory meatus which extends from the base of the auricle to the tympanic membrane (1767).

The tympanic membrane is a sheet of fibrous tissue, 10 millimetres in diameter, almost circular in shape and oblique in position; it separates the external ear from the middle ear (1767,1769).

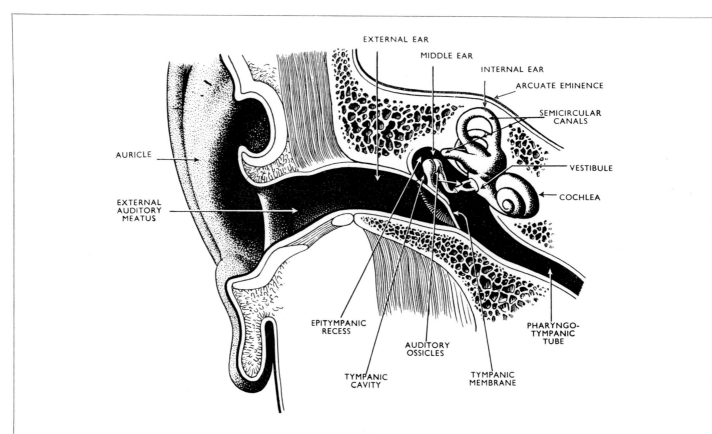

508

1767

Anatomical position and structure

The auditory ossicles are a chain of fragile bones, the malleus, the incus and the stapes, which connect the tympanic membrane with the inner wall of the tympanic cavity, bridging the cavity and transmitting to the internal ear vibrations received from the external ear, by the tympanic membrane (1767,1769).

The middle ear or tympanic cavity, is a small air space between the external ear and the internal ear. It extends above the level of the tympanic membrane to form the epitympanic recess and contains the auditory ossicles (1767,1769).

A triangular opening, the aditus, in the posterior wall of the epitympanic recess, leads to the tympanic antrum. The tympanic, or mastoid antrum, is an air cavity behind the epitympanic recess (1766).

The internal ear or labyrinth consists of a series of bony cavities, named the vestibule, the semicircular canals—superior, posterior and lateral—and the cochlea (1767); contained within the labyrinth is a similarly shaped membranous vessel (1770).

The pharyngo-tympanic tube extending between the pharynx and the tympanic cavity enables the air pressure on each side of the tympanic membrane to be equalized (1767).

The internal auditory meatus, 10 millimetres in length, is almost opposite to the external auditory meatus commencing at the fundus adjacent to the vestibule and cochlea of the internal ear. The canal passes transversely through the petrous part of the temporal bone in a medial direction to terminate posteriorly just above the jugular foramen (1768). It transmits the facial and auditory nerves and the internal auditory artery across the petrous bone.

It is essential to know the anatomy of the temporal bone and its position in the skull in relation to other structures; much can be learned from experimental exposures made on the dry skull, but it is not until the radiographic appearances as shown in the radiographs of living subjects are appreciated that it is possible to carry out the examination of the temporal bones with confidence.

The general relationship of the temporal bones will be appreciated from the three illustrations of the dry skull, external lateral (1771a), a section through the median-sagittal plane (1771b) and the transverse section (1771c), which latter is most helpful in presenting the plan arrangement of the principal base structures.

21

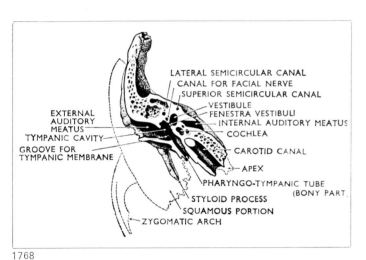

1768

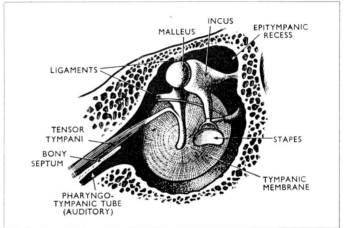

1769

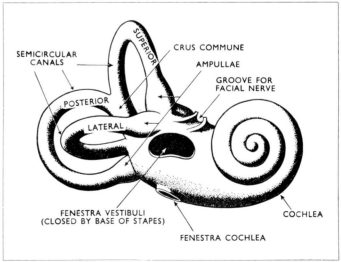

1770

Planes, lines and landmarks

As in previous sections concerned with the skull, observance of the recognized planes, lines and landmarks for guidance in positioning the patient for radiography is most important. The terminology recommended by the Neuroradiological Commission, with appropriate illustrations, is shown in (1772,1773).

These illustrations show the planes and lines referred to in this section for guidance in radiographic projection. Of particular note is the lateral projection accompanied by angulation of the X-ray tube. Thus emphasis is to be placed on the adjustment of the skull with the base line transverse to the axial movement of the tube. On the X-ray couch or vertical stand, the base line should be at right angles to the length of the couch or stand to enable the appropriate tube angulation to be applied with precision for right and left sides in turn.

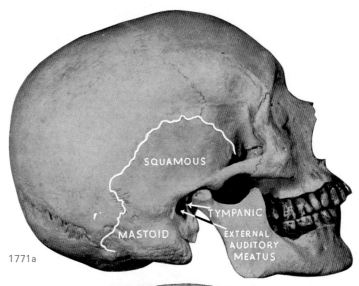

1771a

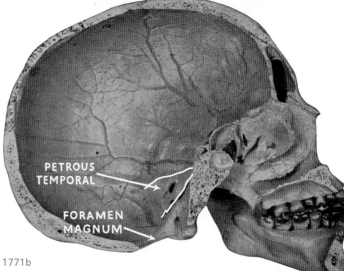

1771b

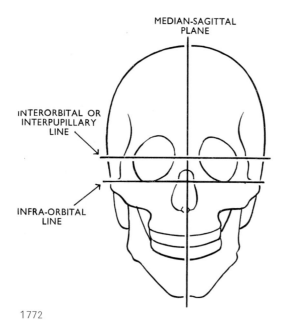

1772

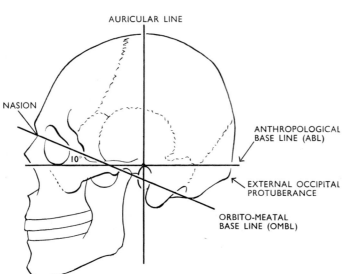

1773

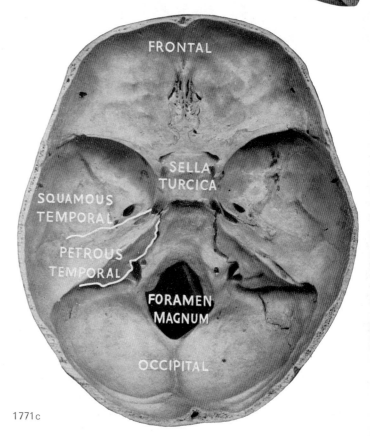

1771c

Technique and equipment

Radiographic investigation is concerned with demonstrating the various cavities and their contents, the cavities being so small and delicately placed within the temporal bone that only the most exacting positioning technique and the finest film definition can demonstrate this region successfully.

To obtain the necessary definition a fine-focus tube is essential, also a small localizing cone and fine grain intensifying screens. Films may be taken either with or without the grid, and the patient may be examined in either the erect or the horizontal position. Both sides are always taken for comparison. Stereoscopic radiographs, macrographs and/or tomograms may also be required.

Important—Each film should be carefully marked as to right and left, using $\frac{1}{4}$ inch lead letters.

The exposure factors quoted in the text refer to an adult subject of average physique.

Several projections are required—lateral, oblique and axial. The method of obtaining these projections depends on whether the special skull table is available, or whether an examination is being made on the standard radiographic couch or with the vertical stand.

The difference in the two methods is that for the skull table the tube can be centred automatically to the intersection of the cross-lines of the skull support for any tube angulation, the desired angle being obtained with precision; also that the position of the head over the cross-lines, by an ingenious arrangement of mirrors and suitable illumination, can be seen from below through the transparent table top. Furthermore, only routine and readily adjustable positions of the head are employed and comparative projections are obtained by precise tube angulation.

With other types of apparatus the head, and frequently both tube and head, are adjusted to obtain the more intricate projections. Centring of the tube is then to the estimated near tube surface of the head, and the cassette is displaced to allow for off-centre projection of the image. To convert the instructions and technique given for the skull table into similar methods for the standard couch or vertical stand, it is necessary to have some means of establishing, on the tube aspect of the head, the position of the intersection of cross-lines shown on the head support. This can be done by using a pointer, or a frame carrying crossed threads, the tube with the necessary degree of angulation being previously centred to the intersection of the cross-lines on the table.

In the following pages, several methods are given for each projection, using both standard equipment and the skull table. There is also a summary of the projection technique for the skull table on page 519, with radiographs on pages 520 and 521.

Examination with the standard equipment is given in two parts, the mastoid and petrous portions of the temporal bone, pages 512 to 518 and 522 to 528 respectively.

For the mastoid region in profile (1) using the angle board is the simplest to carry out, but the vertical projection profile (2) is usually preferred, pages 512, 514.

Lateral projections are made with either the patient's head or the tube tilted in two directions, and again several methods are shown on pages 516 and 517.

Axial and half-axial projections (35 degrees fronto-occipital and occipito-vertical) are used to show both mastoid regions on the one film, page 518.

For the petrous portion of the temporal bone two alternatives are given to the oblique position, (1) Stenver's projection (1804) and (2) a similar projection using the skull table, page 526. Two lateral projections and again the axial and half-axial projections complete the examination.

In using the special skull table the complete examination for the mastoid and petrous portions of the temporal bone is covered by four or five projections. Three projections are taken with the head lateral, two with the tube angled, in turn, 15 degrees and 35 degrees toward the feet, and one with a 30 to 35 degrees angle toward the face. For the latter, the grid is rotated so that the grid slats are in the same direction as the X-ray beam; to obtain a similar projection on the standard X-ray couch, it would be necessary to use a stationary grid.

The axial and half-axial projections are similar on both types of equipment, although adjustment for the base projection on the skull table is both more comfortable for the patient and more convenient for the operator. Both projections may be taken in reverse. Narrow rectangular diaphragms enable the temporal bones to be shown with increased clarity due to the elimination of scattered radiation.

For all projections, care should be taken in adjusting the base line to the correct angle. This adjustment is sometimes overlooked for the lateral projections, and is of particular importance when there is a tube tilt, as this is often the cause of failure to obtain matching projections of right and left sides. This applies also to other examinations of the skull.

Mastoid

The mastoids occupy accessible, mid-lateral positions behind the ears, as seen from the lateral aspect of the skull (1771a). In the true lateral position of the head the right and left mastoids coincide, and it is necessary to use oblique projections in order to obtain separation of the two shadows.

The mastoid process in profile usually presents the greater difficulty. It is necessary to project the process clear of the cervical vertebrae by rotating the head on its axis and at the same time slightly downward in order to project the mastoid tip below the shadow of the occipital bone.

Films may be taken from either antero–posterior or postero–anterior aspect, with or without the angle board and grid. With modern apparatus and suitable accessories the exact duplication of the two sides is a simple achievement.

It is imperative that the walls of the cells should be sharply defined, and that there should also be adequate contrast between actual air cells and walls.

Profile

In these projections the less dense mastoid process is projected clear of the shadows of the base of the skull, with the denser shadow of the mastoid antrum appearing in the same film. In order to demonstrate both densities satisfactorily, it is necessary to compromise in applying the exposure factors. A kilovoltage suitable for the antrum is selected: this should be sufficiently high to reduce the contrast between the two bone densities so that both antrum and tip are equally well shown. A lower kilovoltage, although producing brilliant intimate contrast in the mastoid process, allows either under-exposure of the antrum or over-exposure of the tip, this latter necessitating viewing by local intense spot lighting.

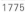

1774

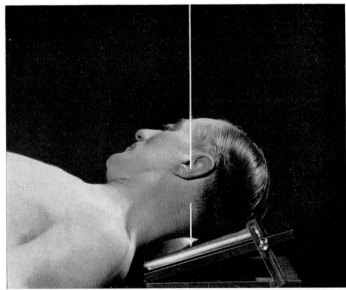

1775

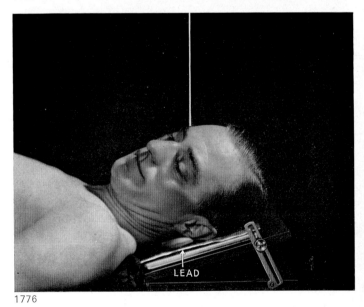

1776

(1) Antero-posterior oblique (basic) Angle board

With the patient supine, the head is placed in contact with the cassette on the 15 to 25 degrees variable angle board, the base line being at right angles to the film border. From this position the head is turned through an angle of 35 degrees away from the affected side, the chin being kept well down toward the chest. The visual view of the head in this position shows the mastoid process in direct alignment with the film and without over-shadowing by adjacent bone structure (1775).

The two sides may be taken on a single film by covering alternate halves with lead as shown in the illustrations, or by using a special cassette tunnel.

■ Centre over the root of the mastoid process remote from the film. A small localizing cone is essential (1774,1775,1776,1777, 1778)

In the resulting radiographs (1777,1778) the mastoid process and antrum are clearly demonstrated. This position is readily obtained and should be within the scope of all workers. The angle board may be replaced by a solid angle block or by suitably placed sandbags.

The angle of the angle board should be varied according to type of subject. A patient with thin shoulders and a long neck will allow comfortable adjustment of the head at a 15 degrees angle, but for a thick shouldered subject, with a short neck, an angle of 25 degrees is essential.

The position of both the patient and the angle board may be reversed to give a similar radiographic result. The patient is then in the prone position and with the angle board open toward the neck. The head is rotated 55 degrees in relation to the film and the tube is centred over the mastoid process nearest the film (1779). Compare with (1774) in the supine position.

21

kVp	mAS	FFD	Film ILFORD	Screens ILFORD	Grid
65	15	36″(90cm)	RAPID R	HD	—

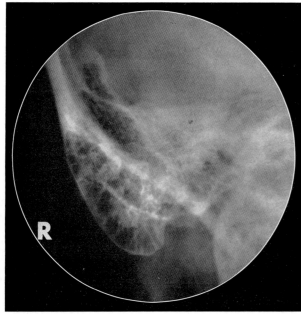

1777

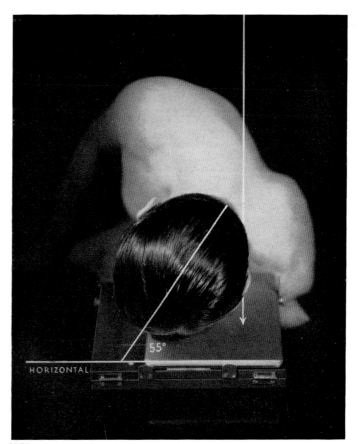

1779

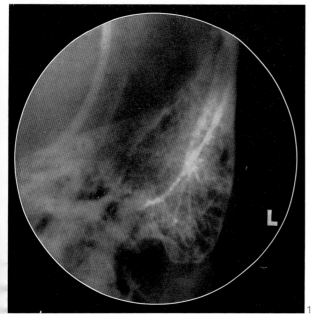

1778

(2) Postero-anterior oblique

This projection may be made with the patient in either the erect or the horizontal position, the Potter–Bucky diaphragm being usually employed.

The head is placed in the occipito-frontal position, with the head-clamp applied to the bi-temporal diameter, and then turned through 35 degrees to the affected side, the base line–film angle being adjusted to 85 degrees. In the horizontal position correct angulation is obtained by applying the protractor to the head from the end of the couch (1784).

■ Centre mid-way between the occipital protuberance and the external auditory meatus of the side nearest the film, with the tube angled 12 degrees toward the head (1780,1783,1784,1785, 1786)

kVp	mAS	FFD	Film ILFORD	Screens ILFORD	Grid
70	40	36″(90cm)	RAPID R	HD	Grid

On examining the head in this position it will be seen that from the tube aspect the mastoid process is in profile and free from overshadowing structures, as also in the previous positions with the angle board.

Comparison for similarity should be made of the two pairs of films taken to show the mastoid process in profile (1781,1782) postero-antero and (1785,1786) antero-posterior oblique.

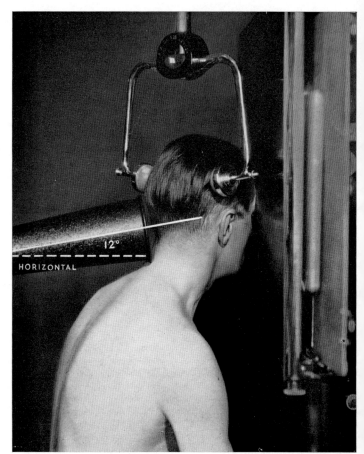

1780

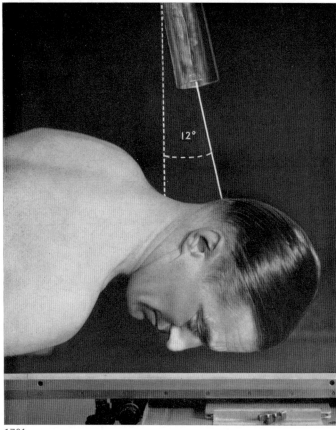

1781

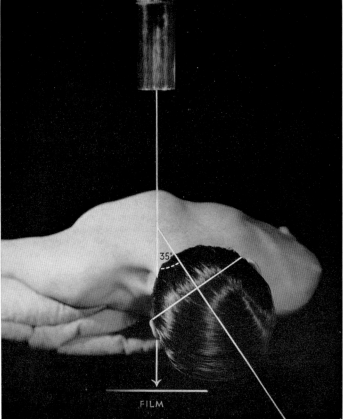

1782

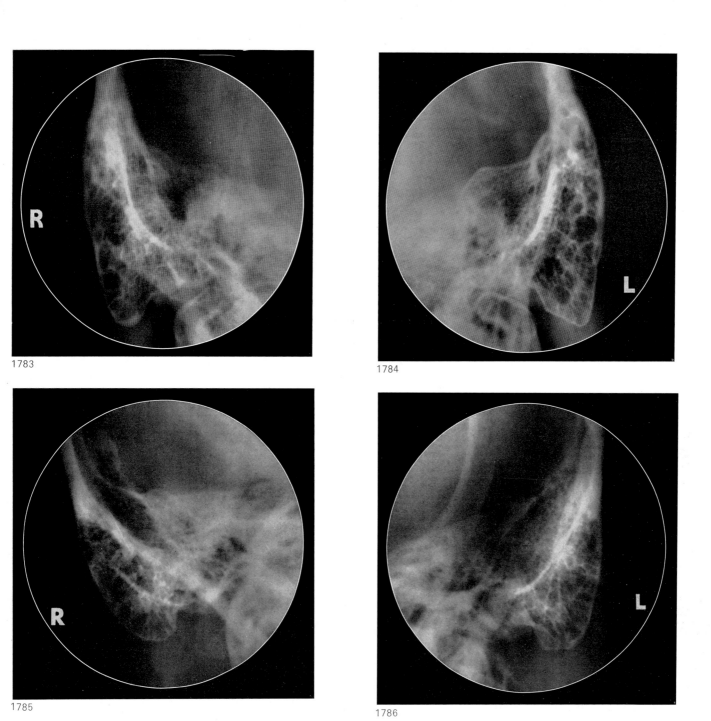

1783

1784

1785

1786

Lateral oblique

For the lateral projection separation of the two sides is obtained either by tilting the head or by angling the tube in relation to the head. The auricle of the ear proximal to the film is folded forward to enable the maximum definition to be obtained, as the air cells are shown superimposed on the cranial bones.

(1) Angle board

In this position the face is rotated 15 degrees forward and inclined 15 degrees downward, using either the angle table shown in (1787), with the patient seated, or the angle block shown in (1788,1791), with the patient either seated or lying full length on the couch.

The auricle of the ear is folded forward (1792) and the head placed with the median plane parallel, and the interorbital line at right angles, to the angle board.

The measurements of a suitable angle block are given in (1791).

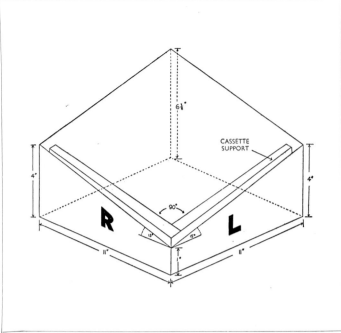

1791

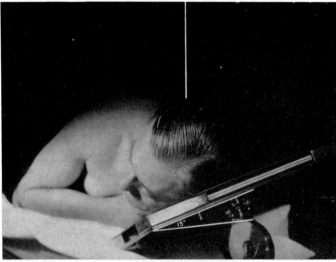

1787

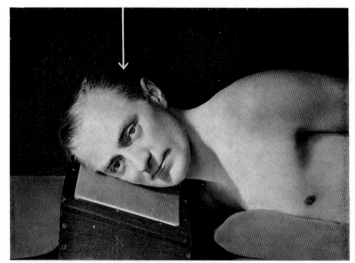

1788

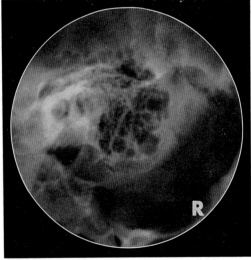

1789

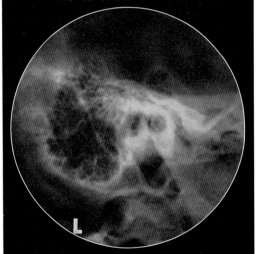

1790

(2) Head tilted

From the lateral position the head is allowed to tilt forward and downward to assume a naturally comfortable position, with the chin and cheek in contact with the film support, the auricle of the ear being folded forward to avoid obscuring the mastoid cells. This position allows the two sides to be well separated from the tube to film aspect.

■ Centre two inches each above and behind the external auditory meatus remote from the film, with the tube straight, using a small extension cone. Both sides are taken for comparison (1792,1793,1789,1790)

(3) Tube angled

For this projection, exposing right and left sides in turn, the head is maintained in the true lateral position, either erect or horizontal, and the tube angled to obtain separation from side to side.

The auricle of the ear proximal to the film is folded forward, as for the two previous projections (1792).

■ Centre two inches above and 2 inches behind the external auditory meatus remote from the film, with the tube angled 15 degrees toward the face and 15 degrees toward the feet, the axial ray passing through the mastoid proximal to the film (1794,1789,1790)

This method, depending entirely on tube angulation, may be found to be more difficult to apply, as the double tube angulation toward the correct centring point is not easy to adjust unless a centre finder or long extension cone is used.

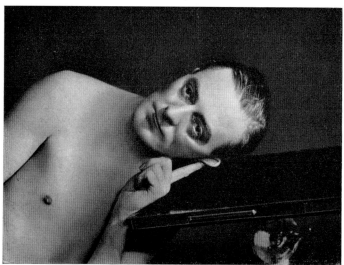

1792

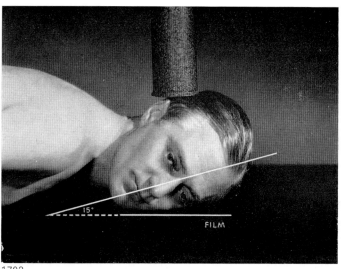

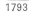

1793

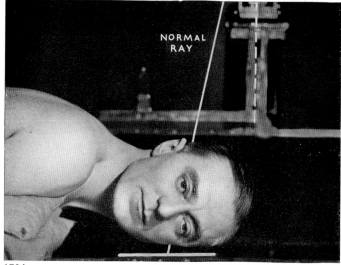

1794

21

Temporal bones
Mastoid

Axial

In each of the following projections the right and left mastoid regions are shown simultaneously and symmetrically following a single exposure.

35° Fronto-occipital

The patient is placed facing the tube, with the chin well down on the chest and with the occipito-cervical region in contact with the film support.

■ Centre in the median line between the mastoid processes, with the tube angled 35 degrees toward the feet (1795,1796)

In this projection, a single exposure shows both mastoids symmetrically, on the same film.

Occipito-vertical

With the patient facing the film, the head is flexed forward, with the chin well down on the chest to bring the vertex of the skull into contact with the film support. The base line to film angle should be approximately 50 degrees.

■ Centre mid-way between the roots of the mastoid processes (1797,1798)

kVp	mAS	FFD	Film ILFORD	Screens ILFORD	Grid
80	80	36″(90cm)	RAPID R	HD	Grid

In the resulting radiograph both mastoid regions are shown, following a single exposure.

For both projections shown on this page the patient may be examined in either the erect or the horizontal position.

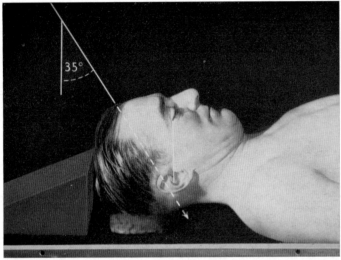

1795

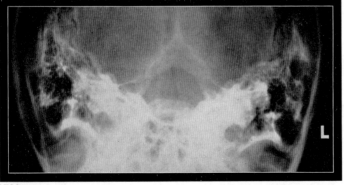

1796

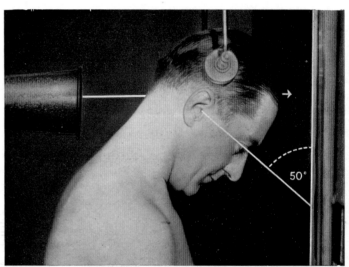

1797

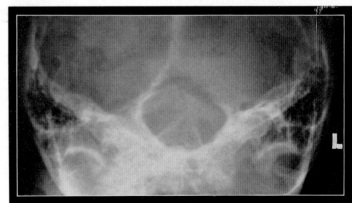

1798

Petrous

Before commencing this examination of the middle and internal ear, reference should be made to the illustrations and anatomical description of this region on pages 508 to 510. Reference should also be made to pages 520 and 521 where the technique for the petrous bone is illustrated by radiographs and tracing diagrams as described later on this page. The technique in the following pages is adapted to the use of the general X-ray couch, the vertical stand and the skull table.

Radiographs are taken of each side separately; laterally, with two different tube angles and either from the posterior oblique or lateral oblique aspects. In films exposed from the fronto-occipital and submento-vertical aspects both sides are shown following a single exposure.

The patient may be examined in either the horizontal or erect position. A fine-focus tube and small localizing cone are essential and, with the use of the moving grid, every effort is made to obtain good contrast and definition, while, owing to the great density of this region, a fairly high kilovoltage is employed.

Auditory nerve tumour

Investigation for the purpose of demonstrating the presence of an auditory (eighth) nerve tumour should include radiographs showing the petrous portion of the temporal bone, and particularly the internal auditory meatus, both sides being exposed for comparison, either separately, or simultaneously as shown in the radiographs and tracing diagrams on pages 517 and 518.

The axial projection of the temporal bones of a stillborn infant (1832b) is of interest to compare with the adult subject (1832a).

The series of radiographs and tracing diagrams on pages 520 and 521 were taken under the following conditions:

(1799, 1800)
Head lateral, auricle folded forward and with the external auditory meatus centred to the intersection of the cross-lines on the head-rest, base line parallel to the transverse line, tube angled 15 degrees toward the feet and centred to the cross-lines (1821) page 525. On the standard couch (1811), page 522.

(1801, 1802)
Head lateral, auricle folded forward and a point 2 centimetres below the external auditory meatus placed over the intersection of the cross-lines, base line parallel to the transverse line, tube angled 35 degrees toward the feet, and centred to the cross-lines (1823), page 525. On the standard couch (1811), page 522.

(1803, 1804)
Head lateral and bent forward so that the base line is at an angle of 5 degrees to the transverse line, or with the tube tilted 10 degrees toward the head as in (1825,1826), page 526. A point 2 centimetres in front and 1 centimetre above the external auditory meatus is placed over the intersection of the cross-lines, tube angled 30 to 35 degrees toward the face and centred to the cross-lines.

(1805, 1806)
Stenver's projection as shown on page 523. It should be noted that the radiographs compare very closely with (1803,1804).

(1807, 1808)
Half-axial 35 degrees fronto-occipital with slit diaphragm; the patient is supine with the nape of the neck placed over the intersection of the cross-lines and with the base line vertical, tube angled 30 to 35 degrees toward the feet and centred to the cross-lines, page 527.

(1809, 1810)
Axial or base projection, submento-vertical, with slit diaphragm; with the base line parallel to the film, the tube is centred between the angle of the jaw and with the axial ray at right angles to the base line (1831), page 527.

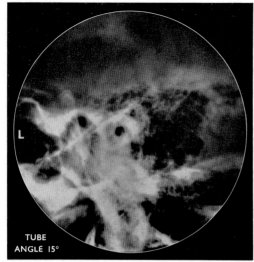

1799

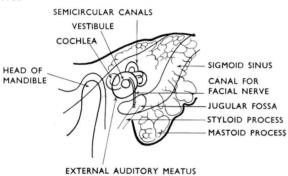

SEMICIRCULAR CANALS
VESTIBULE
COCHLEA
HEAD OF MANDIBLE
SIGMOID SINUS
CANAL FOR FACIAL NERVE
JUGULAR FOSSA
STYLOID PROCESS
MASTOID PROCESS
EXTERNAL AUDITORY MEATUS

1800

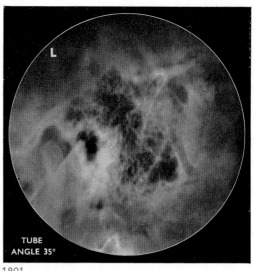

1801

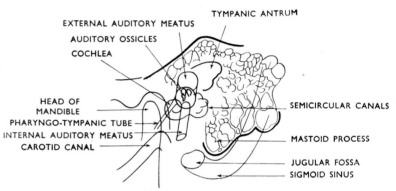

EXTERNAL AUDITORY MEATUS
TYMPANIC ANTRUM
AUDITORY OSSICLES
COCHLEA
HEAD OF MANDIBLE
PHARYNGO-TYMPANIC TUBE
INTERNAL AUDITORY MEATUS
CAROTID CANAL
SEMICIRCULAR CANALS
MASTOID PROCESS
JUGULAR FOSSA
SIGMOID SINUS

1802

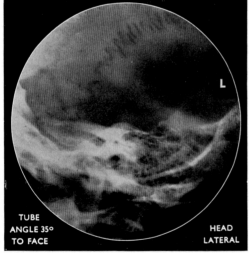

TUBE ANGLE 35° TO FACE   HEAD LATERAL

1803

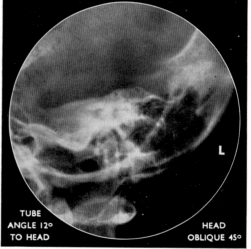

TUBE ANGLE 12° TO HEAD   HEAD OBLIQUE 45°

1805

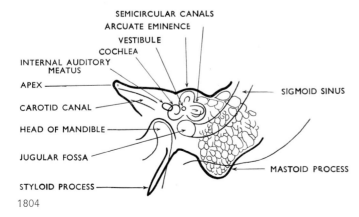

SEMICIRCULAR CANALS
ARCUATE EMINENCE
VESTIBULE
COCHLEA
INTERNAL AUDITORY MEATUS
APEX
CAROTID CANAL
HEAD OF MANDIBLE
JUGULAR FOSSA
SIGMOID SINUS
MASTOID PROCESS
STYLOID PROCESS

1804

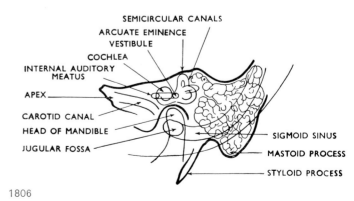

SEMICIRCULAR CANALS
ARCUATE EMINENCE
VESTIBULE
COCHLEA
INTERNAL AUDITORY MEATUS
APEX
CAROTID CANAL
HEAD OF MANDIBLE
JUGULAR FOSSA
SIGMOID SINUS
MASTOID PROCESS
STYLOID PROCESS

1806

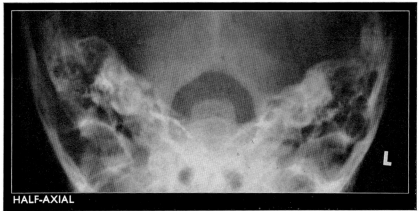

HALF-AXIAL

1807

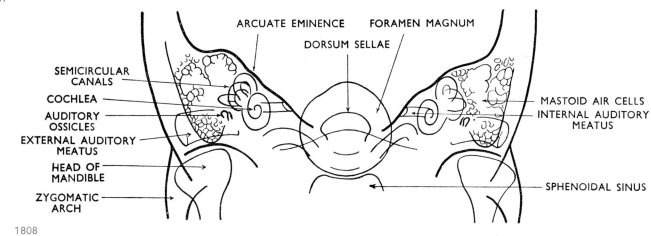

SEMICIRCULAR CANALS
COCHLEA
AUDITORY OSSICLES
EXTERNAL AUDITORY MEATUS
HEAD OF MANDIBLE
ZYGOMATIC ARCH

ARCUATE EMINENCE
FORAMEN MAGNUM
DORSUM SELLAE

MASTOID AIR CELLS
INTERNAL AUDITORY MEATUS
SPHENOIDAL SINUS

1808

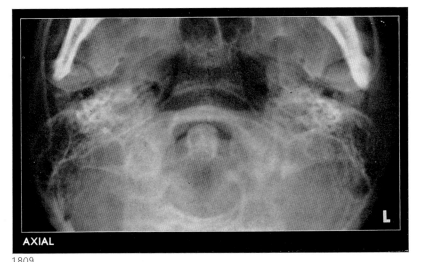

AXIAL

1809

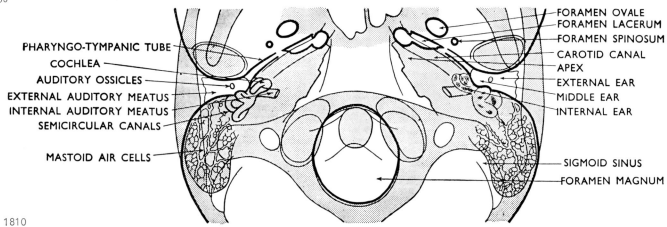

PHARYNGO-TYMPANIC TUBE
COCHLEA
AUDITORY OSSICLES
EXTERNAL AUDITORY MEATUS
INTERNAL AUDITORY MEATUS
SEMICIRCULAR CANALS
MASTOID AIR CELLS

FORAMEN OVALE
FORAMEN LACERUM
FORAMEN SPINOSUM
CAROTID CANAL
APEX
EXTERNAL EAR
MIDDLE EAR
INTERNAL EAR
SIGMOID SINUS
FORAMEN MAGNUM

1810

kVp	mAS	FFD	Film ILFORD	Screens ILFORD	Grid
70	50	36"(90cm)	RAPID R	HD	Grid

General purpose couch or stand
Lateral

Two projections are made with the head in the true lateral position and with the auricle of the ear folded forward. To ensure that comparable projections are obtained of right and left sides the base line of the skull must be at right angles to the direction of the tube angulation. For the first projection the tube is angled 15 degrees toward the feet and centred 1 inch above the external auditory meatus (1811,1812). For the second projection the tube is angled 35 degrees toward the feet and centred 3 inches above the external auditory meatus (1811,1813). Reference should be made to tracing diagrams (1800,1802) shown on page 520.

For these projections, to show the labyrinth it is necessary to use high penetration and close coning; the increased tube angulation from 15 to 35 degrees necessitating an addition of 10 milliampere-seconds for the latter.

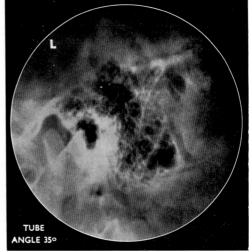

1812

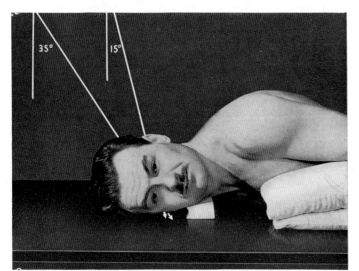

1811

1813

Oblique—Postero-anterior

The patient is placed with the head in the occipital-frontal position. The patient is adjusted in position so that the central line of the table is under the middle of the supra-orbital margin of the eye on the side being examined. The radiograph base line is at right angles. Rotate the head 45° to the affected side to bring the superior border of the petrous temporal parallel to the film. This position can be checked by applying a protractor from the end of the couch.

■ Centre with the tube angled 12° toward the head mid-way between the external auditory meatus and the occipital protuberance. A small diaphragm aperture should be used and both sides taken for comparison

This is a modification of Stenver's view.

The illustration of the transverse section of the dry skull (1815) is positioned and lined to show the relationship of the petrous portion of the temporal bone to the film and tube, and to emphasize the necessity for exact head adjustment to bring the petrous temporal parallel to the film to enable satisfactory projections to be made.

kVp	mAS	FFD	Film ILFORD	Screens ILFORD	Grid
85	60	36″(90cm)	RAPID R	HD	Grid

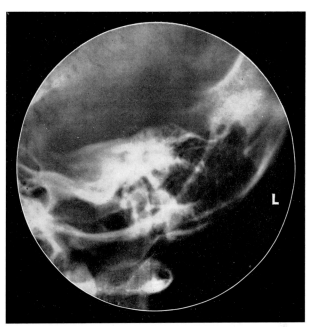

1816

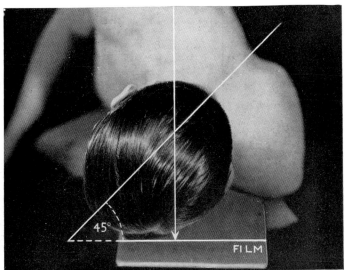

1814

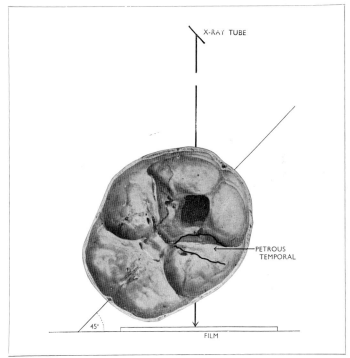

1815

Simultaneous comparison of petrous
Fronto-occipital

The head is placed in the fronto-occipital position, the base-line is at right angles to the film. Centre in the mid-line over the vertex so that the petrous is projected directly within the orbital cavities. The frontal-occipital position is preferred to the occipital-frontal position in that the orbital cavity area being remote from the film is considerably magnified allowing a more intensive area of the petrous on either side to be seen. This view is particularly suited to children (1817,1818).

Modified Stenver's adapted to skull table

The patient is placed with the head in the occipito-frontal position. The base line is at right angles. The head is adjusted so that the central cross lines are over the middle of the supra-orbital margin of the eye on the side being examined. The head is then rotated 45° to bring the petrous of the side being examined parallel with the film.

■ Centre mid-way between the external auditory meatus and the occipital protuberance with the tube angled 12° cephaled. A small diaphragm aperture is necessary to maintain contrast. Both sides are taken for comparison (1819).

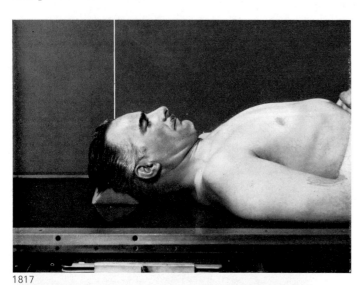

1817

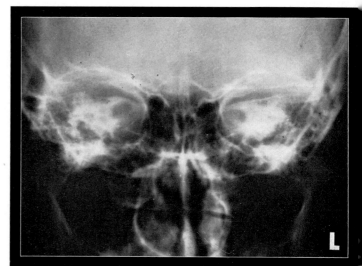

1818

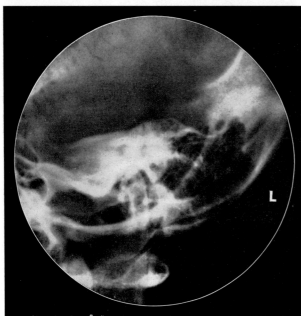

1819

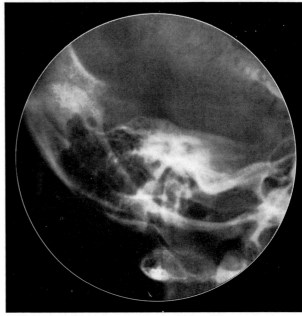

1820

Skull table

Lateral (1)

Taking right and left sides in turn, with the patient prone and with the auricle folded forward, the head is turned to assume a lateral position with the cross-lines, as seen in the mirror, just behind the external auditory meatus. Careful adjustment is necessary to enable the interorbital line to be at right angles to the film and the base line to be at right angles to the direction of tube angulation.

■ Centre with the tube angled 15 degrees toward the feet; the central ray is directed to a point just behind the external auditory meatus to correspond to the position of the cross-lines as seen in the mirror (1821,1822)

kVp	mAS	FFD	Film ILFORD	Screens ILFORD	Grid
75	150	36″(90cm)	RAPID R	HD	Grid

Lateral (2)

With the head lateral and the auricle folded forward, the cross-lines in the mirror should be at a point just behind and 1 centimetre below the external auditory meatus. Again, the interorbital line is at right angles to the film and the base line is at right angles to the tube angulation.

■ Centre with the tube angled 35 degrees toward the feet, corresponding with the position of the cross-lines as seen in the mirror—1 centimetre below and just behind the external auditory meatus (1823,1824)

Note—These two lateral projections (1822,1824) combine to give valuable detail of anatomical structures as shown in the radiographs with tracing diagrams (1799,1800) and (1801,1802).

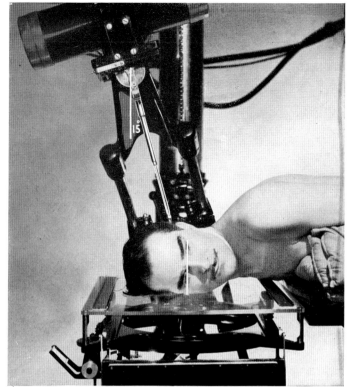

1821

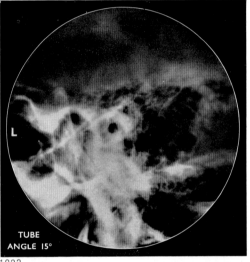

1822

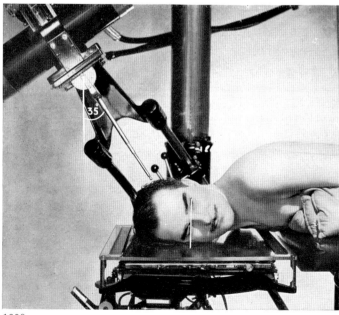

1823

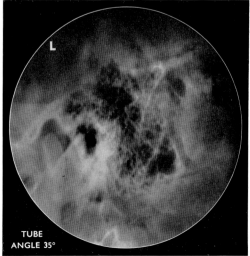

1824

			Films	Screens	
kVp	mAS	FFD	ILFORD	ILFORD	Grid
85	100	36″(90cm)	RAPID R	HD	Grid

Oblique—lateral

With the patient prone, the head is placed in the lateral position as for the lateral projection, but with the cross-lines as seen in the mirror 2 centimetres in front and 1 centimetre above the external auditory meatus. The head is flexed forward to enable the base line to be at an angle of 5 degrees to the transverse cross-line.

■ Centre with the tube angled 30 degrees toward the face and 10 degrees toward the head, with the point of entry of the angled beam coincident with the mirrored position of the cross-lines. The grid is rotated to enable the grid slats to be parallel to the direction of the angled beam (1825,1826,1827,1828)

Note—The direction of the beam is at right angles to the long axis of the petrous bone and the resulting radiograph is similar to that produced by the modified Stenver's projection (1816). Reference should be made also to radiographs and tracing diagrams (1803,1804) as compared with (1805,1806).

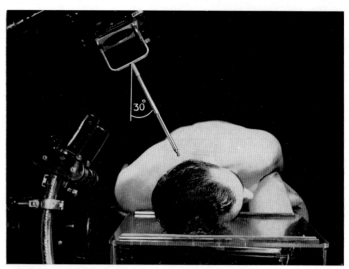

1826

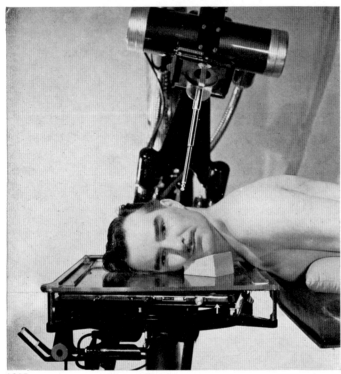

1825

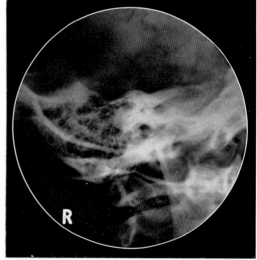

1827

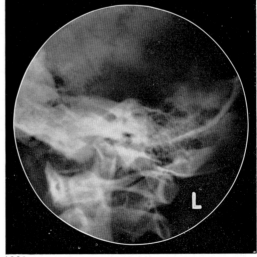

1828

The right and left temporal bones may be shown for comparison on a single exposure, being made in either the half-axial or axial positions. Reference should be made to the tracing diagrams of these projections (1808) and (1810) on page 521. A narrow rectangular diaphragm is used for these projections.

35° Fronto-occipital (half-axial)

With the patient supine, the skull table is angled to bring the base line at right angles to the film and with the mirrored cross-lines at the nape of the neck.

■ Centre with the tube angled 35 degrees toward the feet (1829,1830)

kVp	mAS	FFD	Film ILFORD	Screens ILFORD	Grid
80	120	36″(90cm)	RAPID R	HD	Grid

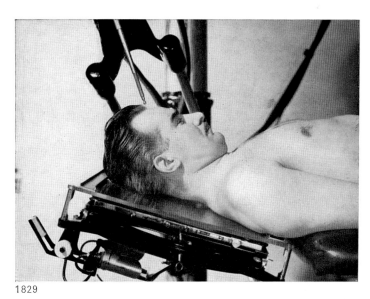

1829

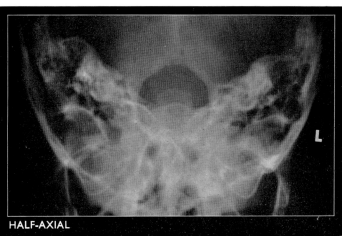

HALF-AXIAL

1830

Submento-vertical (axial)

The patient is placed in the supine position with the head extended to bring the vertex of the skull into contact with the skull table which is lowered and angled when necessary for the patient's comfort, the ideal position being attained when the base line is parallel to the film.

■ Centre between the external auditory meatuses, from below the mandible with the tube angled at 95 degrees to the base line (1831,1832a)

kVp	mAS	FFD	Film ILFORD	Screens ILFORD	Grid
85	150	36″(90cm)	RAPID R	HD	Grid

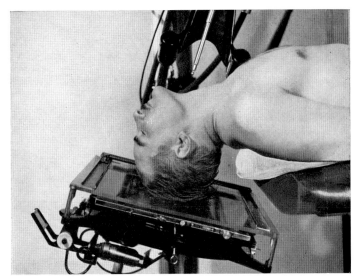

1831

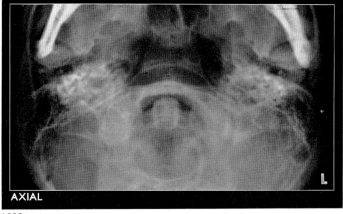

AXIAL

1832a

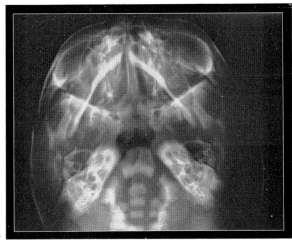

1832b

21 Tomography

Although the position of the auditory ossicles can be seen in a standard radiograph of the temporal bones, tomography enables these tiny individual bones to be more readily identified. Layers are taken at 1–2 mm intervals throughout the shallow depth occupied by this chain of minute bones, the malleus, the incus and the stapes. Trisection multisection is also suited to this technique. The 1 mm thickness of the card backing of the intensifying screens provides the necessary interval between the film levels. Three exposures divided over a 10 × 12 film ensures that adequate coverage and location have been achieved.

Pluridirectional movement will provide the greatest distinction between subject levels and is recommended for this multisection procedure.

For the subject demonstrated in (1833) three levels are included on right and left sides in turn, at

11 centimetres
10·9 centimetres and
10·8 centimetres

Technique

The patient is supine, the head in the fronto-occipital position with the base line at 90 degrees to the couch-top. The head is immobilized by using a head band or clamp.

Spaced diaphragm apertures 15 mm diameter are used and the tube is centred over the glabella, or if each side is localized separately, centre through each orbit with a single 15 mm diaphragm aperture.

The recommended angle, is the greatest available, whichever of the three movements linear, circular or hypocycloidal is in use.

The initial level is the table-top to tragus distance, thereafter with trisection this height is dropped 3 millimetres for each of the two successive exposures.

Other structures which may be shown within the depth recorded are the internal auditory meatus, the cochlea, the semicircular canals, the internal, auditory canal and the antrum.

Two patient positions are in general use:
(1) The anterior-posterior projection (described above)
(2) Lateral oblique (both sides being exposed separately).

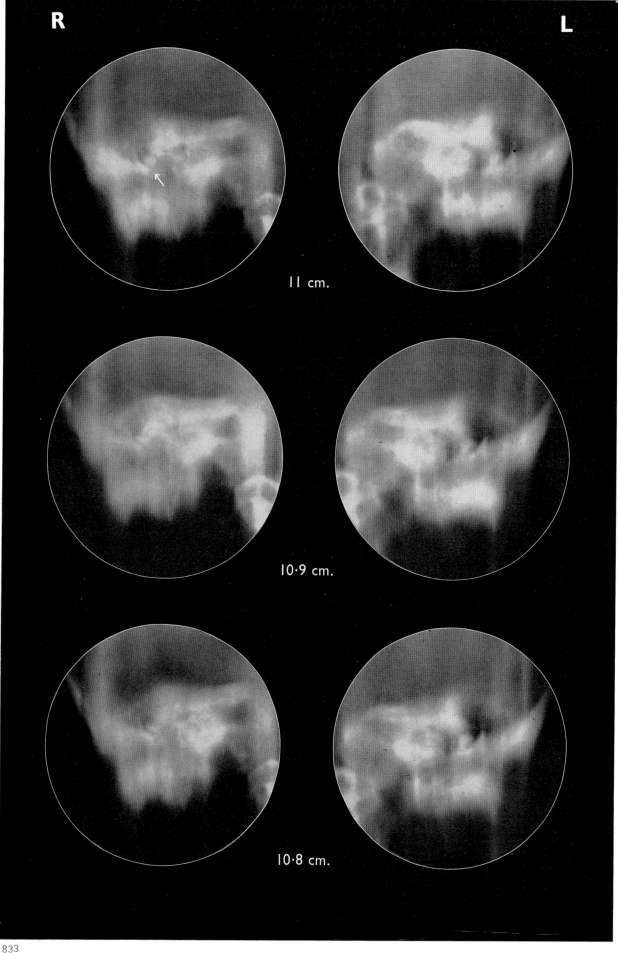

11 cm.

10·9 cm.

10·8 cm.

Macroradiography

Employing enlargement technique results showing the delicate internal structure of the middle ear are particularly rewarding.

The patient is supine with the base-line at 90° to the film and carefully immobilized, the tube with a narrow slit diaphragm is centred over the mid-orbital region. The use of a 0·3 mm focal spot is essential and the level of the petrous is situated mid-way between focus and film. Standard screens are used for this ×2 enlargement.

The grid is removed, allowing the space-gap to attenuate the scattered radiation and improve contrast.

The enlarged structures of the middle ear are shown with clarity within the boundaries of the orbits.

Illustration (1834) shows how readily the skull unit may be adapted for enlargement technique.

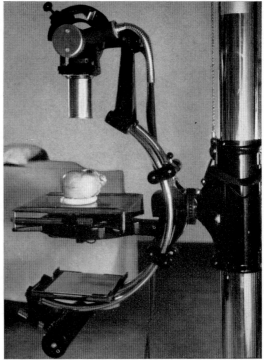

1834

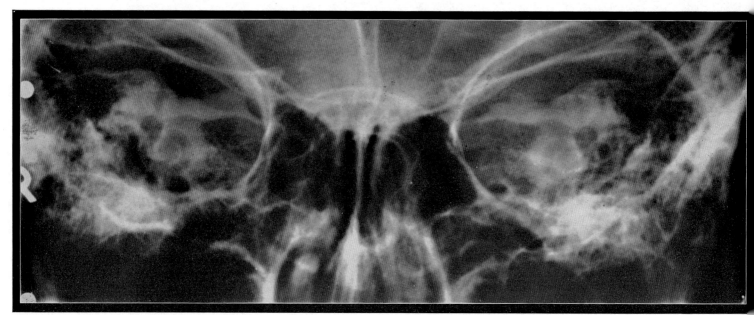

1835

Optic foramen

The two short canals forming the optic foramina transmit the optic nerves from the cranium to the orbits, passing in a forward direction (1836), downward (1837), and obliquely outward (1838), to terminate above and medially to the apex of each orbit. Radiographically, the foramina appear as nearly circular apertures within the orbital cavity. In the three radiographs of the dry skull, a coil of lead foil has been inserted into the foramen on the right side, to enable the aperture to be visualized from the lateral (1836), anterior (1837), and plan (1838) aspects. From these radiographs the necessary projections to see through the foramina can well be appreciated.

Another series of exposures on the dry skull taken at different degrees of rotation shows that at 35 degrees rotation of the head the foramina appear to be circular (1839), that at 25 degrees the foramina are oval in shape (1840), and likewise at 45 degrees rotation of the head the foramina appear as oval-shaped apertures (1841). Hence the adoption of 35 degrees rotation of the head.

Two methods are shown, (1) for the general couch and (2) for the skull table.

The general couch method depends largely on the adjustment of the head in relation to the tube, whereas the skull table method provides for the adjustment of the tube centring in relation to the head on the head being placed in a symmetrical standard position.

On referring to a third series of exposures on the dry skull, it will be seen that provided the head is positioned correctly for the general couch method, there is little change in the appearance of the foramina, whether the tube is centred 1 inch forward (1846), backward (1847), upward (1848), or downward (1849), in relation to the recommended centring point.

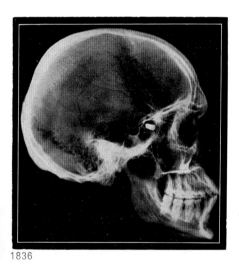

1836

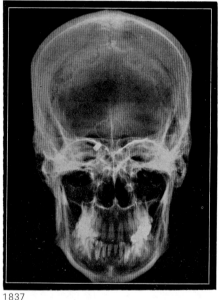

1837

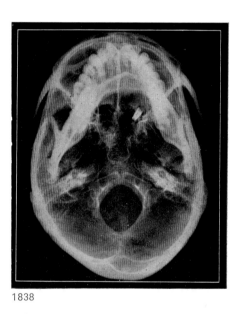

1838

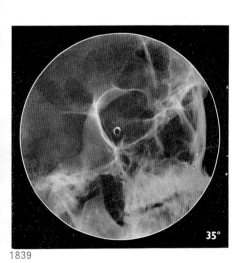

1839

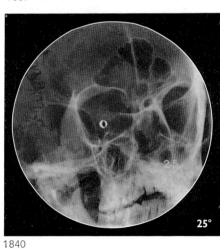

1840

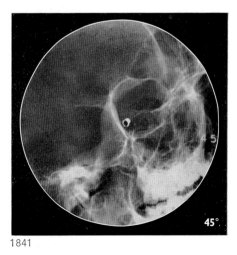

1841

General couch method

With the patient in the prone position, the head is placed with the base line at an angle of 35 degrees to the couch, and then rotated 35 degrees to right and left sides in turn to bring the orbital margin concerned parallel to the film.

■ Centre three inches above and two-and-a-half inches behind the uppermost external auditory meatus and directly through the orbit of the side being examined (1842,1843,1844,1845)

kVp	mAS	FFD	Film ILFORD	Screens ILFORD	Grid
70	100	36″(90cm)	RAPID R	HD	Grid

The radiographs (1845) should be compared with similar projections taken of the same subject on the skull table (1852).

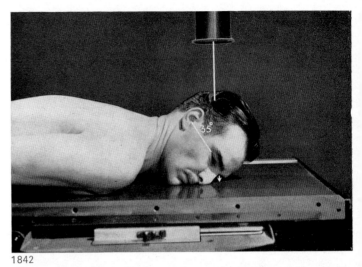

1842

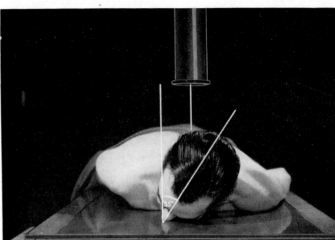

1843

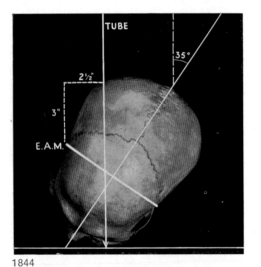

1844

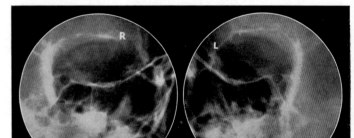

1845

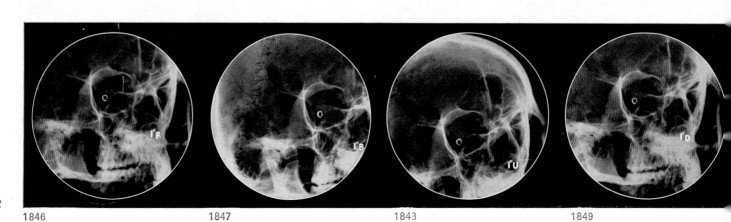

1846   1847   1843   1849

Skull table method

With the patient prone, place the head with the median sagittal plane and the baseline at right angles to the film and with the cross over the inner canthus of the orbit examined, as viewed from the mirror aspect. Adjust the cassette one inch toward the side to be examined and one inch toward the feet. Rotate the grid to enable the slats to be parallel to the direction of the X-ray beam, use the eccentric diaphragm to confine the beam to the side being examined.

■ Centre automatically to the centre of the skull table. Angle the tube 20 degrees toward the feet and 20° to the centred optic from the opposite side to that being examined. Both orbits should be examined for comparison

On taking the opposite side, remember to move the grid, eccentric diaphragm and film to the appropriate displaced positions.

The radiographs (1852) should be compared with similar exposures made on the general couch (1845).

Abnormalities

Two radiographs show the difference from side to side with an abnormal condition reported on the right side (1853).

Tomography

With tomography by the multisection method, assuming the thickness of the backing of the intensifying screens as 1 to 2 millimetre separators, rewarding results are obtained particularly when a suspected defect is difficult to define.

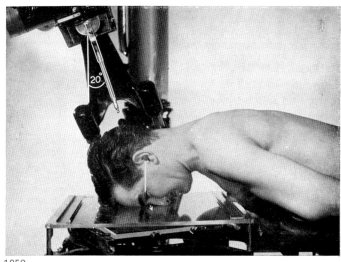

1850

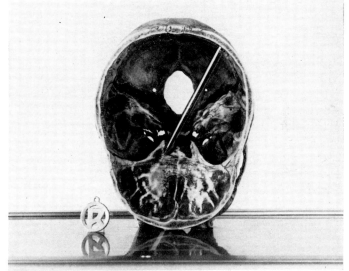

1851

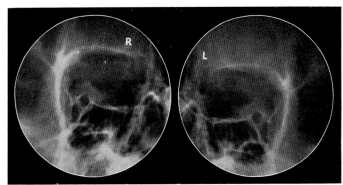

1852

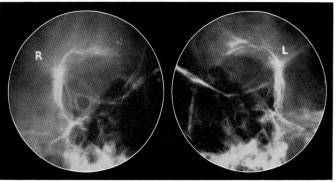

1853

Alternative skull positioning

Conventional skull positioning is with a view to ensuring that the subject interest is in its closest proximity to the film. The extended rating of both the 0·3 mm–0·6 mm, however, permit alternative skull procedure wherein although the subject matter is more remote from the film, the resulting magnification is obtained with acceptable definition. In a number of instances this permits adapting positioning, primarily with a view to the comfort and convenience of the injured patient.

Further advantages are that difficult location of centring may be more readily facilitated, and the increased obliquity of the radiation due to the extended part-film displacement; may produce greater dissociation of closely adjoining subject areas.

The following are a number of skull positions where, for one or other of these reasons, they may be considered to be a more satisfactory procedure.

Reversed optic foramina technique

With the head in the antero–posterior position the chin is raised to bring the radiographic baseline at an angle of 35°, the head is then rotated 35° away from the affected side. The superior and inferior orbital cavity margins of the affected orbit are now parallel with the plane of the film.

■ Centre directly over the eye with the X-ray beam perpendicular to the film

Both orbits are taken for comparison, and in the initial set-up, the head is displaced 1 inch to the left and right side of the centre line of the table in turn to centralise the respective orbital cavity.

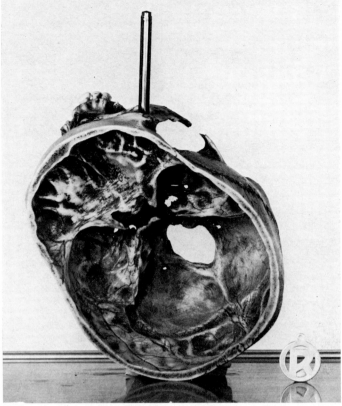

1854

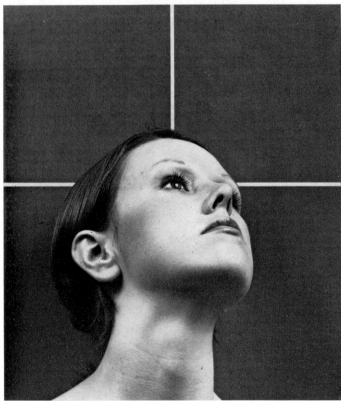

1855

Antero-posterior oblique

From the antero-posterior position, with the baseline perpendicular to the film, rotate the head 45° *away* from the affected side.

■ Centre one inch (2·5 cm) in, and above the EAM with the central ray directed 10° caudally (1856, 1857)

Both sides are taken for comparison.

45° Antero-posterior oblique

From the antero-posterior position, with the baseline perpendicular to the film, rotate the head 45° *to* the affected side.

■ Centre two inches (5 cm) above the fronto-zygomatic suture closest to the tube with the central directed 45° caudally (1858)

As can be seen from the dry skull illustration (1859) the petrous on the side to which the skull is orientated, is projected in a vertical direction, and this aspect may provide additional information to the conventional transverse projection.

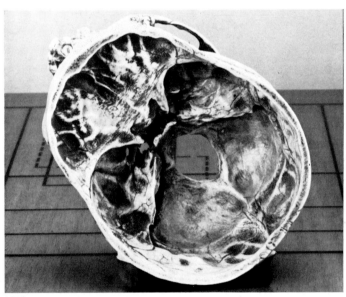

1856

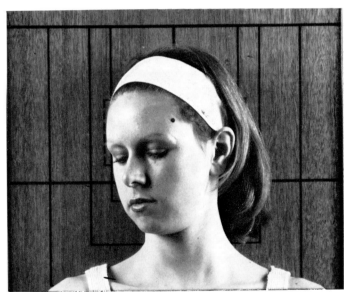

1858

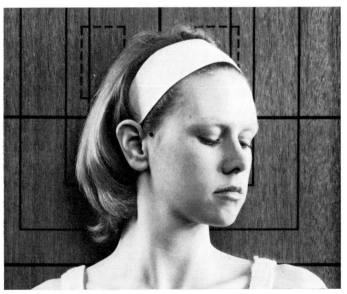

1857

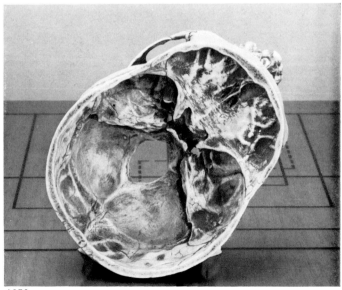

1859

25° Occipito-frontal

With the patient in the lying or sitting erect posture, the head is positioned postero-anterior with the radiographic baseline at right angles to the film.

Centring—The X-ray beam is directed with a 25° cephaled tilt to the nasion (1860)

This view is particularly useful in demonstrating the palate, the styloid processes, the orbital floor and intra-orbital fissure.

Cribiform plate (Ethmoidal bone)
Postero-anterior oblique

From the true postero-anterior position

(1) rotate the head 45° to the affected side.

(2) with an upward inclination of the face, adjust the radiographic base-line 35° to the horizontal.

■ Centre through the orbit in contact with the film, directing the central ray 10° caudally (1861)

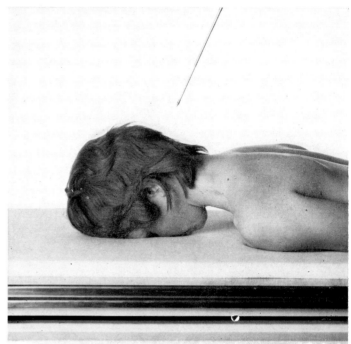

1860

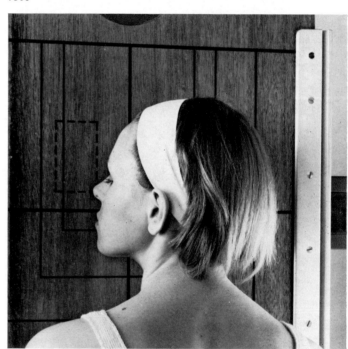

1861

22

VENTRICULOGRAPHY AND ENCEPHALOGRAPHY

STEREOTAXIS

VENTRICULOGRAPHY AND ENCEPHALOGRAPHY

The central nervous system extends from the brain to the termination of the spinal cord at the level of the first to second lumbar vertebrae. The ventricular system is situated in the mid and hind brain within the skull and the spinal cord within the spinal canal. The ventricles and cord are connected through the canalis centralis of the fourth ventricle and the central canal of the spinal cord.

The ventricular system consists of four ventricles—two lateral ventricles and two others named, respectively, the third and the fourth ventricle. Normally they contain cerebro-spinal fluid, which is of the same density as the brain substance. For the purpose of radiographic examination, some of this cerebro-spinal fluid is replaced by air in order to obtain the necessary contrast for demonstration. Since the position of the air varies as the patient is moved, a complete examination of the ventricles may be carried out by changing the position of the head so that each part of the ventricular system is, in turn, filled with air.

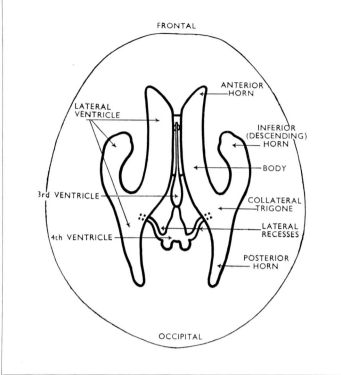

1862

The diagrams (1862,1863) show the ventricular system within the bony cranium from the lateral and superior aspects.

The lateral ventricles, one in each hemisphere of the brain, are separated in the mid-line and communicate by way of the interventricular foramen with the third ventricle. Each lateral ventricle consists of a body and anterior, posterior, and inferior or descending horns.

The third ventricle in the mid-line is between and below the level of the anterior horns, and above the level of the inferior horns, of the lateral ventricles. It communicates with the lateral ventricles, which are above and in front, by the interventricular foramen (of Monro), and with the fourth ventricle, below and behind, by the aqueduct of the midbrain (of Sylvius).

The fourth ventricle, also in the mid-line, is below the inferior horns of the lateral ventricles. It communicates above, by the aqueduct of the midbrain, with the third ventricle; laterally, through the apertures to the lateral recesses and posteriorly through the median aperture, all of which protrude into the subarachnoid space in the region of the cisterna magna and pontis; and below, the canalis centralis is continuous with the central canal of the spinal cord.

The introduction of air or oxygen into the ventricles for the purpose of their demonstration may be made directly, following a trephining operation, when it is termed ventriculography, or by means of a lumbar or cisternal puncture, when it is known as encephalography.

When an opaque medium is used 2 to 3 millilitres of ethyl iodophenylundecylate (Myodil) are injected into a lateral ventricle during pneumoventriculography and the patient is postured under screen control until the opaque medium is seen to be blocked or to have reached the fourth ventricle.

For ventriculography, as a theatre procedure two burr holes are made in the posterior parietal regions, a position in which

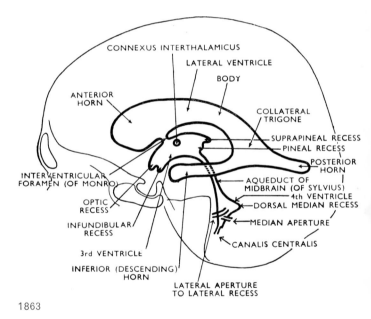

1863

damage to the brain is avoided. On transferring the patient to the X-ray department, a balanced cerebro-spinal fluid air replacement is made in the ventricles, by aspiration and injection. The smallest possible dressings are strapped to the head wounds to facilitate correct positioning for radiography.

For encephalography the patient is maintained in the seated posture during the lumbar or cisternal injection in order that the air introduced may rise to fill the ventricles (1930,1931).

The patient usually suffers more discomfort following the injection for encephalography than for ventriculography. Radiographic projection is identical.

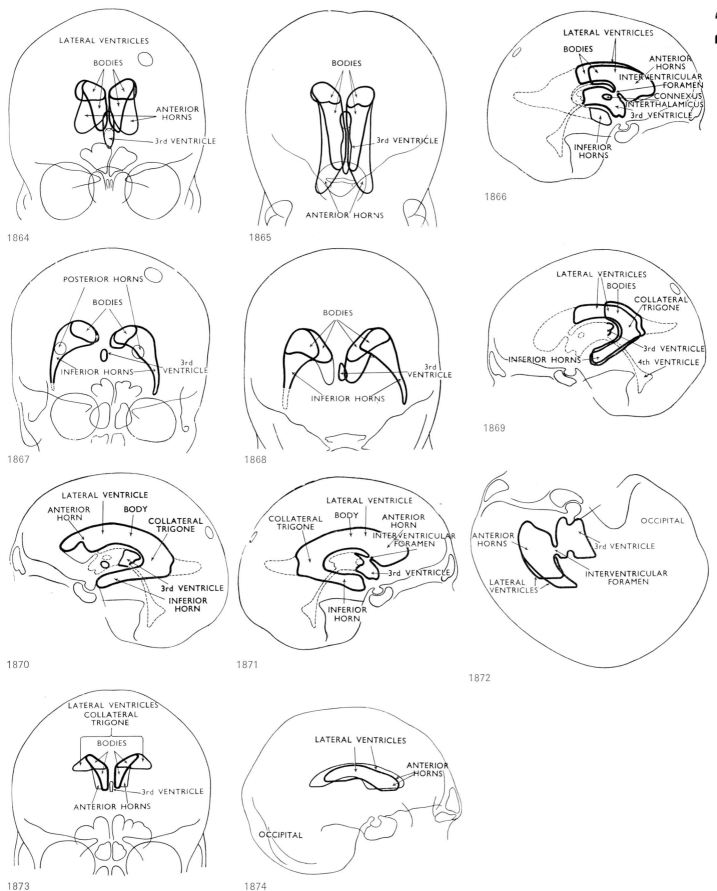

LATERAL VENTRICLES

BODIES

ANTERIOR HORNS

3rd VENTRICLE

1864

BODIES

3rd VENTRICLE

ANTERIOR HORNS

1865

LATERAL VENTRICLES

BODIES

ANTERIOR HORNS

INTERVENTRICULAR FORAMEN

CONNEXUS INTERTHALAMICUS

3rd VENTRICLE

INFERIOR HORNS

1866

POSTERIOR HORNS

BODIES

INFERIOR HORNS

3rd VENTRICLE

1867

BODIES

INFERIOR HORNS

3rd VENTRICLE

1868

LATERAL VENTRICLES

BODIES

COLLATERAL TRIGONE

3rd VENTRICLE

4th VENTRICLE

INFERIOR HORNS

1869

LATERAL VENTRICLE

ANTERIOR HORN

BODY

COLLATERAL TRIGONE

3rd VENTRICLE

INFERIOR HORN

1870

LATERAL VENTRICLE

COLLATERAL TRIGONE

BODY

ANTERIOR HORN

INTERVENTRICULAR FORAMEN

3rd VENTRICLE

INFERIOR HORN

1871

OCCIPITAL

ANTERIOR HORNS

3rd VENTRICLE

INTERVENTRICULAR FORAMEN

LATERAL VENTRICLES

1872

LATERAL VENTRICLES

COLLATERAL TRIGONE

BODIES

3rd VENTRICLE

ANTERIOR HORNS

1873

LATERAL VENTRICLES

ANTERIOR HORNS

OCCIPITAL

1874

This series of radiographic tracing diagrams (1864–1874) shows how the ventricular system is recorded positionally with air filling and should be studied in conjuction with the general anatomical diagrams (1862–1863). The original radiographs from which these collectively tracings were made are shown on pages 540 and 541, with a summary of the positions tabled for reference.

The radiographs resulting from the ten positions described and illustrated in this section are repeated on these two pages, with tabulated details of positioning and ventricles shown, in order that comparisons may be facilitated. Radiographs (1877, 1880,1882) are placed in the positions occupied during exposure.

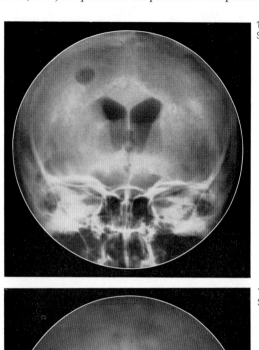

1875
Supine

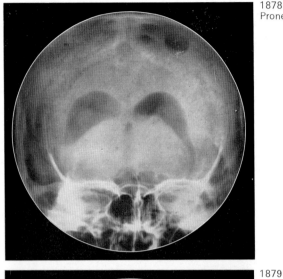

1878
Prone

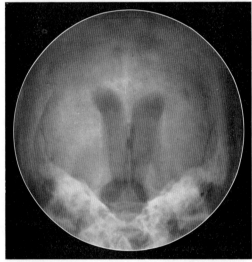

1876
Supine

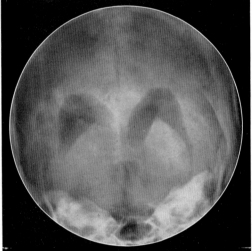

1879
Prone

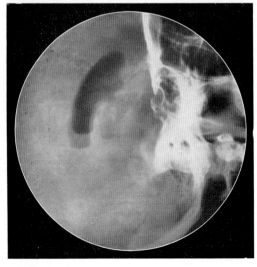

1877
Supine

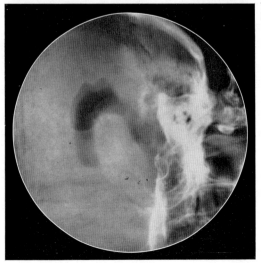

1880
Prone

No.	Patient	Position	Tube	Ventricles shown
1875	Supine (1893)	Fronto-Occipital	Straight	Lateral-Anterior Horns, and Bodies. Third.
1876	Supine (1896)	Fronto-Occipital Half-Axial	Angled 25° to 30° (OMBL)	Lateral-Anterior Horns, and Bodies. Third.
1877	Supine (1899)	Lateral	Horizontal	Lateral-Anterior Horns. Interventricular Foramen. Third.
1878	Prone (1903)	Occipito-Fronta.	Straight	Lateral-Inferior and Posterior Horns, and Bodies. Third.
1879	Prone (1906)	Occipito-Frontal Half-Axial	Angled 25° to 30° (OMBL)	Lateral-Inferior and Posterior Horns, and Bodies. Third.
1880	Prone (1909)	Lateral	Horizontal	Lateral-Inferior and Posterior Horns, and Bodies.
1881	Lateral Left and Right (1913) (1916)	Lateral	Straight	Lateral-Interventricular Foramen. Third. Aqueduct of the Midbrain. Fourth.
1882	Supine Head Lowered (1919) (1920)	Lateral	Horizontal	Lateral-Anterior Horns. Interventricular Foramen. Third. Aqueduct of the Midbrain. Fourth.
1883	Erect (1924)	Fronto-Occipital	Horizontal	Lateral-Upper Anterior Horns and Bodies.
1884	Erect (1927)	Lateral	Horizontal	Lateral-Upper Anterior Horns and Bodies.

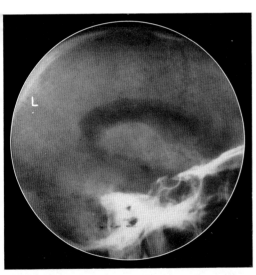

1881
Lateral

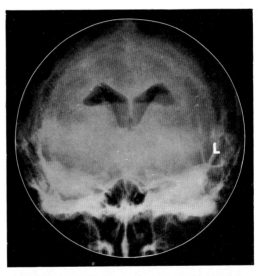

1883
Vertical

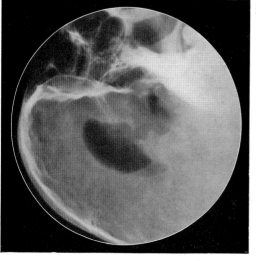

1882
Supine Head
Lowered

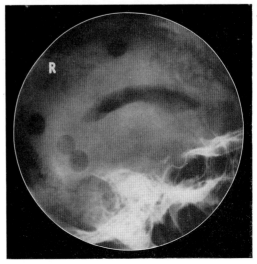

1884
Vertical

22 Apparatus

The skull table, used throughout the illustrations in this section, is particularly suitable for the examination of the ventricles as the position of tube and film can be readily varied without undue movement of the patient. With a little care and forethought, however, satisfactory results may be obtained with the ordinary couch, vertical stand and mobile tube support, and particularly in conjunction with the readily adjusted pedestal Bucky diaphragm.

It is not possible to give full details of the skull table, but the following selected features should be noted.

The unit consists of a small area grid table attached to a special tube mounting, which allows for precision adjustment of the tube focus in relation to the subject and film. The unit is mounted on a substantial vertical column and is quite separate from the trolley-type couch.

At all angles of the tube, the tube focus is automatically centred to the moving grid and film, unless the tube is decentralized for a special purpose. In the illustrations, the centre-finder is shown pointing in the direction of the central ray; it is hinged, and is moved to one side before making an exposure. From the central position the tube moves through 90 degrees in each of three directions so that additional projections can be made without moving the patient. A special fitting is used to enable the cassette and stationary grid to be held at right angles to the working position of the moving grid. Tube and grid table may also be moved simultaneously through 90 degrees to accommodate both erect and horizontal positioning.

Vertical movement of the complete unit in relation to the couch provides for the additional dropped head positions used in ventriculography (1920).

The grid can be rotated to enable the grid slats to be adjusted to the direction of the X-ray beam when unusual tube angulation is required.

The positioning of the head in relation to the film is facilitated by the use of reflecting mirrors (1886), placed beneath the transparent table top, which operate when the hinged grid is removed or allowed to hang vertically beside the table (1889).

Immobilization is by a linen band attached to spring rollers which can be tightened from both sides simultaneously (1889).

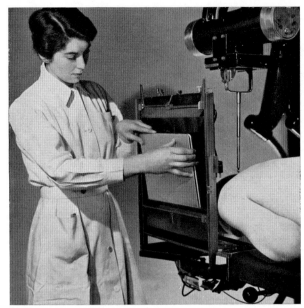

1885

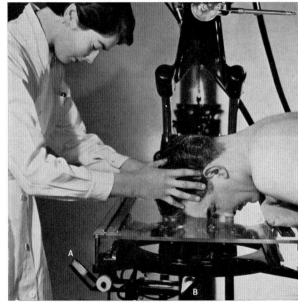

1886

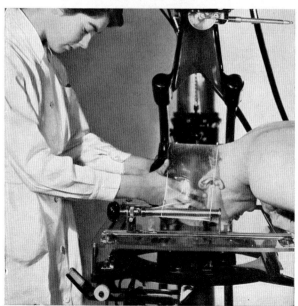

1887

A temporary plastic band is demonstrated in the earlier illustrations, but the band has been discarded later to avoid obscuring the actual positions of the head.

A slot near the tube aperture accommodates the flat-type primary diaphragm (1888). A set of eight diaphragms provides a series of circular and rectangular apertures to suit the various projections of the skull.

A preliminary series of photographs (1885 to 1890) illustrates some of the special features of the skull table.

(**1885**) Shows the cassette being placed in position beneath the grid, which has been withdrawn from the table and hinged upward for this purpose.

(**1886**) The grid assembly has been removed to disclose details of the visual positioning device. Two small electric bulbs illuminate the subject through the transparent table top. Two mirrors (A) and (B) are so placed as to enable the operator to see the actual positioning of the patient and also to see the effect of any necessary adjustments to the head relative to the cross-lines on the table top.

(**1887**) Two metal runners have been added to accommodate the attachments for the immobilizing band. The operator adjusts the head beneath the band.

(**1888**) With one hand the operator steadies the head while the band is tightened from one side.

(**1889**) Shows the usual practice of tightening the immobilizing band from both spring rollers simultaneously while checking the position of the head in the mirror. The moving grid assembly has been replaced and is hinged downward after inserting the cassette as shown in (1885).

(**1890**) The grid is now in position beneath the transparent table top with the immobilizing band finally tightened over the head.

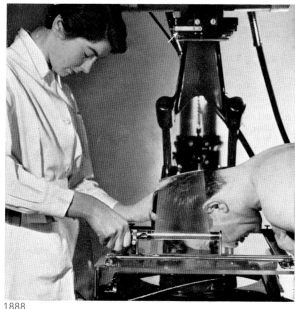

1888

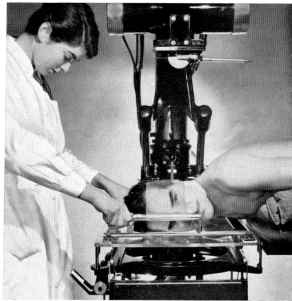

1889

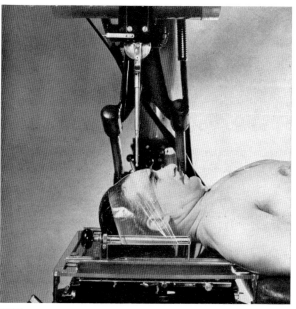

1890

Positioning

In the following order of positioning it should be noted that for each position of the head, films are taken from the several aspects of the air-filled portions of the ventricles. It should be appreciated, however, that the precise positioning of the head given below will be varied to accommodate specific local conditions. Also, each positional series of three radiographs will be examined by the radiologist or neuro-surgeon before moving the patient and proceeding with the examination.

PATIENT SUPINE: Fronto-occipital—tube straight; fronto-occipital—tube angled 30 degrees to feet (half-axial); lateral.
PATIENT PRONE: Occipito-frontal—tube straight: occipito-frontal—tube angled 30 degrees to head; lateral.
PATIENT LATERAL: Lateral right; lateral left.
PATIENT SUPINE: Head lowered; lateral.
PATIENT VERTICAL: Fronto-occipital; lateral.

In changing the position of the head a gentle rocking movement assists the filling of the ventricles, but jerky movements should be avoided or the patient's sensation of nausea will be intensified, and in some positions of the head the air may pass out of the ventricular system. A brief interval between each movement of the patient should be allowed to enable the air to move to the new position within the ventricles.

The cerebro-spinal fluid-air replacement in the ventricular system may vary from 10 to 200 millilitres; less than 10 millilitres of air is unsatisfactory, 30 to 40 millilitres being the average quantity introduced.

In the text a photograph, radiograph and diagram are shown for each projection of the ventricles, and on pages 540 and 541 a complete set of radiographs is shown for comparison, with a set of complementary diagrams on page 539.

Autotomography enables the third and fourth ventricles to be visualized, page 557.

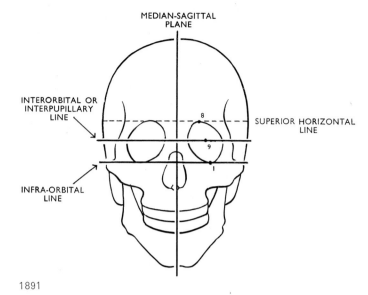

1891

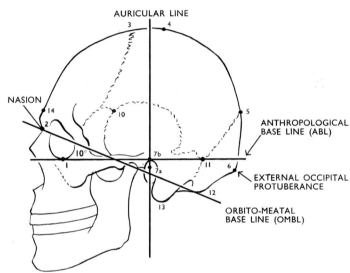

1892

Planes, lines and landmarks

To make full use of the skull table meticulous care is necessary in positioning the patient to the cross-lines on the base. Positioning is aided by following the lines, planes and landmarks recommended by the Commission of Neuroradiology, Milan 1961, under the title of Projections and Nomenclature in Neuroradiology (Report of World Federation). The two illustrations from the report are included for the frontal and lateral aspects of the skull (1891, 1892), with the numbered regions given below.

(1) Infra–orbital point. (2) Nasion. (3) Bregma. (4) Vertex. (5) Lambda. (6) Inion. (7a) Centre of the external auditory canal or axis of the external auditory meatus. (7b) Superior border of the meatus. (8) Superior border of the orbit. (9) Centre of the orbit. (10) Pterion. (11) Asterion. (12) Lowest point of the occiput. (13) Mastoid tip. (14) Glabella.

Positioning and centring for this section are based on the use of the orbito-meatal base line (OMBL). On using the anthropological base line (ABL) tube angulation is adjusted accordingly.

(1) Supine—fronto-occipital

With the patient supine, the head is carefully adjusted with the base line and median plane at right angles to the table and with the centre pointer 1½ inches above the level of the nasion to be coincident with the centre of the grid.

■ Centre 1½ inches above the nasion (1893,1894,1895)

A primary diaphragm of suitable aperture is selected in advance and the moving grid is set for the appropriate length of exposure. On tightening the immobilizing band, the centre pointer is hinged to one side and the exposure is made.

Note—In this position of the head the air rises to fill the bodies and anterior horns of the lateral ventricles, and sometimes a part of the third ventricle, as may be seen in radiograph (1894) and in the tracing diagram (1895).

kVp	mAS	FFD	Film ILFORD	Screens ILFORD	Grid
75	25	36" (90cm)	RAPID R	FT	Grid

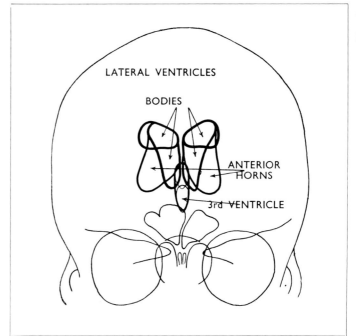

1895

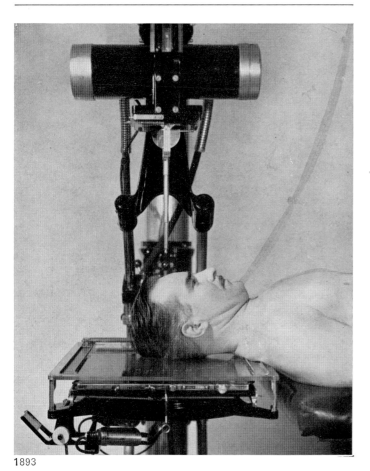

1893

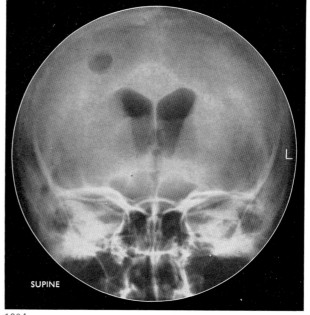

1894

(2) Supine—fronto-occipital with tube angled (half-axial)

With the patient in the same position as for the previous projection, the tube is angled from 25 to 30 degrees toward the feet. Since in using the skull table the tube is automatically centred to the small-area grid it is necessary to move the patient toward the tube to enable the centre pointer to be directed to the level of two inches above the nasion. The film is displaced 2 inches toward the feet to accommodate the effect of tube angulation.

■ Centre two inches above the nasion, with the tube angled 25 to 30 degrees toward the feet. The centre pointer is moved to one side before making the exposure (1896,1897,1898)

Note—The tube adjustment allows the air-filled anterior horns, the bodies of the lateral ventricles, and the third ventricle to be seen from a different angle, as shown in the radiograph (1897) and also in the tracing diagram (1898).

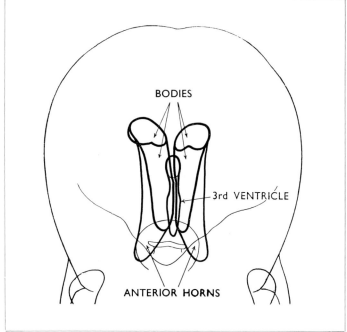

1898

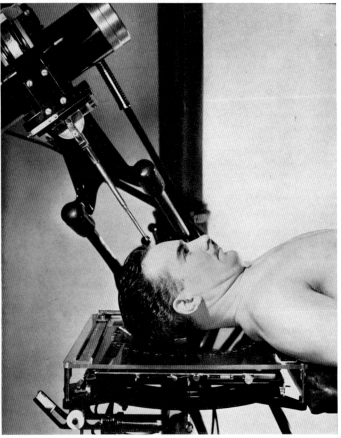

1896

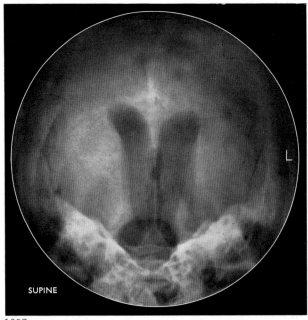

1897

kVp	mAS	FFD	Film ILFORD	Screens ILFORD	Grid
80	25	36″(90cm)	RAPID R	FT	Grid

(3) Supine—lateral

The head may be moved gently backward and forward to encourage the passage of the air into the third ventricle, and then placed in the same position as for the two previous projections, with a small pad under the head. The tube on its arcuate support is moved round the head through 90 degrees to the horizontal position, and is then rotated on its axis until the centre pointer is horizontal. On sliding the vertical cassette support into position on the rails, provided also for the immobilizing band attachment, the cassette is placed with the stationary grid vertically against the lateral aspect of the head. To enable the beam to be centred to the anterior horns of the lateral ventricles, the head and tube are adjusted to bring the centre pointer to a position $2\frac{1}{2}$ inches above and 1 inch anterior to the external auditory meatus.

■ Centre $2\frac{1}{2}$ inches above and 1 inch in front of the external auditory meatus. The centre pointer is moved to one side before making the exposure (1899,1900,1901,1902)

The exposure factors are shown on page 550.

Note—The anterior horns of the lateral ventricles and part of the third ventricle are demonstrated. Radiograph (1900) is shown in the position in which it was exposed, as indicated by the air level in the ventricles. Radiograph (1901) is viewed in the conventional position for the skull to coincide with the tracing diagram (1902).

This projection completes the supine series, the adjustment in the tube centring having allowed the air-filled portion of the ventricular system to be seen from an aspect at right angles to the two previous projections. This is also the 'key' film to the antero-posterior projections should there be any doubt as to the actual portion of the ventricular system shown.

This series of three radiographs taken with the patient in the supine position will be viewed by the radiologist or neuro-surgeon before the patient is moved into the prone position.

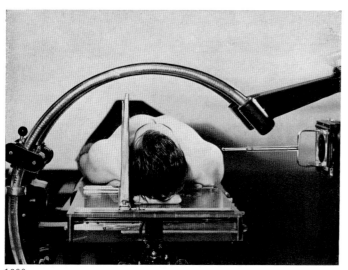

1899

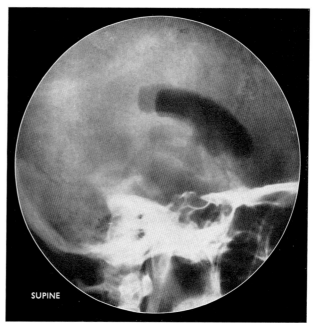

SUPINE

1901

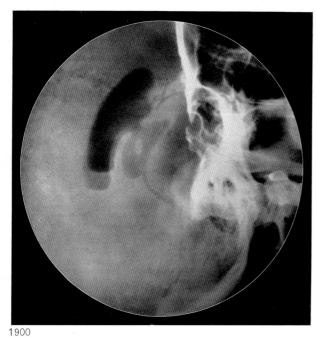

1900

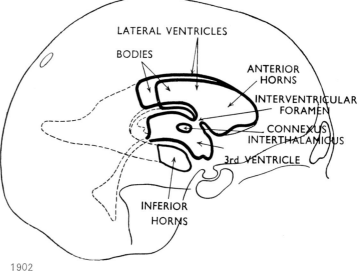

LATERAL VENTRICLES

BODIES

ANTERIOR HORNS

INTERVENTRICULAR FORAMEN

CONNEXUS INTERTHALAMICUS

3rd VENTRICLE

INFERIOR HORNS

1902

(4) Prone—occipito-frontal

The grid assembly is withdrawn from the table top and after removing the cassette it is hinged downward to enable the viewing device to be used. The patient is gently turned from the supine to the prone position. The head is again adjusted with the base line and median plane at right angles to the film, with the nasion $1\frac{1}{2}$ inches below the cross-lines on the table top, as seen in the viewing mirror. On tightening the immobilizing band, this visual guidance safeguards any further displacement of the head. The hinged centre pointer is moved to one side for the exposure to be made.

■ Centre to $1\frac{1}{2}$ inches above the nasion, the tube being centred automatically to the cross-lines indicating the centre of the grid (1903,1904,1905)

Note—With the head in this position the air rises from the anterior horns to fill the inferior and the posterior horns of the lateral ventricles, and a part of the third ventricle, as will be seen in the radiograph (1904) and tracing diagram (1905).

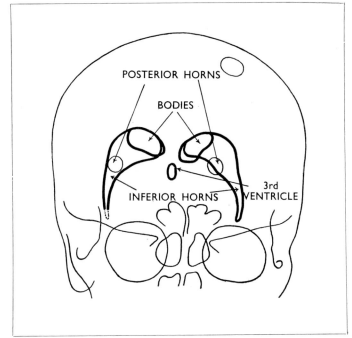

1905

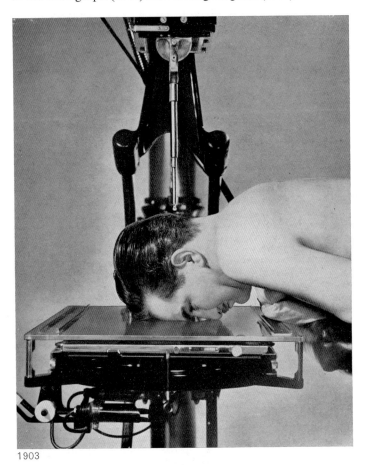

1903

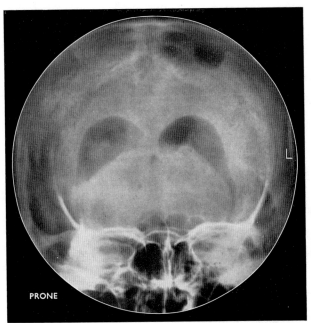

1904

kVp	mAS	FFD	Film ILFORD	Screens ILFORD	Grid
75	25	36″(90cm)	RAPID R	FT	Grid

(5) Prone—occipito-frontal with tube angled (half-axial)

With the head in the same position as for (1903), the tube is angled 25 to 30 degrees toward the vertex; as centring to the grid and film is automatic with the skull table, the patient is moved toward the tube and positioned with a point 2½ inches above the nasion toward the cross-lines, as seen in the mirror. The cassette is moved 2 inches toward the head to accommodate the effect of angling the tube.

■ Centre the cross-lines to 2½ inches above the nasion as seen in the mirror. The tube is angled 25 to 30 degrees toward the head. After tightening the immobilizing band, remember to set the grid and to hinge back the centre pointer before making the exposure (1906,1907,1908)

Note—This tube adjustment allows the air-filled inferior horns and usually the posterior horns of the lateral ventricles to be seen from a different angle—although in this subject the right posterior horn is not visible—as shown in the radiograph (1907) and tracing diagram (1908).

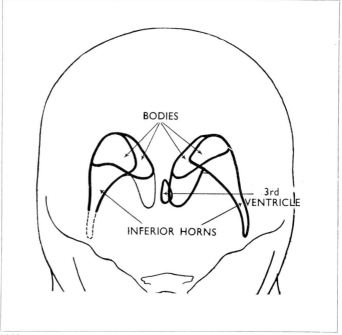

1908

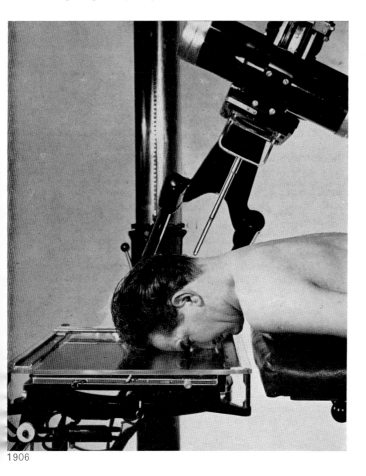

1906

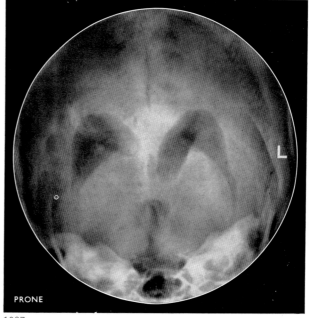

1907

kVp	mAS	FFD	Film ILFORD	Screens ILFORD	Grid
80	25	36″(90cm)	RAPD R	FT	Grid

(6) Prone—lateral

With the patient in the same position, the tube is moved round the head, through 90 degrees, for horizontal projection. The tube is also rotated on its axis to enable the centre pointer to be directed at right angles to the cassette and stationary grid placed in the vertical support against the side of the head.

■ Centre from the horizontal position, $2\frac{1}{2}$ inches above and $1\frac{1}{2}$ inches posterior to the external auditory meatus (1909, 1910, 1911, 1912)

Note—In this projection, the posterior horn of the lateral ventricles is usually seen, but with this particular subject filling of the posterior horn is incomplete. The inferior horns are seen, however, and also a small part of the third ventricle. The fourth ventricle may also be shown in this projection. Radiograph (1910) is given in the position in which it was exposed and (1911) in the conventional lateral viewing position to coincide with the tracing diagram (1912).

This projection completes the prone series of exposures and enables the filling of the ventricles shown in the complementary postero-anterior projections to be appreciated. Reference for comparison with the supine position should be made to page 547.

Again, the series of three radiographs taken in the prone position is seen by the radiologist or neuro-surgeon, usually before moving the patient for a decision to be made with regard to further necessary projections.

kVp	mAS	FFD	Film ILFORD	Screens ILFORD	Grid
80	25	36″(90cm)	RAPID R	FT	Grid

1909

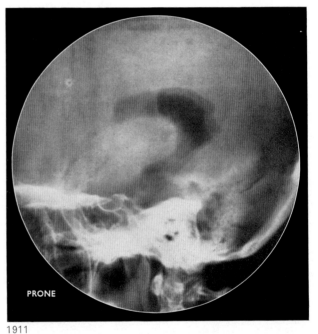

PRONE

1911

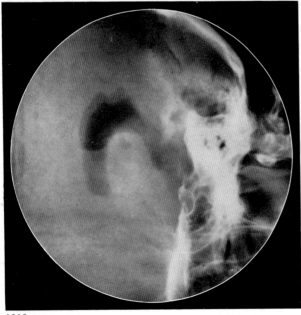

1910

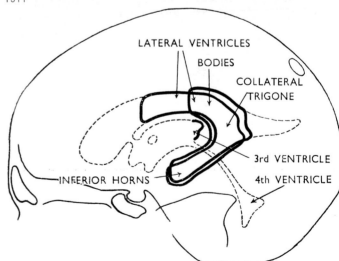

LATERAL VENTRICLES
BODIES
COLLATERAL TRIGONE
3rd VENTRICLE
4th VENTRICLE
INFERIOR HORNS

1912

(7) Lateral—right and left

From the occipito-frontal position, the head is gently moved through 90 degrees to right and left sides in turn, to occupy the true lateral position for each exposure, with the interorbital line at right angles and the median line parallel to the film (1913, 1916). A short lapse of time should be allowed between positioning and exposure to enable the air to rise to the new position. Using the viewing mirror, the head is adjusted under the immobilizing band to the cross-lines on the tabletop.

■ Centre 2 inches above and 1 inch in front of the external auditory meatus (1913, 1914, 1915, 1916, 1917, 1918)

The exposure factors are shown on page 550.

Note—With the head in the lateral position the air rises to fill the lateral ventricle remote from the film, and also the third and fourth ventricles; the interventricular foramen and the acqueduct of the midbrain may be shown. See radiographs (1914, 1917) and tracing diagrams (1915, 1918) showing right and left sides respectively.

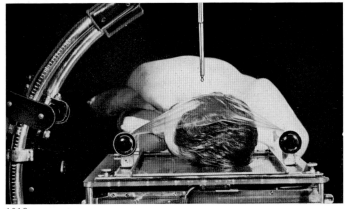

1913

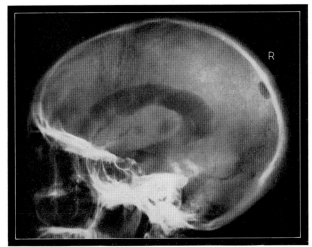

1914

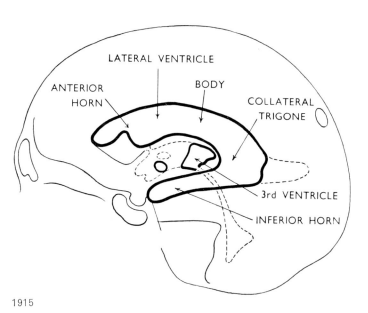

1915

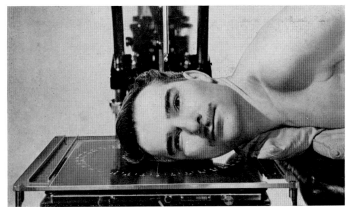

1916

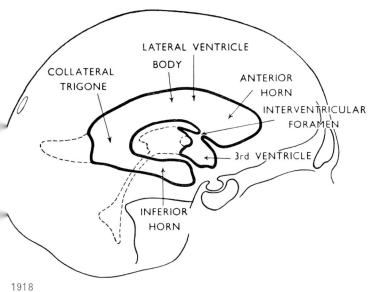

1918

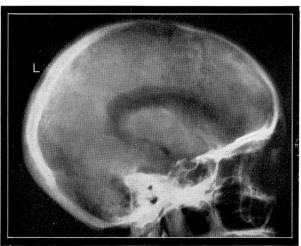

1917

(8) Supine—lateral head lowered

With the patient supine and the skull table lowered in relation to the couch, the neck is allowed to extend until the vertex of the skull rests on a wool pad in contact with the Perspex table top. The pad should raise the head sufficiently to include the essential area on the film for the lateral projection.

Gentle movements are essential and the extension of the neck should not be excessive, as with the head in this position the air is inclined to pass out of the ventricular system through the fourth ventricle. This position, therefore, usually terminates the examination.

The cassette and stationary grid in the vertical support are placed against the lateral aspect of the head and the tube is moved through 90 degrees to enable this projection to be made from the horizontal position.

■ Centre 2 inches above and 1 inch in front of the external auditory meatus (1919,1920,1921,1922)

The exposure factors are shown on page 550.

Note—As the head is moved into position, the air rises toward the third and fourth ventricles. This projection shows, therefore, the anterior horns of the lateral ventricles, the interventricular foramen, the third ventricle, and it is hoped to include the fourth ventricle. Radiograph (1921) is shown in the conventional viewing position for the general skull to coincide with tracing diagram (1922), and radiograph (1923) is shown in the position in which it was exposed.

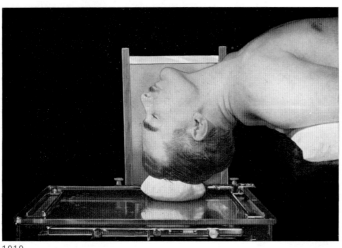
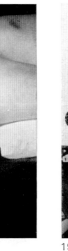

1919

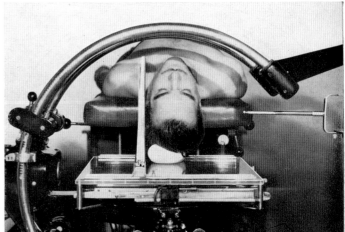

1920

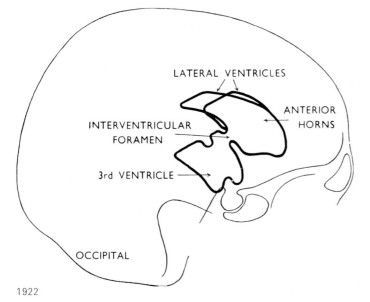

LATERAL VENTRICLES

ANTERIOR HORNS

INTERVENTRICULAR FORAMEN

3rd VENTRICLE

OCCIPITAL

1922

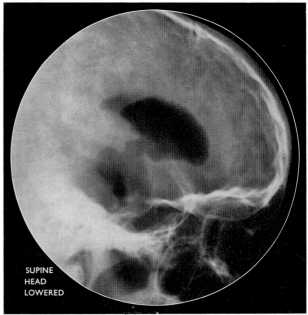

SUPINE HEAD LOWERED

1921

(9) Erect—fronto-occipital

With the patient seated against the supporting back-rest of the couch, the grid table and tube are moved simultaneously through 90 degrees for vertical projection of the ventricles. Again, the tube is adjusted on its axis to enable the centre pointer to be directed horizontally. The patient faces the tube with the chin well down to bring the base line and median plane at right angles to the film and with a point 1½ inches above the nasion toward the centre pointer.

■ Centre 1½ inches above the nasion, with the tube horizontal (1924, 1925, 1926)

kVp	mAS	FFD	Film ILFORD	Screens ILFORD	Grid
75	25	36″ (90cm)	RAPID R	FT	Grid

Note—The erect position of the head allows the air to rise to fill the uppermost portions of the lateral ventricles, showing chiefly the bodies, anterior horns, and the collateral trigone, as in the radiograph (1925) and tracing diagram (1926).

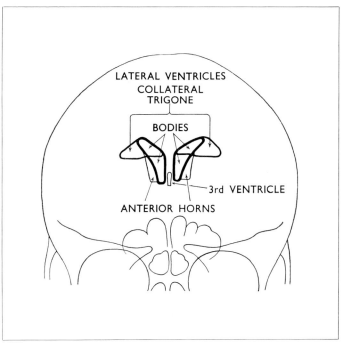

1926

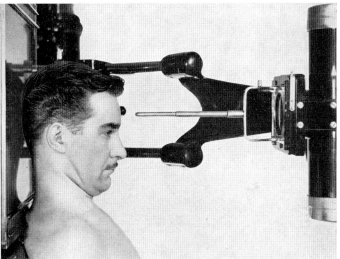

1924

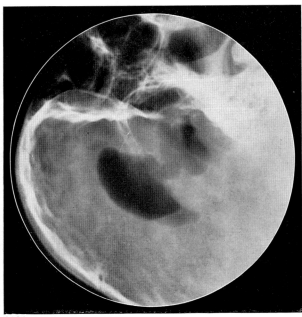

1923

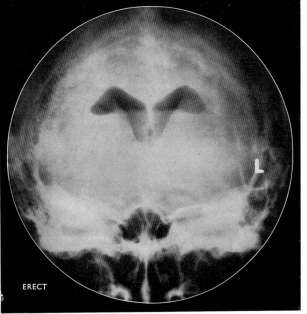

1925

(10) Erect—lateral

With the patient in the same position, the tube is moved on its arcuate arm through 90 degrees and, as previously, adjusted on its axis to enable the centre pointer to be directed horizontally for the lateral projection. The cassette and stationary grid in the special fitting are placed against the head, which is adjusted to enable the centre pointer to be directed to a position two inches above and one inch in front of the external auditory meatus.

■ Centre 2 inches above and 1 inch in front of the external auditory meatus (1927,1928,1929)

Note—This position shows the uppermost portions of the anterior horns and bodies of the lateral ventricles (1928,1929), and serves to confirm what the previous erect position may have shown.

kVp	mAS	FFD	Film ILFORD	Screens ILFORD	Grid
70	15	36"(90cm)	RAPID R	FT	Grid

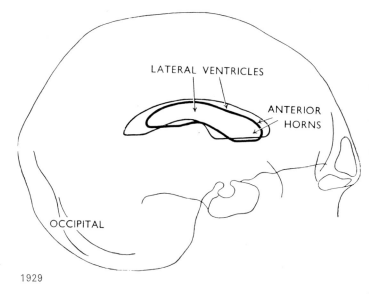

1929

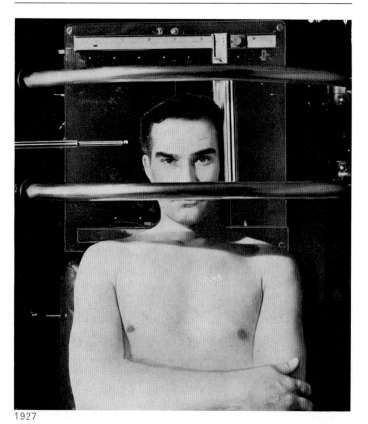

1927

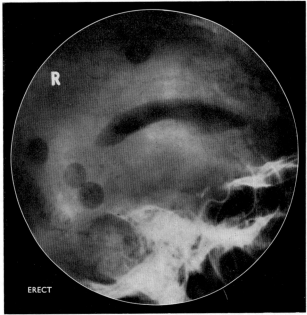

1928

Encephalography

Photograph (1930) shows the position of the patient for the lumbar injection which may be used as an alternative to the cisternal injection, the examination being described as encephalography. The two photographs (1930,1931) show positions occipito-frontal and lateral such as could be used in place of the two erect positions, antero-posterior (1924) and lateral (1927). However, when it is necessary to show the posterior fossa, with the exposure made during injection, the head is adjusted by dropping the chin to enable the base line to be at an angle of 80 degrees for the two exposures.

A series of radiographs of a child (1932 to 1939) shows eight

positions for encephalography which, as previously stated, coincide with the positions used in the preceding pages for ventriculography, respectively.

(1932), page 545   (1936), page 549
(1933), page 546   (1937), page 550
(1934), page 547   (1938,1939), page 551
(1935), page 548

The absence of burr holes should be noted as indicating the encephalography series (1932 to 1939) as compared with the burr holes shown in the ventriculography series.

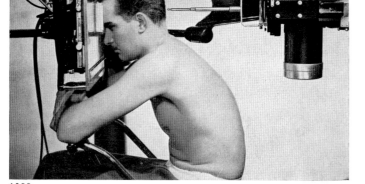

1930

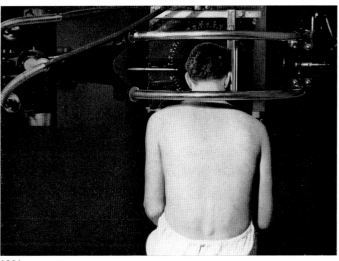

1931

1932, 1933, 1934   1938

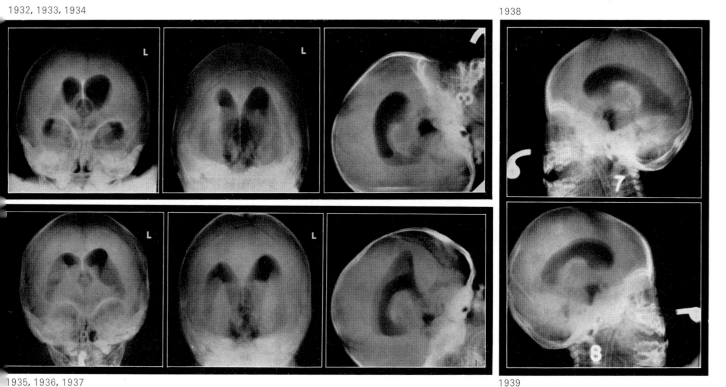

1935, 1936, 1937   1939

Opaque injection

When it is necessary to confirm a block, together with its position within the ventricular system, an opaque medium is injected following the conventional air study. Using the opaque medium ethyl iodophenydecylate (Myodil), approximately 2 millilitres are injected through an existing burr hole into a lateral ventricle. The procedure is followed visually on the fluorescent screen or television monitor, when controlled movement in raising the head enables the opaque medium to pass normally from the lateral ventricle, through the interventricular foramen to the third ventricle, and through the aqueduct of the midbrain to the fourth ventricle (1940b).

Radiographs recording the movement, in part, may be made in the lateral, antero-posterior and half axial positions (1940a). Alternatively, a block or other abnormality in the system will be further investigated by additional adjustments of the head, in particular to promote the directional flow of the opaque medium within the system. This is recorded in radiographs selected from

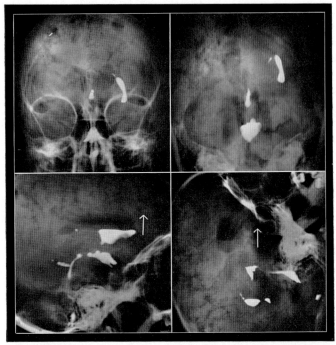

1940a

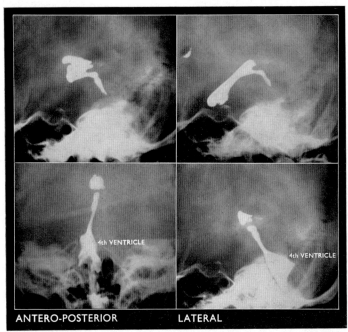

1940b

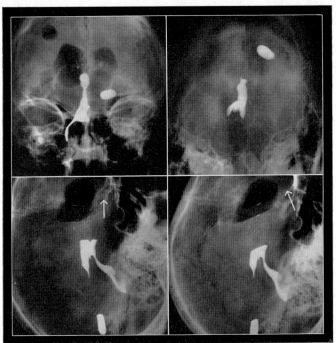

1940c

the considerable series of a subject reported as pathological (1940c) and in a normal subject (1940a). These embrace the three projections, as previously, and in series (1940a,b,c) the additional lateral projection to show by comparison the backward adjustment of the head to facilitate the downward flow of the opaque medium. The arrows indicate the related lateral positions of the head.

In the event of obstruction the site would be indicated possibly necessitating further radiographic investigation.

Autotomography

Autotomography is the production of a tomogram by making small arcuate movements of the subject in relation to a stationary tube and film, the reverse of conventional tomography, but having the same effect of blurring all tissues on each side of the objective layer. In particular, autotomography serves to demonstrate the third and fourth ventricles and is important for the more difficult to define fourth ventricle. Although special attachments are becoming available for autotomography which establish the sagittal axis of movement and regulate the plane and degree of rotation, results obtained have justified the manual method controlled movement by the operator.

The patient is seated facing the skull table with the neck flexed forward by 10 to 15 degrees to produce a base line to film angle of approximately 80 degrees (OMBL). The film cassette and tube are placed for lateral projection centring to the fourth ventricle approximately 1 centimetre behind the pinna of the ear. Movement of the head on the odontoid process, related by the position of the head to the centralized fourth ventricle, is about 5 degrees to right and left sides, in all an arcuate movement of 10 degrees which is continued smoothly on the one horizontal plane (1941).

An injection of approximately 5 millilitres of air is made immediately before the commencement of movement to ensure that air is present in the third and fourth ventricles.

Having instructed the patient and rehearsed the procedure, the gentle and controlled arcuate movement of the head is continued several times to allow some latitude in selecting the ideal moment of exposure, to provide a satisfactory autotomogram (1943b). A sling bandage around the head in conjunction with the head harness used for the unco-operative or unconscious patient, enables the necessary rotation to be carried out by the operator from a minimum distance of $1\frac{1}{2}$ metres.

The diagram (1941) shows the position of the head from above with the axis and the direction of the arcuate movements indicated. Radiographs (1942a,1943a) are the controls and (1942b,1943b) the autotomographs of the same patients presenting satisfactory projections of the fourth ventricle.

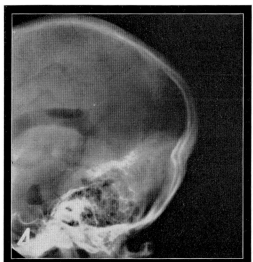

1942a

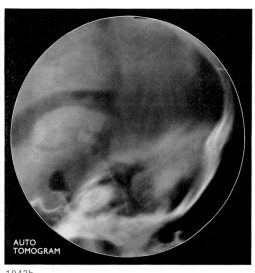

1942b

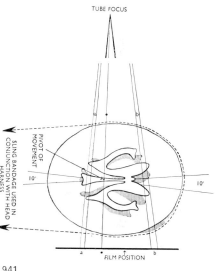

1941

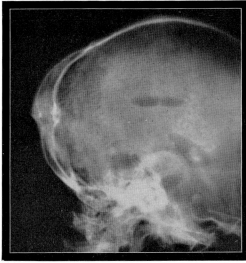

1943a

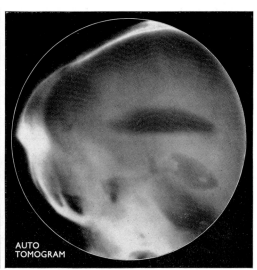

1943b

22 Stereotaxis

Stereotaxis is a system for the accurate insertion of a cannula, needle or electrode into the cranium by the safest route to a specific point, or a small area, within the cranial viscera, mainly used in neurosurgery. The surgical approach and depth are accurately determined by radiography in conjunction with measuring apparatus immovably secured to the skull. Measurements on radiographs taken in two or more planes at right angles enable the depth and the angle approach to be accurately plotted. Several designs of craniostat localizer have been used.

The radiographer has an important but limited role in stereotaxis being responsible for the efficient functioning of the X-ray equipment, and correct exposure for suitable quality radiographs produced in the minimum of time for wet film interpretation by the surgeon. The actual exacting positioning of the patient is prearranged to include correct centring in accordance with the localization equipment employed, any necessary modification being made by the surgeon.

Brief descriptions for two methods of stereotaxis serve to convey an appreciation of three dimensional radiography which subconsciously is the background to so many radiographic investigations.

1. This method, employed chiefly for Parkinson's disease, involves localization and an injection into the thalamus. The patient's head is marked out to include centring positions for antero-posterior and lateral radiographs.

The surgical operation involves a single screw hole in the cranium for the attachment of the localizing instrument. This carries a small external protractor which is adjustable in position by rotation through 90 degrees for the antero-posterior and lateral projections to show on the radiographs for guidance in adjusting the needle, or cannula, to the exact direction within the cranium in three dimensions. The needle is notched in centimetres and a prepared table shows the enlargement factor involved in accordance with the standard distances employed. On injecting a small amount of air into the ventricles as an aid to establishing the objective, radiographs are taken at 30 inches focus–film distance with the median-sagittal plan at 7 inches

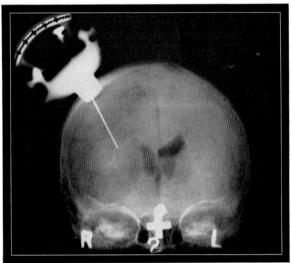

1944a

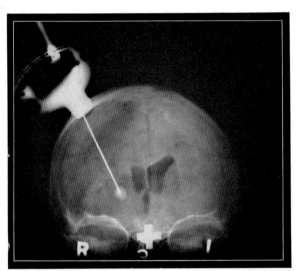

1945a

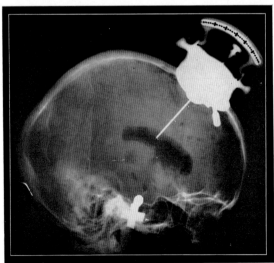

1944b

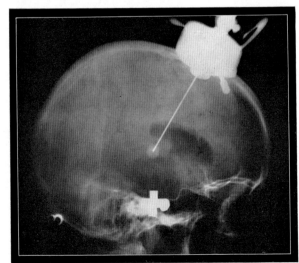

1945b

from the lateral film position and centring to the marked positions on the head (1944a,b). On the two radiographs the position for the direction of the needle is carefully checked against the protractor in the three dimensions and in the event of an adjustment being necessary further radiographs are taken. Finally, the injection is made followed by two more radiographs (1945a,b) in which the involved area is shown. As a matter of interest, the moment of injection for Parkinson's disease brings an immediate and spectacular relief of the patient's symtoms.

2. This method enables any pre-selected objective within the cranium to be reached both directly and with precision. Two adjacent burr holes in the cranium are covered by a double metal cap and ball apparatus (1946a), which allows for the insertion of a needle or probe in the correct direction toward two alternative objectives.

The craniostat, consisting of a rectangular framework of metal tubing and light metal castings, is fixed to the cranium by four screws placed symmetrically to hold the head securely in position (1946b) in relation to the arcuate localizing instrument (1946c). This instrument is eventually attached to the framework and is adjustable in relation to the burr holes in the cranium (1946a,c).

With the head positioned, chin down with a base-line angle of 30 degrees to the horizontal, an injection of Myodil into the frontal horn of a lateral ventricle passes into the third ventricle enabling the selected landmarks to be visualized, for instance, the posterior margin of the foramen of Munro and the posterior commissure.

In adjusting the framed head for radiography, a double grid of wires forming 1 millimetre squares (1946b) is placed on the proximal side of the skull against the selected area of the cranium. Meticulous care is taken in adjusting the relationship of head, craniostat and X-ray tube, including the frequent aid of spirit levels. The focus–film distance is twelve feet to minimize perspective distortion. In the region of the central ray the error is nil, increasing to about 0·25 millimetre, 5 millimetres away from the central ray. The X-ray beam is directed to the centre of the wire grids by means of a telescopic centring devise so that the error is negligible, especially as the grids are over a selected area. Double grids are used to confirm that the centring has been correct; their images should be superimposed. The grids are shown in position in antero-posterior and lateral specimen radiographs (1946d). A point is selected by reference to the 1 millimetre squares and its distance relative to the zero lines noted. On these measurements the trunnions of an arcuate instrument director are placed so as to coincide with the selected point, the wire grids having been removed from the head frame. The arcuate director can also be moved to the left or right of the median plane by an amount measured on the antero-posterior radiograph. The target will now be at the centre of the radius of the arc and can be approached from any point on a hemisphere, the most suitable angles in the sagittal and coronal planes being measured on the radiographs.

Three radiographs (1947a,b,c) show the grids in position with the probe inserted through a burr hole to terminate at the selected objective in (1947a,c). For confirmation of the position two lateral radiographs are taken (1947b), with direct centring and (1947c) with a lateral tube displacement. The actual therapeutic injection may take place some days later, the cap and ball apparatus having been retained in the cranium (1947a).

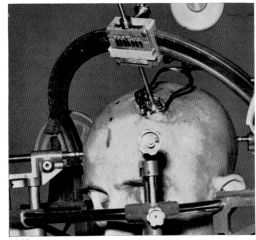

1946a

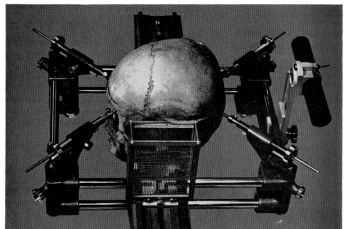

1946b

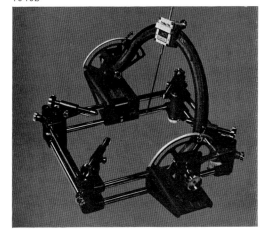

1946c

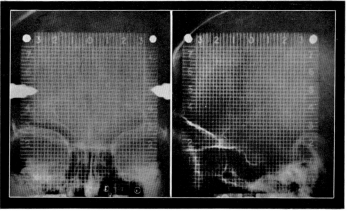

1946d

559

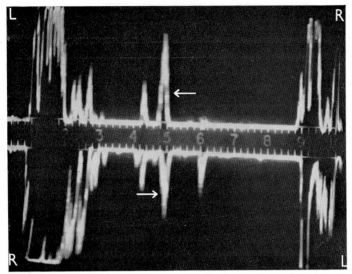

1948a

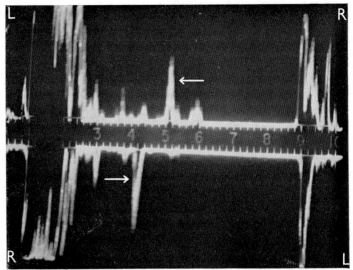

1948b

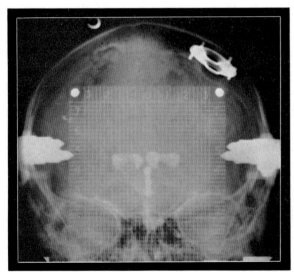

1947a

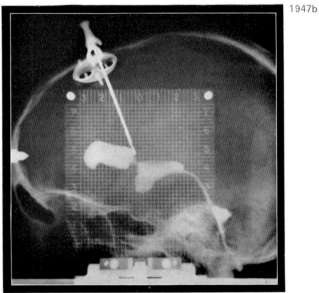

1947b

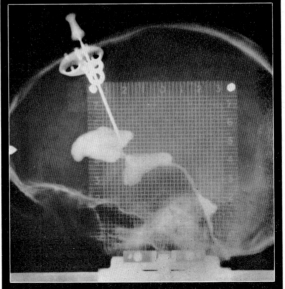

1947c

Ultrasound investigation

Ultrasonics is defined as the science of mechanical vibrations of frequencies greater than those normally audible to the human ear.

Briefly, the equipment consists of an oscillator producing ultrasound vibrations; an applicator incorporating two crystals, one each for the passage and return of the reflected vibrations, or echoes; an amplifier; a cathode ray oscilloscope for visual guidance in scanning for target level, and a Polaroid camera providing concurrent selective oscillographs (1948a,b). The camera is brought into use with an offset viewing device to enable the selected stage in scanning to be recorded simultaneously.

To avoid an air gap which would give misleading reflections, for cerebral investigations the probe contact area is periodically well lubricated with oil or glycerine; for investigation of the trunk and limbs immersion in water is desirable.

Scanning the cranium by ultrasound is used as a preliminary to radiological investigation to record changes in contour and, in particular, to show the midline division of the brain. Small displacements can be recorded, possibly indicating an abnormal pressure within the brain. Confirmatory scannings from right and left sides show a normal condition with the midline coincident in (1948a) and with a space lag between right and left indicating displacement of the midline in (1948b).

Ultrasound may be used for other regions and purposes; for instance, to record the size and shape of the heart; in obstetrics to indicate the presence and dimension of the foetal head, and possibly the shape and size of the maternal pelvis; to confirm the presence of a non-opaque foreign body; and as a technique for layer radiography.

Gamma ray scanning

Gamma (gamma ray) scanning is a means of disclosing abnormal conditions in various parts of the body by virtue of the selective concentration of injected radio-active material in abnormal tissue, which is recorded by the scanner either directly by stylo pencil on paper or photographically on film.

For the scintillograms illustrated in (1949a,b), reported as showing a meningioma, 10 microcuries of radioactive mercury per kilogram of body weight, were injected intravenously 6 hours before the scanning procedure.

With the scanner in action, gamma rays from the mercury activate the scintillation counter and a pulse is generated which operates a recording light internally and a thermo-elastic marker externally activating a thermal sensitive paper. The internal light flashes are recorded on a sensitive photographic film held in a darkslide.

The patient is immobilized in position in turn for antero–posterior and lateral scanning using a retaining band to hold the position. The machine is first used manually to plot the outline of the head including the external auditory meatuses in the form of a series of dots, which joined by pencil line gives a general limiting outline of the cranium. The scanner is then set in motion to operate automatically with a stop in two directions to cover the extreme limits of the skull or particular locality of the skull. Loaded with X-ray film the scanner travels backward and forward with about one-tenth inch raster divisions until the skull or other region is completely covered. Films are processed under department conditions (1949a,1949b).

Note—A further development in the equipment enables a radiograph and superimposed scintillogram to be recorded in turn on the one film. X-ray film is used without intensifying screens and selected under-exposure is employed for the radiograph to provide background identification features for the scintillogram.

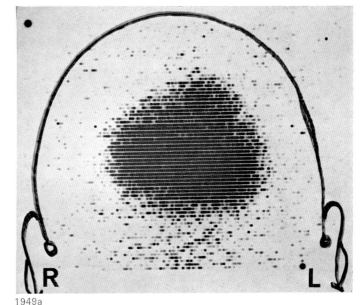

1949a

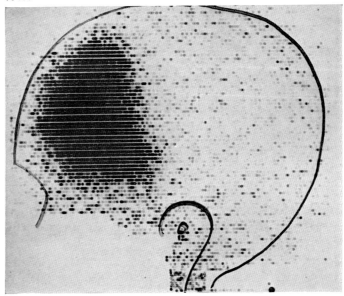

1949b

23

MYELOGRAPHY

MYELOGRAPHY

Continuing the central nervous system, the spinal cord is surrounded by three membranous coverings having between them two spaces of unequal shape and size. Between the innermost membrane, or pia mater, and the second, or arachnoid mater, is the subarachnoid space containing cerebro-spinal fluid; the smaller space between the arachnoid and the outer membrane, or dura mater, is termed the subdural space. The dura mater is separated from the wall of the vertebral canal by the extradural space, containing loose connective tissue, veins and fat shown diagrammatically in (1950).

Myelography, the radiographic investigation of the spinal canal, is undertaken for the purpose of demonstrating the condition of the membranes and of examining any encroachment upon or obstruction of the spaces between and about them. The investigation is made after injection of a contrast medium into the subarachnoid space.

The contrast medium may be an opaque organic iodine preparation which gravitates to the lowest level, or it may be transradiant, either air or oxygen, which rises to the uppermost level.

Either form of contrast medium is used for the subarachnoid space, but the opaque medium is the more frequently employed.

The opaque medium used for myelography is the organic iodine compound ethyl iodophenolundecylate; for proprietary names such as Myodil refer to Supplement 1. The injection is in the order of from 5 to 10 millilitres, but it may reach 20 millilitres. The preparations of iodized oil are no longer used for routine myelography but when used the injection is usually limited to 5 millilitres.

The Subarachnoid space

On using either a suboccipital or more often a lumbar point of entry, the injected contrast medium follows the tilting of the patient longitudinally (1956 to 1961), and also rotationally through 360 degrees (1953,1954,1955). The heavy opaque medium gravitates to the lowest level of the subarachnoid space; on the other hand the light contrast medium rises to show the higher levels. Thus, in positioning the patient, the part to be examined must be so arranged as to be enveloped by the contrast medium, when any intruding abnormality may be shown in profile. A partial or complete obstruction to the flow within the space may be demonstrated in any position. Under normal conditions, by tilting the patient longitudinally the opaque globule may be seen moving from end to end of the subarachnoid space (1956 to 1961).

The two longitudinal sectional diagrams show the gravitation of the opaque medium with the patient in the prone position (1951) and in the supine position (1952).

In the series of cross-sectional diagrams of a single vertebra, positioning required for the heavy opaque medium is clearly indicated and the light area above serves to illustrate the region which would be occupied by injected oxygen. Thus, for the two methods, reverse positioning is required to show similar regions.

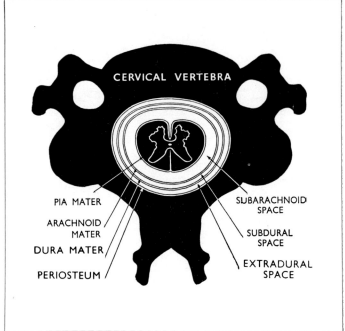

CERVICAL VERTEBRA

PIA MATER
ARACHNOID MATER
DURA MATER
PERIOSTEUM

SUBARACHNOID SPACE
SUBDURAL SPACE
EXTRADURAL SPACE

1950

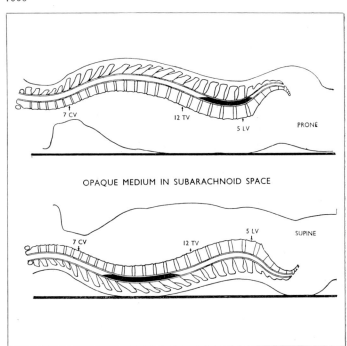

7 CV   12 TV   5 LV   PRONE

OPAQUE MEDIUM IN SUBARACHNOID SPACE

7 CV   12 TV   5 LV   SUPINE

1951 (top) 1952 (above)

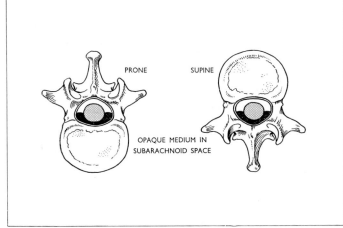

PRONE   SUPINE

OPAQUE MEDIUM IN SUBARACHNOID SPACE

1953

The six diagrams show a single vertebra placed in prone and supine (1953), right and left lateral (1954), and anterior and posterior oblique (1955) positions and, in each position, the section of the neural canal to be enveloped by the contrast medium.

Although, diagrammatically, the space is half-filled with the opaque medium, in practice the injected material is concentrated by positioning manipulation to each small area in turn, to demonstrate the space completely.

Following the injection of the opaque medium, it is essential to the success of the examination that the opaque globule remains intact: separation is avoided by maintaining the patient in a position to enable the opaque medium to gravitate to the region to be examined, when, being heavier than the cerebro-spinal fluid, the medium will sink slowly to the lowest level of the cavity (1956) to (1961).

When oxygen is used for this examination (1976), from 30 to 50 millilitres replaces a similar quantity of cerebrospinal fluid. The injection is made with the patient horizontal and in the subsequent positioning manipulation during screening, every care is taken to avoid the passage of the gas into the ventricular system of the brain, which tends to occur as the patient approaches the upright position.

A tilting couch provides smooth control of the longitudinal movement of the patient through erect, horizontal, and reverse tilting positions, pages 563, 564.

Exacting screening by the radiologist is the essential part of this examination during a gradual tilting of the couch and rotation of the patient, as found to be necessary. On showing the lesion in profile, small films are exposed from the appropriate aspects. Further radiographs may be taken the following day. Identification of sequence radiographs with the subject and from right to left sides must be infallible.

A convenient arrangement is for the image intensifier to be movable over 90 degrees or more, or for two intensifiers to be incorporated for screening and filming.

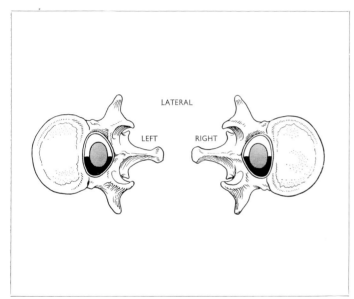

1954

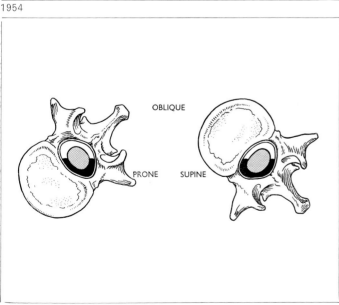

1955

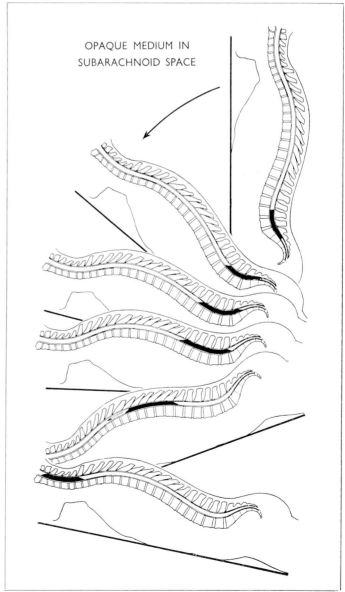

OPAQUE MEDIUM IN SUBARACHNOID SPACE

1956, 1957, 1958, 1959, 1960, 1961

Owing to the curvature of the vertebral column, the prone position is suitable for the lower region, with a small tilt toward the feet to contain the opaque medium in the lumbar concavity; further limited longitudinal couch tilting is used for the necessary detailed screen examination from vertebra to vertebra. The position is similar for the cervical region, but considerable tilting is necessary following a lumbar puncture because the opaque column must pass over the convexity of the thoracic vertebrae. For the thoracic region, very careful tilting is required to examine the individual vertebral levels in the prone position; the supine position provides the gravity pool for posterior localized screen examination.

As the examination reaches cervical level (1961), the head is placed with the median plane in line with the trunk, the neck being extended with the chin resting on the couch. This will prevent the opaque medium from passing into the cranial system. An example of this positioning is shown in radiograph (1973). Once the opaque medium has reached the cervical region, the couch is returned to the horizontal position and then gentle tilting is used to examine each vertebra in turn. A slight rotation of the head assists in the controlled movement necessary to show the upper cervical level of the opaque medium.

Diagrams (1956) to (1961) show the progress of the tilting couch from the erect to the reversed tilting, prone position, with the appropriate movement of the opaque medium within the subarachnoid space.

A series of photographs shows the patient rotated into the left oblique position (1962), the left lateral position (1963), the supine position with the pelvis lowered (1964), and with the head lowered (1965). Also, (1966) with the patient in the prone position on reverse tilting shows the usual screen and serial device being moved into place. For any position, horizontal tube projection may be necessary (1967).

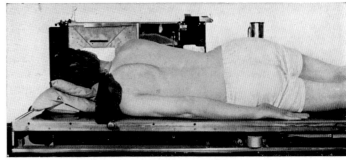

1962

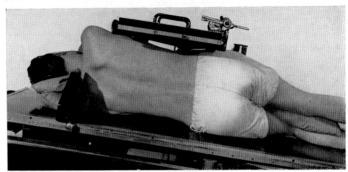

1963

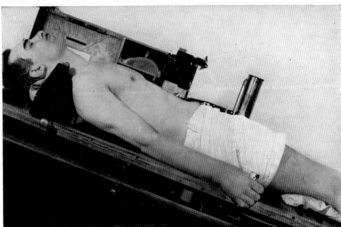

1964

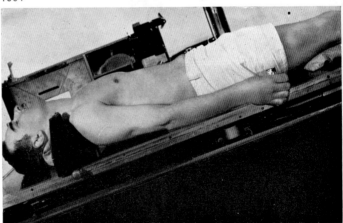

1965

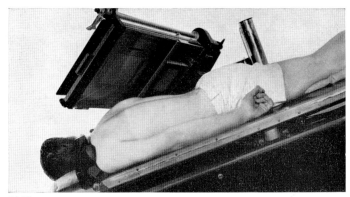

1966

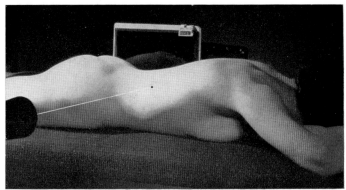

1967

When a lesion is found to block completely the flow of the opaque column, a second injection is made at a higher level to enable the extent of the lesion to be determined, as shown between the two columns of contrast medium. Opaque preparations such as Myodil may be aspirated on completing the radiographic examination (1975) and this course is considered to be advisable.

General projections of the vertebral column are usually taken in addition to the localized serial device exposures.

The radiographs on pages 567, 568, show the application of myelography to various regions of the neural canal. Serial exposures of the cervical region following a cisternal injection are shown in postero-anterior (1968) and lateral (1969). Three regions of the neural canal using the serial cassette, include lumbar (1970), thoraco-lumbar (1971) and thoracic (1972). The lateral cervical radiograph (1973) was taken with the neck extended and using horizontal tube projection.

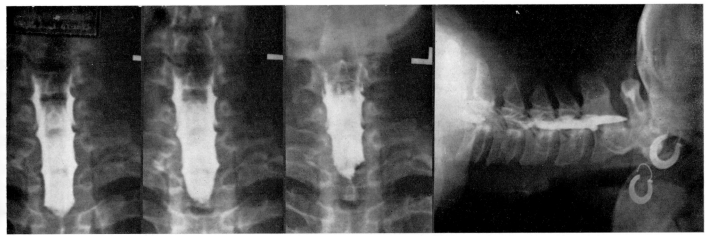

1968   1969

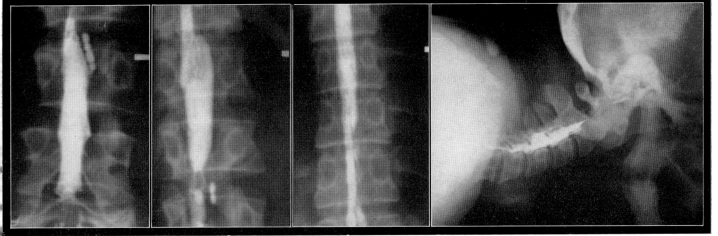

970   1971   1972   1973

23

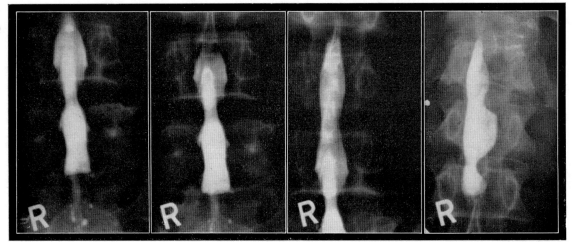

1974

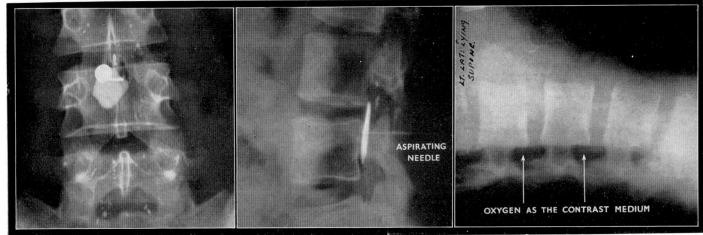

ASPIRATING NEEDLE

LT. LAT. LYING SUPINE.

OXYGEN AS THE CONTRAST MEDIUM

1975

1976

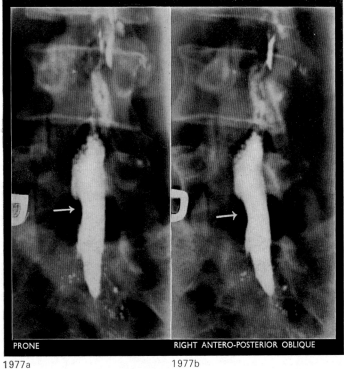

PRONE

RIGHT ANTERO-POSTERIOR OBLIQUE

1977a

1977b

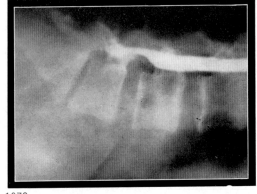

1978

Serial exposures of the lumbar region are shown in (1974). Aspiration of the opaque medium is shown in postero-anterior and lateral projections (1975).

The dorsal decubitus radiograph (1976) was taken following an injection of oxygen, which shows as a dark area in the lumbar region.

When opaque medium reaches the extradural space, usually inadvertently, it mingles with the fatty substance in the cavity and eventually tends to pass through the intervertebral foramina to show the nerve sheaths (1979a).

Intervertebral discs

The foregoing technique includes the examination for a slipped intervertebral disc, which usually occurs in the fourth and fifth lumbar, and the lower cervical regions.

Following the injection of the opaque medium into the subarachnoid space, with the patient facing the tube in the erect screening position, the couch is gradually lowered to enable the opaque medium to cover the region of each disc in turn as the patient approaches the prone position (1977a). The screen examination also follows the right and left rotation of the patient to confirm the presence of an irregularity of the outline of the opaque column as in (1977b), indicating, as reported in this instance, that there is an intrusion of the disc into the neural canal. A confirmatory lateral projection may be taken in the prone position, as in (1978). These small area radiographs must be carefully identified as to location and also as to right and left sides.

Radiographs (1979b) show an intervertebral disc made visible by calcification of the nucleus. Direct opaque injection of the disc has been described as discography.

General Note—Examinations by stereography or tomography may be included.

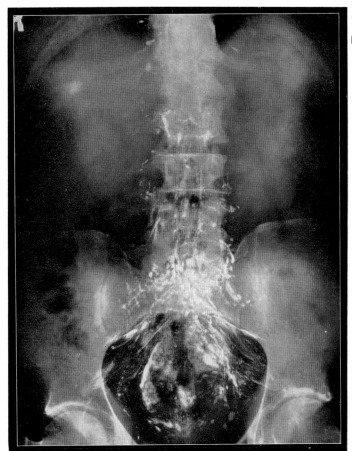

1979a

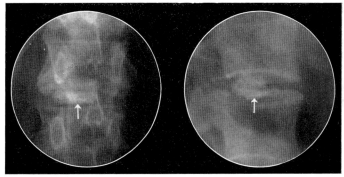

1979b

24

ANGIOGRAPHY

SECTION 24

ANGIOGRAPHY

The term angiography indicates the radiographic examination of the circulatory system. As the system is largely transradiant, it is necessary to introduce an opaque medium into the blood stream to enable the blood vessels to become visible for radiological investigation. Angiography embraces both the arterial system—arteriography, and the venous system—venography, or phlebography. The closely allied lymphatic system is also included. Descriptive titles for the technique as applied to the various regions concerned include:

Cerebral angiography, pages 575 to 579;
Cardiac angiography, pages 580 to 586;
Abdominal angiography, aortography, pages 590 to 595;
Peripheral angiography, pages 596 to 595;
Lymphangiography, pages 601 to 602.

Opaque media

The opaque medium used is one of the water soluble organic iodine compounds such as: Angiografin, Cardio–Conray, Conray 280, 420, Hypaque 65%, 85%, Triosil 75%, Urografin 76%, Vasiodone.

The patient is always tested for sensitivity to these preparations usually on the day preceding the examination.

As appropriate, the opaque medium may be introduced intravenously, either by percutaneous injection or following an incision to disclose the artery or vein for direct injection. It may also be introduced by selective catheterization or occasionally by interosseous injection. The method may be descending or retrograde. The injection may be arranged to give maximum concentration of the opaque medium in the shortest possible time or, for certain purposes, over a slightly delayed period coinciding with carefully timed pre-arranged exposures. The radiographic equipment, particularly film changing mechanism, is designed accordingly.

Film changers

The type of film changer employed depends on the particular region involved and the speed at which film changing is required. In its simplest form, the film changer is manually operated and the speed of exposure does not exceed two per second, which is adequate for certain investigations. Simple mechanization enables the films to be exposed at the rate of four per second and this is suitable when exposures are limited to six or eight. When high speed work is necessary and exposures are made at from six to twelve per second, with up to twenty or more exposures per subject position at a predetermined and variable speed rate, the equipment becomes more specialized, particularly when two planes of the subject are exposed simultaneously. Simultaneous biplane projection is desirable for certain investigations as the use of the opaque medium is then limited to a single injection and, at the same time, similar phases are shown on complementary exposures.

The specialized equipment employed for film changing ranges from relatively simple apparatus for handling a series of loaded cassettes, to automatic magazines designed either for cut films, in which the feed mechanism is so arranged that each film in turn rests momentarily between a single pair of intensifying screens. Other methods include indirect radiography using 70 millimetre film in a motorized cassette and cineradiography on 35 millimetre film. For the simultaneous biplane method, the X-ray tube and the cassette or film changer are duplicated.

In addition to these various film-changing methods, scanography may be applied to the limbs using a single long 14 × 36 inch film for both lower limbs as described in Section 3, and using a narrower film or series of films in a cassette measuring 8 × 40 inches for a single limb.

All of these methods have individual problems of taking, processing and viewing. Furthermore, the question of protection from excessive radiation is a very special problem—for the patient, for the surgeon making the injection, for the radiologist, for the radiographer, and for other personnel, particularly when the cassettes are manually operated.

Manually operated cassette changers for four or six cassettes are available in various forms and are often designed and made in the individual hospital. The cassettes, 12 × 15 inches or 14 × 14 inches, may be moved transversely as in (1980), or they may be moved longitudinally, from end to end of the couch (1982) when the operator is able to work at a greater distance from the X-ray tube. With either method, it may be desirable to follow up an injection for abdominal aortography by having a 14 × 36 inch cassette in position, with a second tube centred over the limbs to enable an exposure to be made immediately on completing the abdominal exposure (1981).

A unit which provides for abdominal and peripheral angiography in serial form is shown on page 591.

The placing of the manually operated cassettes for the skull table is shown in (1989). Three exposures are made for the lateral projection and two following a second injection for the antero-posterior position. Handles on the cassettes facilitate their rapid removal. Cassettes used in this way are backed with lead or other suitable material to prevent radiation-fogging of other films in the cassette magazine. The magazine may be completely automatic with more films available for both projections.

A mechanically operated cassette changer with the cassettes moving longitudinally is shown diagrammatically in (1982). Exposures are at the rate of up to four per second. Made in various forms, these cassette changers are adequate for the majority of examinations by angiography. Other types of film changer can be used in duplicate for simultaneous biplane technique.

For high speed work, a special film changer is required. There are two main types for direct radiography, (a) using separate films and (b) using roll film:

(a) Up to thirty cut films, usually 10 × 12 inches or 14 × 14 inches, are placed without wrapping in a slotted light-proof magazine. In action, each film in turn passes between a pair of intensifying screens, with compression applied during the exposure; the exposed films then pass into a light-tight container for removal to the darkroom (1983). Exposures are made at the rate of up to six per second and a predetermined rate and grouping of exposures can be pre-set to operate automatically. On completing the exposures, the light-tight container is taken to the darkroom and the films are processed.

24

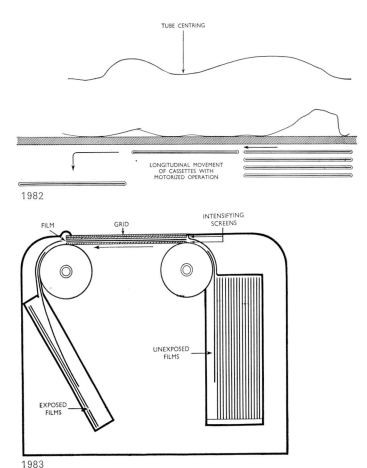

MANUAL OPERATION

CASSETTES 1—3

TRANSVERSE FILM CHANGER 4 CASSETTES

STATIONARY GRID

CASSETTES 2—4

1980

TUBE CENTRING

LONGITUDINAL MOVEMENT OF CASSETTES WITH MOTORIZED OPERATION

1982

2nd X-RAY TUBE CENTRE

1st X-RAY TUBE

14″ × 36″ CASSETTE FOR PERIPHERAL ARTERIOGRAPHY

14″ × 17″ CASSETTES FOR ABDOMINAL AORTOGRAPHY

1981

FILM

GRID

INTENSIFYING SCREENS

UNEXPOSED FILMS

EXPOSED FILMS

1983

Two of these cassette changers placed at right angles provide for simultaneous biplane technique as with the roll film unit (1984), the patient being positioned to record either antero-posterior and lateral, or right and left oblique projections, with the X-ray tubes and high tension equipment arranged accordingly.

(b) Similar equipment provides for the use of roll film, twelve inches wide, in lengths of up to fifty feet (15 metres). As previously, the film passes between a pair of intensifying screens, with compression applied during the exposure period. Exposures may be made at the rate of up to eight, or even twelve per second and, again, a prearranged plan of exposure grouping can be set in motion to operate automatically for up to forty exposures. Two such units provide for simultaneous biplane technique (1984). On completing the series of exposures, the film spools are lifted from the film changer in complete darkness and placed in light-tight containers for carrying to the darkroom. The rolls of film are threaded on to large spirals which enable the films to be conveniently processed through automatic processors.

Both half cycle ($3\frac{1}{2}$ minutes) and 90 second processing are extremely complementary to this type of examination, in that the information from the series of films is available in a brief interval, allowing appraisal as to the necessity or not of continued examination. Special panorama type viewing facilities are provided to afford sequence viewing of the series.

Subtraction

Subtraction technique is included for cerebral angiography on page 588, for cardiac angiography on pages 587, and also for abdominal aortography on page 589.

Indirect methods of angiography are in the form of miniature radiography and cineradiography.

Miniature angiography

The equipment for indirect radiography using 70 millimetre film and employing the mirror optical system is described in Section 34 and the two units are shown in position for simultaneous biplane technique. The exposure rate is at up to six per second using the Rapidex cassette which provides for up to forty exposures. A pre-arranged programme of speed and spacing of exposures can be operated automatically. For cerebral angiography, the optical system is modified to enable the cranium to fill a 10 × 10 inch screen, thus providing the maximum size of image to fill the 70 millimetre film. Viewing is direct or with 50 per cent magnification.

Cineangiography

Cineradiography with the image intensifier is described in Section 35. Simultaneous biplane technique is not readily applicable. The exposure rate can be at up to fifty frames per second, but a speed of twenty-five frames per second is usually sufficient. Viewing is by cinematograph projection.

Precautions

These investigations are most exacting, particularly for cardiac angiography involving the possible adverse effects of the opaque medium and considerable radiation exposure to the patient, in addition to the expenditure of a large quantity of film costing approximately £15 per patient. Much depends on the care and efficiency of the radiographer to ensure that the end result is in every way successful. All possible emergencies must be anticipated, with the X-ray unit and accessories in perfect working order including the preparation of the film magazines, checking exposure conditions and finally the processing and handling of the long lengths of roll film.

For these angiographic procedures exacting and comprehensive team work is essential.

Protection from unnecessary radiation must be scrupulously observed for both the patient and for all personnel concerned.

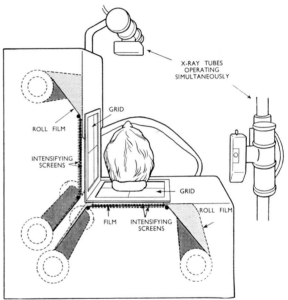

1984

Cerebral angiography

Three tracing diagrams, which have been prepared from a series of angiograms of one side of the head, show the vessels involved in cerebral angiography. The lateral projections (1985, 1988) and the anterior projection (1986) show the principal arteries, and the lateral projection (1987) shows the principal veins and sinuses.

Opaque medium

The opaque medium used for cerebral angiography may be; Angiografin, Conray 280, Hypaque 45%, Urografin 45% or 65%.

The patient is tested for sensitivity to one or other of the above preparations on the previous day. 10 millilitres of the opaque medium are injected for each stage of the examination. Each injection is completed within 2 seconds and the exposures are made within a further 5 seconds. The patency of the needle is

maintained throughout the entire examination by the infusion of saline. Following local or general anaesthetic 10 millilitres of the opaque media is injected rapidly into the internal carotid artery; although for a suspected lesion of the internal carotid, the injection site would be at the lower level of the common carotid artery. Towards the end of the injection of the opaque media the first exposure is taken followed by further films over a 5 second period to embrace the arterial capillary and venous phases. A minimum of 3 films is necessary.

The route through the internal carotid artery is to show the anterior and middle cerebral vessels (2001); an injection into the vertebral artery is used to disclose the posterior cerebral and cerebellar arteries (2002). These two radiographs are of the one subject.

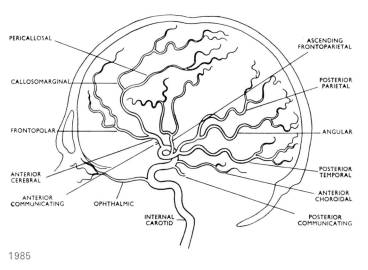

1985

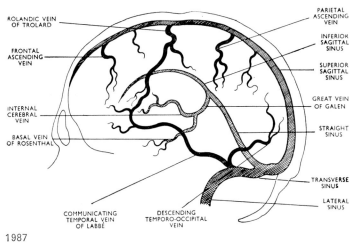

1987

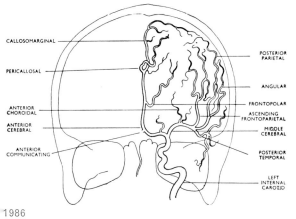

1986

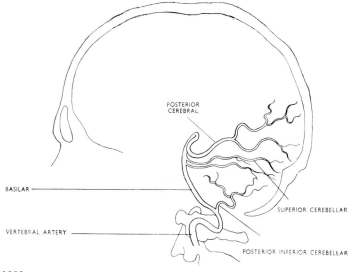

1988

Technique with the skull table

Team work in the radiographic department is particularly desirable for this investigation, where freedom of movement for the radiologist whilst making the injection, adequate protection from radiation, and speed of exposure following the injection, are essential.

The patient is placed in the supine position with the neck hyper-extended by placing foam pads under the shoulders or by lowering the head support of the skull table. The immobilizing band is placed loosely over the forehead to be tightened at a later stage. The X-ray tube is lowered for horizontal projection. The special magazine containing three cassettes is prepared in advance; this, by spring control, enables each cassette in turn to be brought into position with great rapidity for the next exposure. For the lateral projections, the magazine is fixed vertically against the side of the head which is remote from the side being injected. A second magazine for two cassettes is fitted below the head rest to be loaded at a later stage for the antero-posterior projections (1989).

Although the technique described is that employed with the skull table using the manually operated lateral, three-cassette and anterior two-cassette magazine, the two magazines may be completely automatic and of greater film capacity for both projections thus eliminating radiation exposure to the radiographer.

Protection for the operator making the injection is provided by lead rubber curtains which, being suspended from above and counter-weighted, can be bought into position without delay.

Immediately before the injection, the patient's head is finally adjusted for the lateral projections and immobilized by tightening the head band. Tube centring is checked, the protective curtains are lowered, and the radiographers are ready to make the exposure as directed, and to remove the exposed cassettes, if manually operated.

The signal for the first exposure is given just prior to, or on, completion of the injection and the 'immediate' exposure is made.

The first cassette (1990) is withdrawn, to be replaced by the second cassette which springs into position in readiness for the second exposure which follows only $2\frac{1}{2}$ seconds after the injection (1991); the procedure is repeated for the third exposure which is made within 5 seconds of the injection being given (1992). The above timing may be modified, and example of this being provided by the series (1995,1996,1997).

Whilst injections of normal saline are continued, the films are processed at speed for inspection by the radiologist who decides on the next stage of the examination.

Exposure timing

Depending on the timing of the exposure the vessels may be shown at three stages, results being designated accordingly as arteriogram, capillary and venogram. Referring to the lateral radiograph, the opaque medium is seen first in the arterial system (1990) at 0·0 seconds, in the capillary stage (1991) at $2\frac{1}{2}$ seconds and in the venous stage (1992) at 5 seconds.

In the antero-posterior projections (1993,1994) the opaque medium is shown in the arterial and venous systems respectively.

To show details of the progress and vascular infiltration of a tumour, films may be exposed at the rate of 6 per second using an automatically operated film changer as described on page 573, or at a still higher rate of exposure by cineradiography.

Exposure time

This should be sufficiently brief to produce sharp outline of the opaque media in the circulatory vessels.

Kilovoltage should be at least 10 kilovolts higher than that for the routine skull position.

In addition to assisting in reduced exposure time it is essential that adequate penetration is obtained to delineate the passage of the carotid vessel over the dense petrous region.

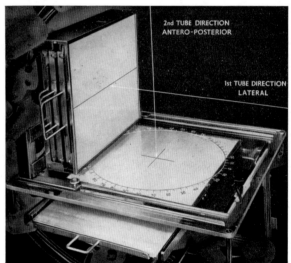

1989

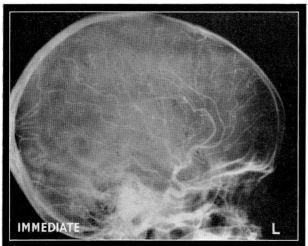

1990

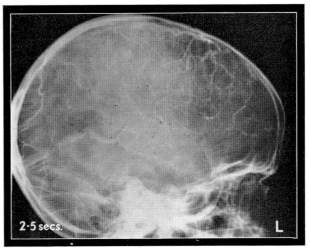

1991

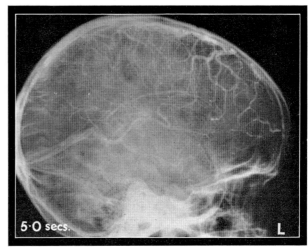

1992

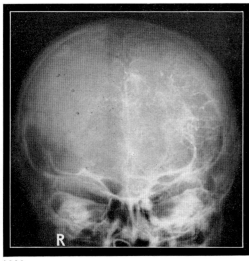

1993

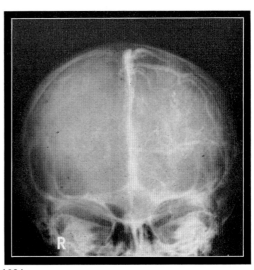

1994

Positioning

Radiographs exposed for a single examination of one side of the head may include the following projections; lateral, antero-posterior with or without 25° caudal tilt or both, and oblique positioning each requiring an injection of 10 millilitres of opaque media.

Lateral view

As previously stated the patient is placed in the supine position with the neck hyper-extended by placing foam pads under the shoulders or by lowering the head support of the skull table. The head is raised on a foam pad to ensure that in the lateral projection the complete area of the skull is included. Exact positioning for symmetry of the skull is very important, the X-ray tube is directed horizontally and centred 1cm above the EAM with the beam aperture confined to the skull area (1995, 1996, 1997).

Antero-posterior

When the radiologist is satisfied with the lateral series of radiographs the tube is rotated 90° and angled 25° caudally. The patient's head is supported while both the shoulder and head foam pads are removed. The head is re-positioned on the table symmetrically over a 15° foam sponge wedge to ensure that the chin is well tucked down and the base line vertical.

Centring with the X-ray beam confined to the localized area and at a level 5 cm above the glabella. A further 10 millilitres of opaque media are injected and the same procedure is followed as for the previous lateral projection (1998).

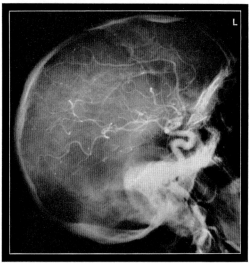

1995

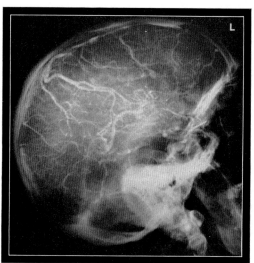

1996

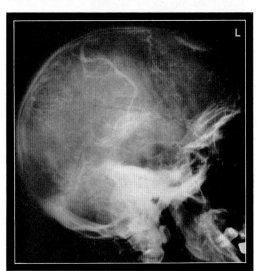

1997

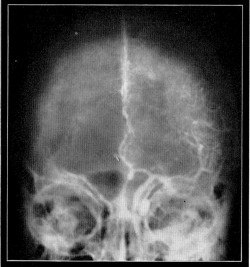

1998

Oblique projections

The head is rotated 30–45° away from the affected side with the tube centred 5 cm above the mid-point of the superior orbital margin of the side being examined, with a 25° caudal tilt. (Depending on the radiologist's preference the tube may also be perpendicular and centred directly over the mid-point of the supra-orbital margin.) The oblique position serves to open up the carotid syphon which otherwise appears as a dense blob on the film (1999,2000).

Vertebral arteriography

Direct puncture

To disclose the posterior cerebral and cerebella circulation by injection of contrast medium into the cervical part of the vertebral artery.

Radiographic procedure is similar to that adopted for carotid angiography, with the exception that it is necessary to augment caudal projection for the antero-posterior position to 30 degrees.

Indirect puncture

An alternative to the above is by the adoption of femoral retrograde technique.

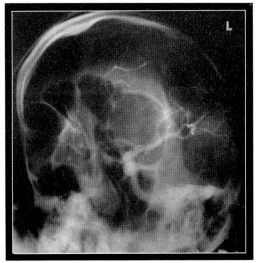

1999

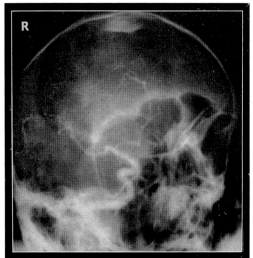

2000

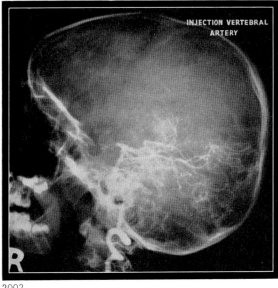

2002

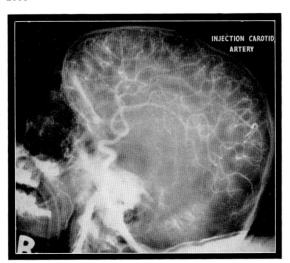

2001

579

24 Cardiac angiography

Opaque medium
The opaque medium in use may be: Hypaque 85 per cent, Urografin 76 per cent, Triosil 75 per cent, Cardio–Conray 420 or, Angiografin.

The injection is repeated when the two planes are exposed separately or when a repeat exposure is necessary. A test for the patient's sensitivity to the chosen organic iodine compound is made on the day preceding the examination, by injection intravenously of one millilitre of the opaque medium selected. Enquiries are also made as to possible allergic tendencies such as a history of hay fever or respiratory conditions such as asthma.

Several methods are employed to introduce the opaque medium, the most favoured being a method of selective angiography.

Cardiac angiography
Caridac angiography is the technique used to show the anatomical features and functioning of the heart and great vessels. The examination entails an injection of an opaque medium and its concentrated movement throughout the cardiac system. Each phase of the movement of the medium is recorded by rapid serial X-ray exposures.

Image intensification and television monitoring are employed for appropriate manoeuvrability and positioning of the catheter. Rapid serial changers, single or preferably bi-plane, with roll film (exposure rate up to 10 per second) or cut film (exposure rate up to 6 per second) allow a pre-arranged plan of exposure grouping which can be set in motion to operate automatically. Alternatively the record can be filmed using the cine angiography method.

Conditions investigated are congenital heart anomalies, rheumatic heart and lung tumours. A section diagram of the heart and great vessels is included for guidance.

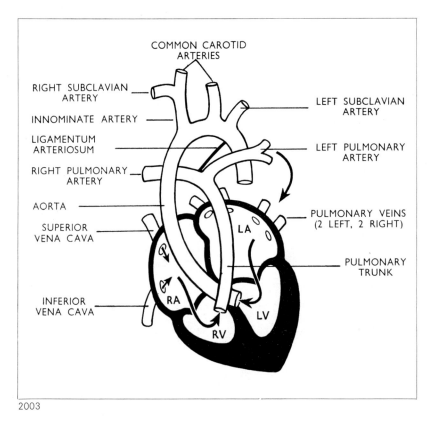

2003

Selective angiography

(a) By catheterization into the median cubital vein at the elbow and manoeuvred by screen control through the venous system to the appropriate chambers of the right or left side of the heart when the foramen ovale is patent (2004).

(b) By catheterization under screening control into the right atrium from the right femoral vein (2005).

(c) Retrograde—Catheterization into one of the femoral arteries and advanced upwards via the aorta, around the aortic arch through the aortic valve, into the left ventricle.

Venous method

Injection by means of a wide bore cannula or plastic catheter into the exposed median cubital vein in the elbow or the saphenous vein in the thigh (2006).

General procedure

A preliminary exposure is usually made on the previous day as a check on exposure technique and for guidance as to the quantity of opaque medium required. The technique for cardiac angiography is exacting in every respect and to enable a satis-

factory diagnosis to be reached the procedure must be planned in advance to suit the condition to be investigated. This embraces the choice of position, the injection site, quantity of medium, injection pressure, the speed and programming of exposures and the actual exposure required on seeing the preliminary film. These radiographs are denser than for routine work as the heart substance must be penetrated sufficiently to show the passage of the opaque medium. Positioning and programming of exposures will vary with the condition under investigation and will be decided by the radiologist or cardiologist.

The actual procedure of injection and exposure of films occupies not more than 10 seconds, but this follows a great deal of preparation. Every detail must be arranged in advance, cassettes or film magazines loaded and placed in position, exposure conditions checked and tested, tubes centred, radiation protection arrangements in order, and processing equipment ready for use; finally the patient, either under local or general anaesthetic, is positioned appropriately in relation to the X-ray tubes, and film area. Large foam–sponge blocks are used to raise the patient to the correct height relative to the film area.

24

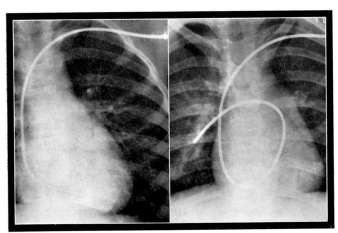

2004a   2004b

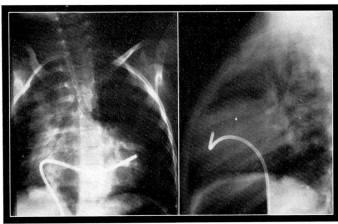

2005

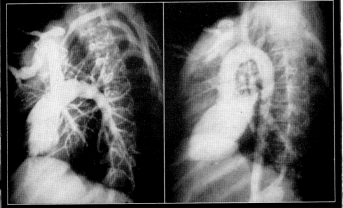

2006

X-ray equipment

Using simultaneous bi-plane film changers two complimentary radiographs are provided at each phase of the examination with one injection.

In simultaneous bi-plane technique two X-ray tubes may be operated from a single six valve high tension unit. The kilovoltage and time are applicable to both tubes, and adjustments for two differing positions of the patient is made by dividing the milliamperage appropriately between the two tubes. For example, postero-anterior 200 MAS, and lateral 400 MAS. Greater advantage, however, is obtained when two transformers, one for each tube is available to provide greater selectivity of all factors.

Cross-hatch stationary grids are let into the two surfaces of the film changer. The elimination of secondary radiation can be further restricted by the use of selective filtration material (for example sheet tin or lead screens placed at the rear of each grid). A small tube aperture restricts radiation to the essential area for each projection.

The speed and spacing of the exposures are important and as previously stated, cardiac units are provided with a programme selector which is set in advance to operate automatically, as shown in the following programmed sequences.

Three exposures per second for 3 seconds (right side); two exposures per second for 2 seconds and four exposures per second for 4 seconds (left side).

Positioning and timing

The radiologist's choice of projections—usually antero-posterior and lateral (2008,2009), or right and left antero-posterior oblique (2013a,b)—depends on the condition to be investigated.

Exposures may be at the rate of from two to ten per second.

For coarctation of the aorta, particularly for the lateral projection, the whole of the thoracic aorta must be shown to include the dome of the diaphragm. Typical exposure is at the rate of one per second for ten seconds. Examples of coarctation near the arch of the aorta are shown in two children, antero-posterior (2010), and antero-posterior (2011) and oblique (2012).

For pulmonary stenosis, the lateral or oblique projections are the more important and, again a typical exposure rate is one per second for ten seconds. An example is shown in the antero-posterior (2008) and lateral (2009) projections.

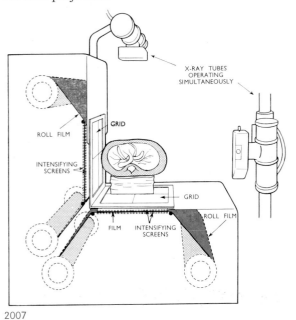

2007

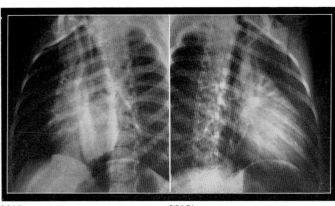

2013a   2013b

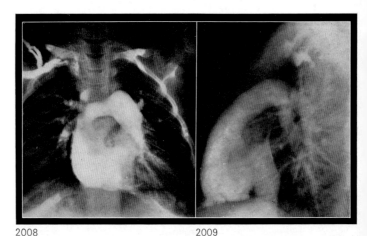

2008   2009

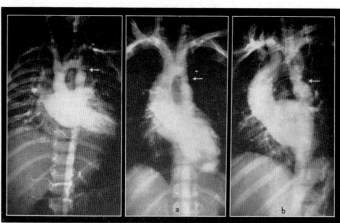

2010   2011   2012

Cardiac angiography selective method

In the current functional method of selective angiography only the essential part of the heart sequence is injected and exposed, thus reducing the possible reactions to the opaque medium to a minimum and avoiding considerable radiation exposure. The catheter is inserted into the median cubital vein at the elbow and passes through the venous system to the region required. The position of the tip of the catheter is checked by visual monitor screening from two positions, antero-posterior and lateral or oblique. Confirmatory films as to position may be taken as in (2014,2015). Two further examples are included (2016) with the tip of the catheter in the right ventricle having passed through the subclavian vein, innominate vein, the superior vena cava and the right atrium to the right ventricle. With the tip of the catheter (2017) in the right pulmonary artery having continued still further through the right ventricle, the main pulmonary trunk and so to the right pulmonary artery.

Preceeding the injection of contrast medium the cardiac catheter is connected to a manometer to record regional heart pressure, and blood samples are withdrawn to determine the oxygen content in the various chambers of the heart and great vessels.

A special high pressure syringe is used for the injection and the opaque media is injected under pressure through the cardiac catheter into the appropriate heart chamber. After injection, exposures are then made at the rate of anything up to 10 per second.

Exposure factors are given below. The opaque medium (OM) employed is Triosil 75 per cent.

(1) Infants 3/4 weeks. Weight 4/6lbs. OM 5/10 millilitres.
(2) Children 5/7 years. Weight 32/47lbs. OM 25/28 millilitres.
(3) Adult. OM 50 millilitres.

24

	kVp AP	Lat	MAS	FFD	Film ILFORD	Screens ILFORD	Grid
(1)	65	85	2	40″ (100cm)	RAPID R	FT	Grid
(2)	75	95	2	40″ (100cm)	RAPID R	FT	Grid
(3)	105	125	5	40″ (100cm)	RAPID R	FT	Grid

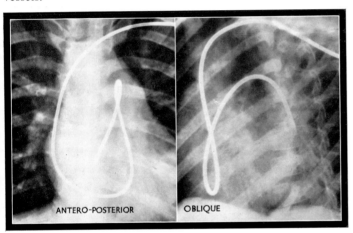

ANTERO-POSTERIOR   OBLIQUE

2014   2015

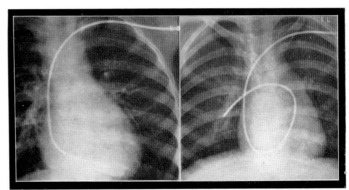

2016   2017

583

Selective cardiac angiography is also shown in the series of antero-posterior and lateral radiographs (2018–2021) taken by the simultaneous bi-plane method. In this instance the catheter is inserted into the femoral vein and passed through the inferior vena cava to the heart. The actual position of the catheter being confirmed (2018).

After injection of the opaque media exposures were made at the rate of 8 per second for two seconds and from the resultant series of simultaneous exposed pairs of radiographs the 8th, 12th and 14th pairs have been selected as follows:

2019 taken at one second.
2020 taken at one and a half seconds.
2021 taken at one and three quarter seconds.

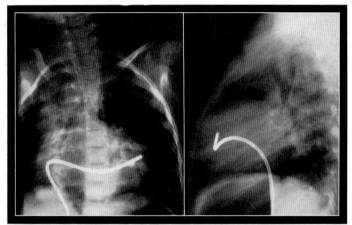

2018

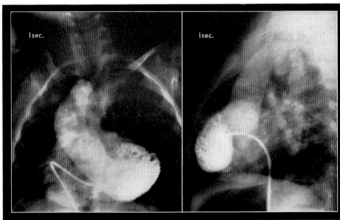

2019

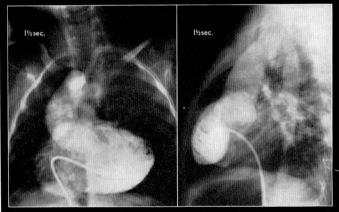

2020

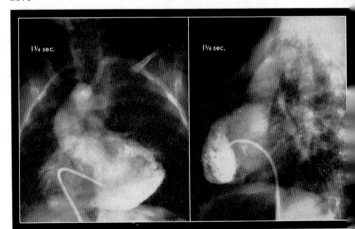

2021

Venous method

For convenience of injection a wide-bore cannula or plastic catheter is introduced a short way into the exposed median cubital vein in the elbow. The terminal end is strapped to the arm to prevent movement of the catheter during the injection, injection is at a rapid rate.

The rate of travel of the opaque medium by this route is $2\frac{1}{2}$–3 seconds to reach the pulmonary artery and 4–5 seconds to reach the aorta. Therefore exposures are usually continued for from 8–10 seconds.

(2022–2029) shows the progress of the opaque medium passing through the heart from the superior vena cava (2022) to the descending aorta (2029). These 8 radiographs have been selected from a series of 28 lateral exposures. The stages selected from this sequence are 1, 2, 4, 6, 8, 10, 21, 28. The approximate timing is shown on each radiograph.

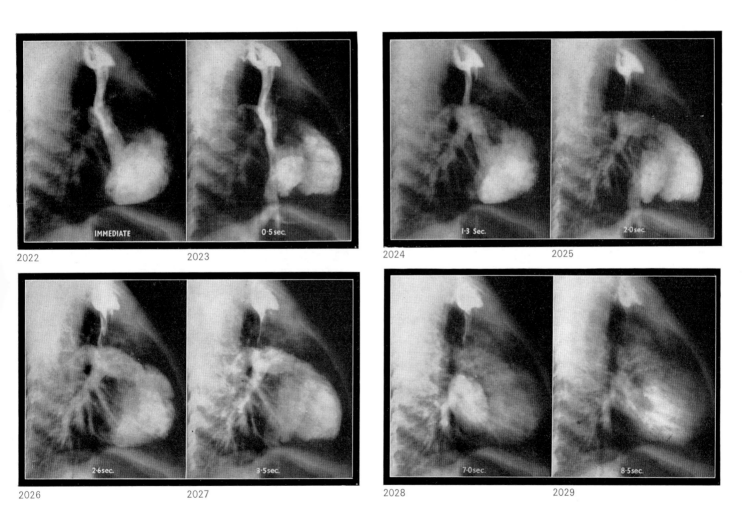

2022 2023 2024 2025

2026 2027 2028 2029

A further series of illustrations of different subjects comprising of radiographs and tracing diagrams is included for guidance.
(2030) antero-posterior, shows the normal outline of the right atrium and ventricle with the pulmonary arteries (3 seconds);
(2031) antero–posterior, shows the left atrium well filled, the left ventricle in systole, poorly filled, and the ascending aorta (6 seconds);
(2032) left anterior oblique, shows the normal right atrium, ventricle and pulmonary arteries (3 seconds);
(2033) left anterior oblique, shows the left atrium and ventricle, the ghost shadow of the right ventricle enables the inter-ventricular septum to be well defined ($7\frac{1}{2}$ seconds).

It will be appreciated that the above examinations are not without danger to the patient both as regards immediate and delayed reactions. Appropos this it is essential that strict aseptic precautions must be observed with constant E.C.G. monitoring, and full facilities for resuscitation immediately available.

Cineangiography

Cardiac cineangiographs are shown in Section 35. These are taken with the image intensifier using a specially adapted 35 millimetre cine camera, and being viewed simultaneously by television monitor. The individual frames have been enlarged selectively but in sequence. The condition is reported as a patent ductus arteriosus.

Subtraction

Subtraction technique

In radiological procedure employing contrast media, information can be lost where there is insufficient distinction between, the opaque vascular pattern and superimposing dense bone structure. If the unwanted image of these structures can be removed it is then possible for the opaque media vascular pattern to be seen without interference, allowing a more positive diagnosis to be made.

Photographic subtraction is a method by which this can be achieved.

The technique involves—

Stage 1

The taking of an initial straight radiograph. This is followed by a series of radiographs taken after the injection of the opaque media has been given.

It is essential that there is complete immobilization of the patient throughout the total sequence of radiographs.

The technical factors should be identical throughout.

The kilovoltage should be such as to give good penetration of the dense bone structures. The essential differences between the first film and the series taken after injection is that the initial film will be minus the recorded opaque media filled vascular pattern on the latter series.

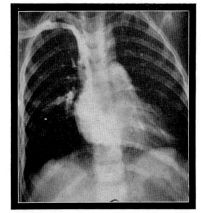
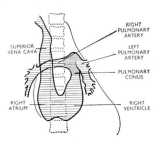

2030

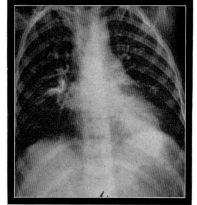
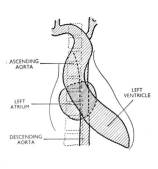

2031

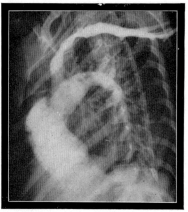
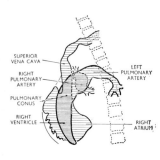

2032

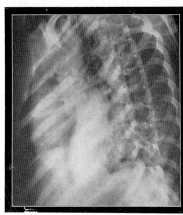
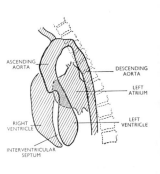

2033

Stage 2

A positive transparency is made of the initial film (the control). This will give an image where all the tones are in reverse of the original radiograph.

A film with a scale of contrast capable of recording the complete tone range of the original radiograph should be used, and Ilford fine-grain ordinary photographic film is recommended. The image should be fully exposed and developed.

Development should be over 2 minutes with agitation in a standard type developer.

Stage 3

The radiograph recording the opaque media and the positive transparency are superimposed in exact register. All detail other than that of the contrast media is then cancelled out due to the masking effect of the positive transparency, and improved clarity of the vascular pattern is established.

Stage 4

Consists of a further exposure of the above composite image, on fine grain ordinary film to reproduce a single film record.

The necessity for the latter procedure is dependent on the required permanency of the record.

Screen method

Printing of Positive Transparency.

Procedure

The initial radiograph in contact with an unexposed X-ray film within a cassette, is exposed to the light of a single screen, the light from the front screen having been rendered ineffective by covering it with black paper.

Exposure Factors

50 kilovolts, 3 mAS, 120 cm.

Processing

2 minute development in standard X-ray developer with agitation.

The mask (positive transparency) is then placed in exact register with the appropriate angiogram and serves to cancel out the unwanted bony and detailed frame of the skull and to leave the clearly defined vessels and thus accentuate any doubtful abnormality.

Bound together the two images in register can be printed on to a further X-ray film to give the subtracted result on a single film by the above screen method if a permanent record is required.

24

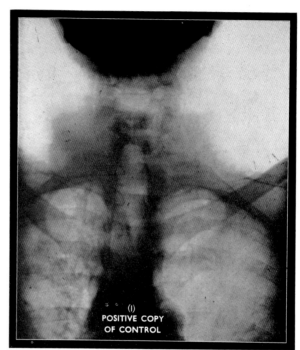

2034a

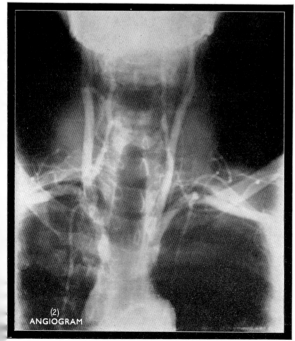

2034b

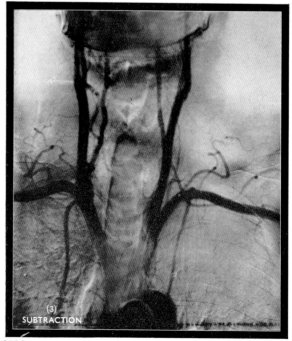

2034c

A male subject of 13 years (2035a,b) is reported as a post-traumatic carotido-cavernous fistula; and a female subject of 53 years (2035c) reported as a meningeoma in the orbit, both shown to great advantage in the subtraction prints.

Note—For comparative purposes, positive reproductions have also been used for the angiograms.

The advantage of employing subtraction technique is again shown in the accompanying illustrations (2036a,b).

(1) A positive reproduction of the original angiogram and (2) the subtraction copy. (2037) in which the renal arteries are shown to considerable advantage as compared with the original radiograph (2038).

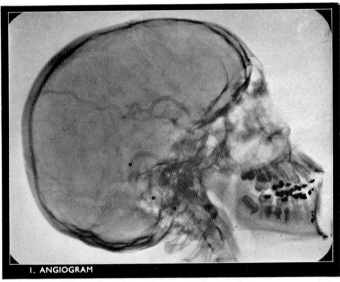

2035a

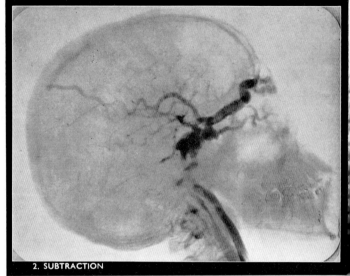

2035b

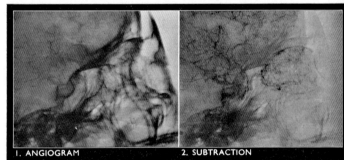

2035c

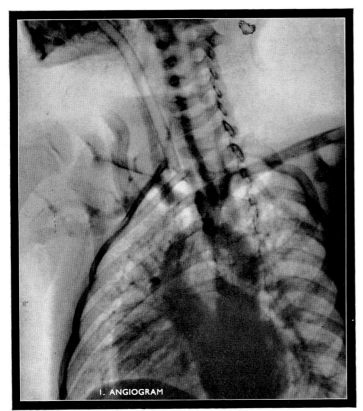

1. ANGIOGRAM

2036a

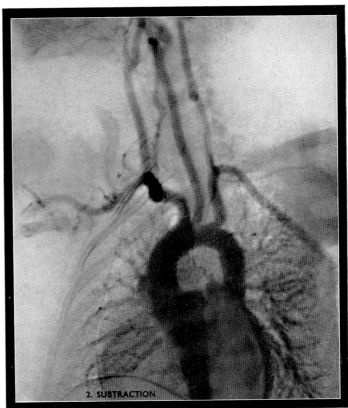

2. SUBTRACTION

2036b

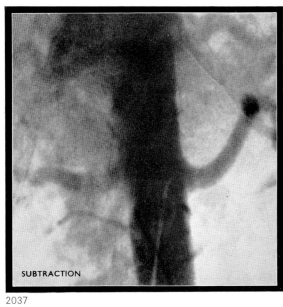

SUBTRACTION

2037

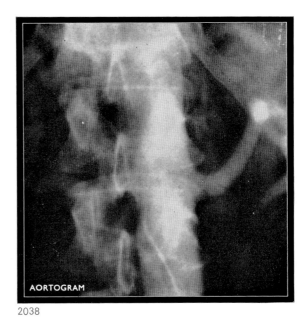

AORTOGRAM

2038

24 Abdominal aortography

The aorta pierces the diaphragm at the level of the twelfth thoracic vertebra to become the abdominal arota. It then passes downward, anterior to the lumber vertebrae, on the left of the mid-line to the level of the fourth lumbar vertebra, where it bifurcates to form the right and left common iliac arteries (2039a,b). As the aorta is not normally visible against the background of the abdominal viscera and the vertebral column, the use of an opaque medium is essential for its demonstration.

Abdominal aortography is used to investigate the aorta and its branches, the vessels of the legs, abnormal abdominal swelling, the kidneys (when it is sometimes combined with retrograde pyelography for renal and supra-renal tumours), cysts causing displacement and, on rare occasions, for the position of the placenta.

(2039a), although by no means a normal subject, is included to show the needle in situ, the general ramifications of the blood vessels and, in particular, the renal vessels, being well demonstrated for the right kidney.

(2039b) shows the bifurcation of the aorta at the fourth lumbar vertebra level to form the right and left common iliac arteris, which continue as the external iliac and thence as the femoral arteries.

Opaque media

The opaque medium employed may be Hypaque 65 per cent, Urografin 60 or 76 per cent, or Triosil 60 per cent, using 30 millilitres for a single injection which is completed in two to three seconds. A test for intolerance is made during the twenty-four hours preceding the examination; it may be made as a preliminary to the main injection.

Procedure—There are two methods of injection, one by the percutaneous translumbar route, and the other, retrograde by catheterization into one of the femoral arteries.

For the translumbar method a general anaesthetic is usually given but in the retrograde method this may be local or general.

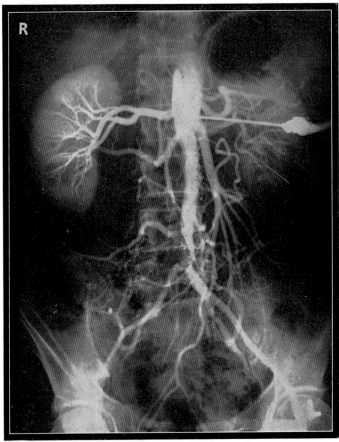

2039a

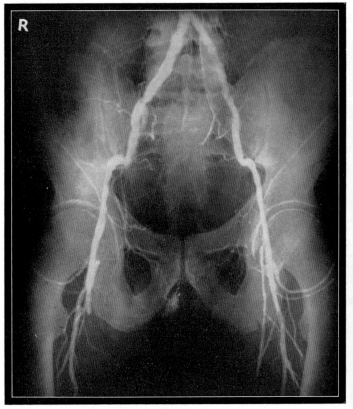

2039b

Cassette and film changers

Many types of manually operated longitudinal cassette changers are in use, page 569. The arrangement for a simple automatic type of cassette changer is shown in (2041). The film changer (2040) to take thirty 14 × 14 inch films (described on page 569) is completely automatic and the exposures can be pre-set for speed and timing at varying intervals to coincide with the injection requirements.

Diagram (2042) shows a cassette changer, described as the Bart's abdomino-peripheral angiography unit, which is designed to include serial exposures of both the abdomen and limbs. Three 14 × 17 inch cassettes and three 14 × 36 inch film-holders are placed in protective brass trays. Two sheets of brass are provided to protect the exposed and reserve films. The cassette trays and brass sheets are attached to cords which enable them to be moved in and out of the exposure field as required, or the movement may be completely automatic. The upper part of the diagram shows the cassette tunnel loaded in readiness for the dual examination, with the tube centred for the abdominal exposures. The lower part shows how each of the

three 14 × 17 inch cassettes has been moved in and out of the exposure field and finally covered by the protective brass sheets. The lower part also shows the tube centred for the limb exposures, for which a wide tube aperture and a long focus–film distance are essential to cover the whole length of the limb. To accommodate the difference in density from hip to ankle, a graduated aluminium wedge filter (2062) is placed at the tube aperture. For the abdominal exposures, a small aperture is provided in the double diaphragm (2043). For the limb exposures, two 14 × 17 inch films may be placed and to end in the cassette in place of the 36 inch length film. The sequence of of events is well-planned in advance. For a similar arrangement of abdominal and peripheral cassettes the movement of the cassettes into the required position is completely automatic.

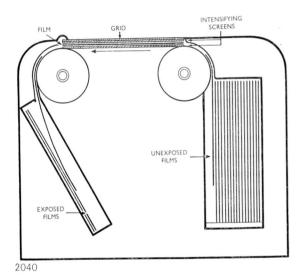

2040

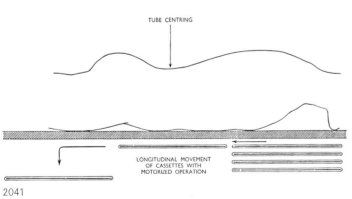

2041

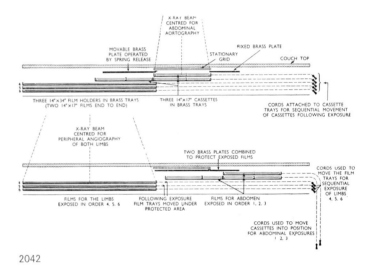

2042

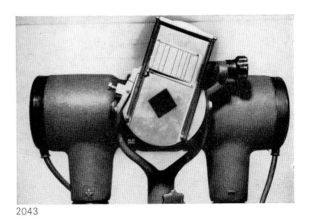

2043

Retrograde

This method tends to be favoured at present. The patient is placed in the supine position over one of the described rapid serial change systems and a preliminary film taken. The examination may then be carried out with the patient under either local or general anaesthesia.

A special needle is inserted into one of the femoral arteries and a flexible guide-wire placed through the needle, the latter is then removed. A radiopaque plastic catheter is threaded over the wire and both are manipulated upwards via the common iliac artery into the aorta. The guide-wire is removed and the position of the catheter checked under monitor screen control.

If the catheter position is satisfactory 20–30 millilitres of the contrast medium is injected manually or with a pressure injector. Films are taken in rapid succession, the sequence and siting being decided by the radiologist.

Abdominal aortography is shown in three stages using the retrograde method of injection—(2043) at ½ second, (2044) at 3 seconds and (2045) at 7 seconds.

Translumbar Aortography

This is generally performed to investigate lesion of the lower aorta and of the iliac arteries. It is particularly useful where an iliac artery block is suspected.

A preliminary film is taken with the patient prone. After general anaesthetic he is again placed in the prone position over one or other of the suitable rapid serial change systems previously described. A special needle is inserted into the aorta to the left of the mid-line at the level of the second to third lumbar vertebra. A control film is taken to show that the position of the needle is satisfactory. A small quantity of the opaque medium may also have been injected to determine dispersal, this film is developed immediately. (Alternatively screen control may be used.) If satisfactory 20–30 millilitres are injected rapidly either manually or with a pressure injector. A rapid succession of films are taken, the sequence and siting being decided by the radiologist.

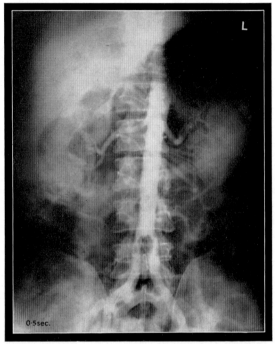

2043

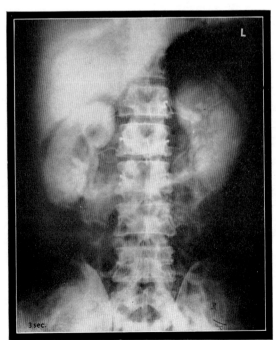

2044

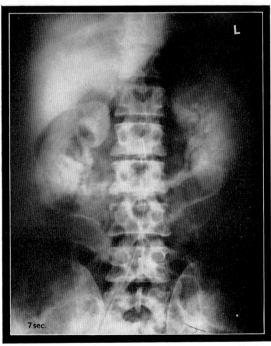

2045

The translumbar route was used for the following:
(2046) taken after half of the opaque medium had been injected and showing as a concentrated blob on the film;
(2047) taken one second later, showing aorta, renal arterial vessels and commencing shadows of the internal iliac vessels;
(2048) showing more vessels and increased opacity of the kidneys;
(2049) showing the venous return referred to as a nephrogram with the renal shadows generally intensified;
(2050) showing the appearances to be similar to those of a late stage kidney opacity of a normal pyelogram.

When the cassettes are manually operated, precise co-ordination of exposure and removal of cassette enables four or more exposures to be made in from four to five seconds. The exposures commence when 20 millilitres of the opaque medium have been injected.

kVp	mAS	FFD	Film ILFORD	Screens ILFORD	Grid
80/90	20	40″ (100cm)	RAPID R	FT	Moving

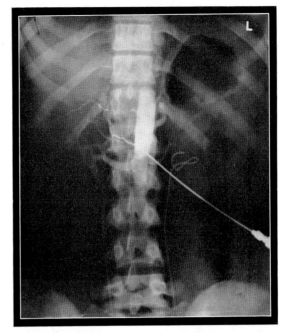

2046

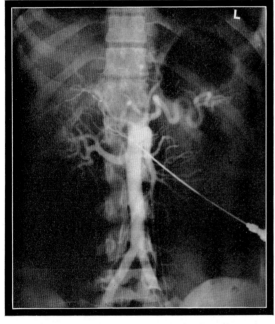

2047

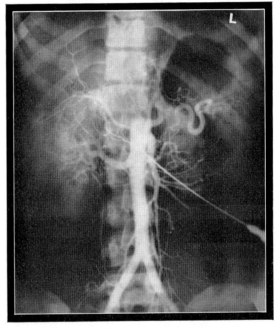

2048

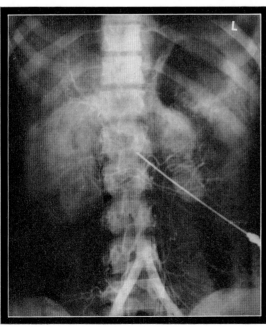

2049

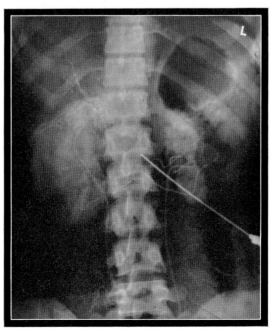

2050

593

Renal arteriography

Investigation of the renal arteries employing the injection of a contrast medium to determine arterial lesions is termed renal arteriography. The examination can be undertaken either using the retrograde method (2055) or alternatively the translumbar injection route (2051,2052) when there is difficulty in the location of either femoral artery. Procedure is similar in either method to that described for aortic angiography, with the exception that the needle or catheter is sighted approximately at the level of the 1st lumbar vertebra above the renal arteries. With a higher injection site the hepatic and splenic arteries may also be demonstrated (2052). Sequence programming and number of films taken is at the instigation of the radiologist varying as to individual preference.

Selective Renal arteriography

Injection into the orifices of selected renal arteries may also be undertaken using a special catheter having a flexible terminal curve. Guidance is under screen control and a confirming preliminary exposure may be made following the injection of a small quantity of the contrast medium.

The first film is exposed during the injection to show the arterial phase—the cassette removed and replaced—and a second exposure taken to show the nephrogram (2053,2054a,b.)

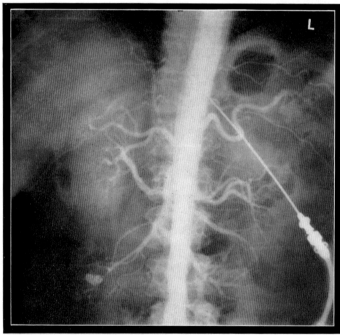

2051

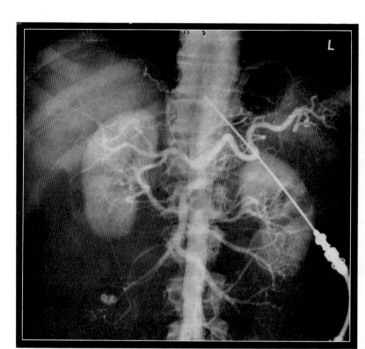

2052

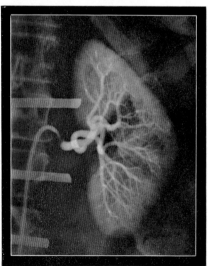

2053

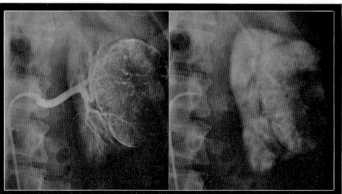

2054a   2054b

Tomographic application

In the single film the arterial pattern will show frequent super-imposition of the vascular network. To demonstrate greater clarity of individual artery branches, multisection radiography employing a three screen unit or a five screen unit with 1 cm and 0·5 cm film spacing intervals respectively will identify the arteries at their own respective levels. In the renal angiogram (2055) the proximal renal arteries are obscured towards their junction with the aorta but are shown in the tomoangiogram (2056).

Film (2056) is the mid-film of a five screen unit series with the fulcrum set at 11 cm.

Exposure conditions

80 kV, 100 mA, 1 second, 40″ FFD, Rapid R film, 90 second processing.

Percutaneous splenography

The X-ray examination of the portal system following direct injection of contrast medium into the spleen to determine the patency of the portal vein and the demonstration of the intra-hepatic venous network. The procedure follows local anaes-thesia and sedation of the patient.

With the patient in the supine position the spleen is punctured at the level of the 10th rib in the mid axillary line. A control film may be taken after injection of a small quantity of contrast medium to determine and confirm the position of the needle. If satisfactory 20 ml of opaque medium is rapidly injected, the needle is then withdrawn. If a serial changer is in use a typical sequence would be one film per second for ten seconds followed by six films at two second intervals.

The results are reviewed following immediate processing to contradict or otherwise, whether a further injection and suc-cession of films are required (2057).

Portal venography (Portophlebography)

With the patient supine and under general anaesthetic, the injection needle is inserted at the level of the eighth to ninth intercostal space and directed upward by 45 degrees into the splenic vein, 20–30 ml of contrast medium is injected slowly and films are exposed at from 1 to 2 seconds after commencement of the injection followed by further films at minute intervals.

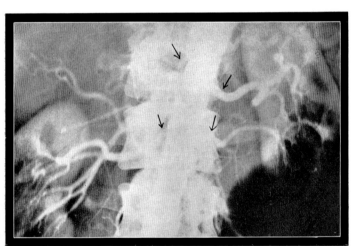

2055

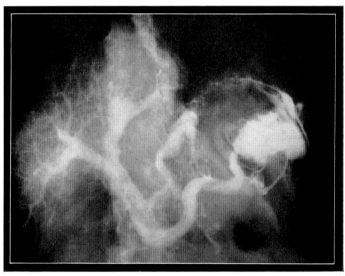

2057

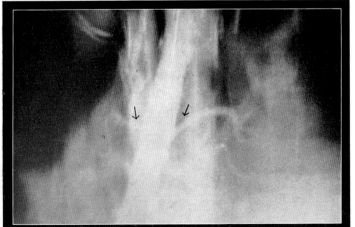

2056

24 Peripheral angiography

As the technique differs for the arterial and the venous part of the circulatory system for the limbs, it is given under the headings arteriography and venography, as applied chiefly to the lower limb.

Arteriography

Arteriography of the lower limb may be a specific examination following injection into the femoral artery for the one limb, or it may be a continuation examination following the injection for abdominal aortography for both limbs. The examination extends from the hip to the ankle. When the injection is into the femoral artery, 20 millilitres of Hypaque 45 per cent., or Conray 280, or Urografin 45 per cent., are injected in from 3–5 seconds.

Scanography method

The tube is fitted with a slit diaphragm having a rectangular aperture one sixteenth of an inch wide. The diaphragm is placed with this narrow slit transverse to the limb and to the direction of the movement and at 40 inch FFD provides a $\frac{1}{2}$ inch film coverage. The density from thigh to ankle can be adjusted during continued exposure by moving the tube slowly over the limb but at different speeds. Over a total 8 seconds exposure interval, 5 seconds are required for the tube movement from hip to knee and 3 seconds from knee to ankle.

The examination may be carried out under general or local anaesthesia. The patient is placed supine on the table with the limb over a 40 × 12 inch cassette which will include the whole of an adult limb. The foot is rotated outwards and immobilized. Following the injection of approximately 10 millilitres of the opaque media the exposure is commenced. Lateral views also may be taken following a further injection.

Alternatively with a moving table-top, where there is sufficient longitudinal table-top excursion, the tube can be centred stationary midway between the hips and the table-top moved at the above rate towards the tube.

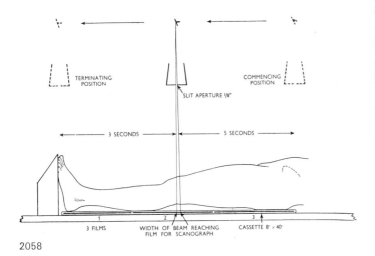

2058

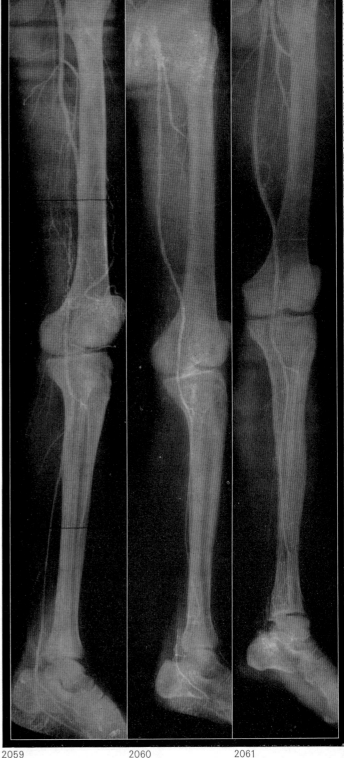

2059   2060   2061

Scanography: Note—Where the long single film is not available, three films can be placed end to end in the cassette (2058).

The depth of the slit should be at least its width to avoid impaired definition due to penumbra.

Additional methods involve the use of separate film exposure and range from,

(a) The simple film changer operated by hand coupled to the moving tube column.

(b) The rapid serial changer used in conjunction with a movable table top, or

(c) a designed changer in the style of the unit described for abdominal and peripheral angiography (2042).

When the appropriate film coverage has been decided the relative film positions can be noted at floor or table top level whichever system is in use practical team work is essential to ensure smooth operation.

With the separate film method the density from thigh to ankle can be suited to the part by,

(a) adjusting the exposure conditions,

(b) by using screens of differing speeds, or

(c) by a balance of screen and non-screen film.

The number of films taken should ensure ample overlap to provide the continuity of information required (2063).

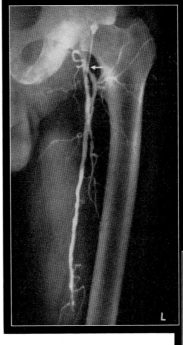

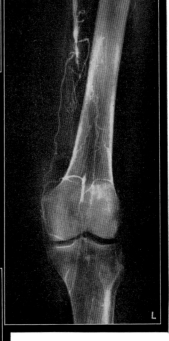

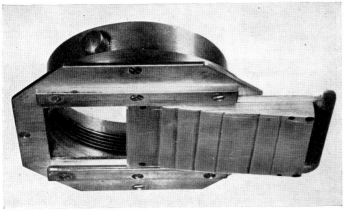

2062

2063

To complete the radiographic appearances of the circulatory system for the lower limb, (2064) shows a positive reproduction of a post-mortem specimen of the foot and ankle in which the blood vessels have been injected to permeate the finest peripheral vessels. A positive impression replaces the current negative impression.

Brachial arteriography

This examination is generally carried out under general anaesthesia. 20–30 millilitres of the opaque media are rapidly injected into the brachial or the subclavian artery.

The film changer method providing rapid sequence separate films, or the "scan" method over a 5 second interval using a single large film are applicable.

Brachial angiograms of the hand and wrist showing the arterial phase in (2065a) and the venous phase in (2065b) are reported as a venous angioma of the hypothenar eminence.

Recently macroradiographic results have proved sufficiently informative compared with contact results to justify its application in angiography. In the examination for congenital heart disease in children the 0.3 mm foci has sufficient load capacity to produce up to ×2 enlargement. Chest and abdominal angiograms can be taken of the adult at a ×1½ enlargement using the 0.6 mm focus. In both instances the "air gap", technique replaces the grid in elliminating scatter. This can be complemented by selective filtration in the form of sheet tin or a lead screen placed on top of the cassette.

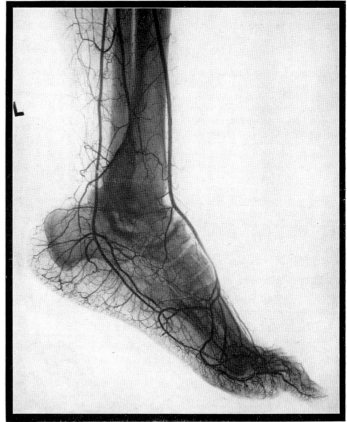

2064

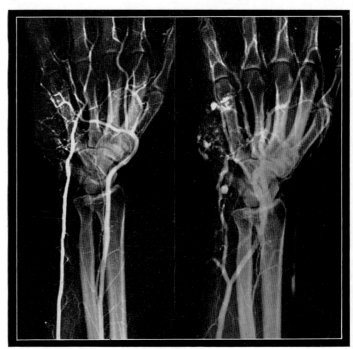

2065a   2065b

Venography

Ascending venography of the lower limbs is undertaken in the investigation to determine the patency of the deep veins, the competence of the valves, and the site of incompetent veins. Generally, the examination is carried out under local anaesthesia and the progress of the contrast medium watched under screening control.

The opaque medium may be Hypaque 45%, or Conray 280, and 30–50 millilitres is injected through a small incision made over a superficial vein on the dorsum of the foot. A previous test of the patient to the opaque media having been undertaken to determine their sensitivity.

The patient is supine, generally with the table tilted 15° downward to the foot and the limb to be examined is rotated slightly outwards. To occlude the superficial veins, compression is applied just above the ankle and on occasion just below the knee.

Under normal conditions, the valves are open, but the application of valsalva manoeuvre ensures that the function of the venous valves are included. This produces a reversal of the direction of the flow of the blood which closes the valve and when the vessels are full of opaque medium the valves become visible on the radiograph.

Valsalva manoeuvre

To this end, practised instruction to the patient, to close the lips and hold the nose during forcible expiration is essential. This procedure is adopted prior to each exposure during the sequence. Timing of the film sequence is at the discretion of the radiologist but generally one or more A.P. films of the lower leg are taken 5–10 seconds after the injection and of the upper thigh film approximately 15–20 seconds later.

Following rapid processing of the above films, a decision may be made to take lateral films and these may be obtained with the patient turned into the lateral position by the same method, following a further injection of 30 millilitres of the contrast medium.

(2066) shows a venal block with collateral circulation and (2067) shows the same subject with the vein repaired, using an arterial graft.

Radiograph (2068) shows the effect of using the Valsalva manoeuvre as compared with (2069) in which no attempt has been made to show the valves.

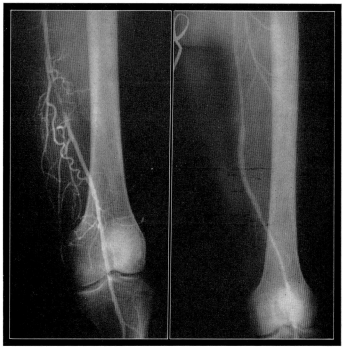

2066   2067

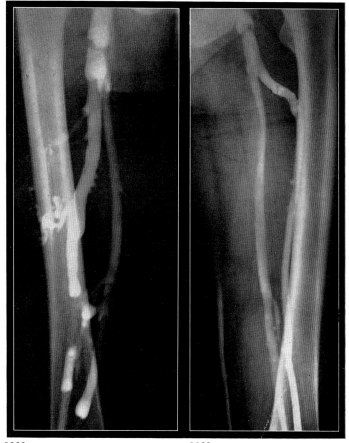

2068   2069

Antero-posterior and lateral radiographs (2070) have been taken with the Valsalva manoeuvre and reported as normal.

Two radiographs, antero-posterior and lateral (2071), are reported as showing an incompetent vein.

With the dorsal foot vein injection poor opacification of the iliac veins is often obtained due to reduced opacification by dilution. When information is sought in this region, generally femoral or at times popliteal vein injection may replace the lower injection site. Films are taken at 1 second intervals and terminated at 5 seconds or at the discretion of the radiologist.

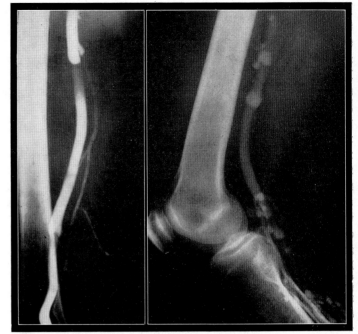

2070

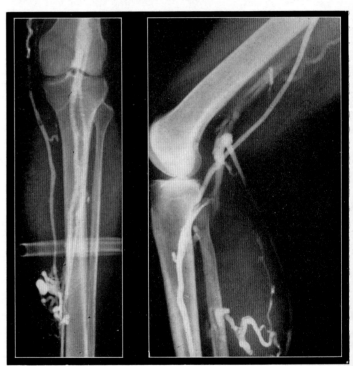

2071

Lymphangiography

Anatomical features

The lymphatic system is closely related to the vascular system; it consists of a network of fine capillary-like lymphatic vessels which commence in the tissue spaces and merge to form larger vessels in both the superficial and deep tissues. Along the course of the lymphatic vessels are localized groups of lymph nodes (or glands). The clear lymph fluid flows through one or more lymph nodes where much of the fluid is reabsorbed. The residual lymph leaves the nodes via the efferent vessels which unit to form the lymph trunks, finally reaching the thoracic duct and the right lymphatic duct. The lymph is returned from the ducts to the venous circulation.

The investigation of the lymphatic system by the injection of an opaque medium into the lymphatic vessels (lymphangiography) or directly into a lymph node, enables pathological conditions of the vessels or of the glands to be demonstrated and in association with radiation therapy provides a record of changing conditions in relation to treatment.

Injection procedures

Lower limb

The patient lies supine on the X-ray table, 2 millilitres of a 10 per cent. aqueous solution of methylene blue is injected subcutaneously into the web between the first and second toes. This is rapidly taken up by the lymphatics, and subcutaneous lymphatics can be seen outlined in blue on the dorsum of the foot. Under local anaesthesia a small transverse incision is made to expose a lymphatic vessel. The tip of a fine needle is inserted into the lymphatic and the needle is strapped to the skin. An injection of up to 10 millilitres of Lipiodol Ultra Fluid (iodized oil) at body temperature, is given with controlled pressure at a very slow rate, through a fine polythene catheter connecting the needle to the syringe, films are taken as required over several hours.

The same procedure is followed to give information regarding the lymphatics in the pelvis and abdomen, with films taken up to 24 hours.

An alternative procedure follows the initial outlining of the lymphatics as previously, by injecting methylene blue dye into the web of the toes and following an interval of approximately fifteen minutes an outlined lymphatic vessel in the groin is exposed and the contrast medium injected directly, films are taken up to 24 hours.

Lymphangiograms of a normal lower limb of two subjects (2072), were exposed each with two 6 × 15 inch films placed end to end in a long cassette, employing the wedge filter, (2062); (2300) was reported as a grossly abnormal condition.

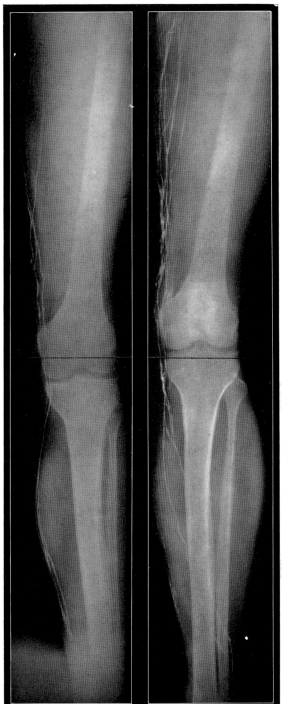

2072

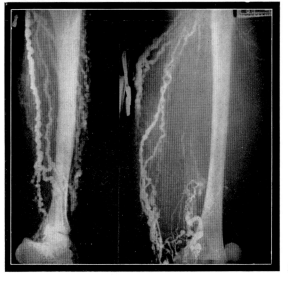

601

2073

Radiographic sequence

On the day of the injection, in addition to the lower limb a well penetrated postero-anterior of the chest is taken, both femora, the abdomen to include the upper femora, and the lateral lumbar region to include two inches in front of the vertebral bodies. On the day after the injection, the exposures are repeated for the chest, abdomen and lumbar spine with in addition oblique projections of the pelvis.

Upper limb

A similar technique to that described for the lower limb is performed on the upper limb, the incision being made in the axilla after injection of the due in the web of the fingers, 5 millilitres of Lipiodol Ultra Fluid is sufficient for the injection of the upper arm. This, however, is a less frequent examination.

Opacified lumbar lymph nodes are shown in (2074a) and pelvic and inguinal nodes in (2074b).

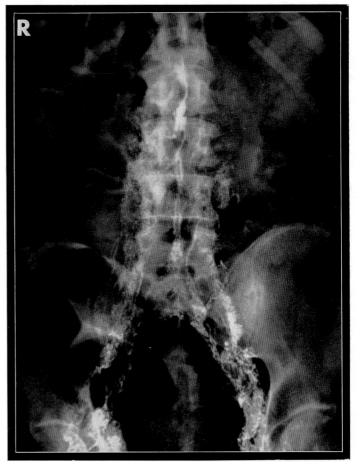

2074a

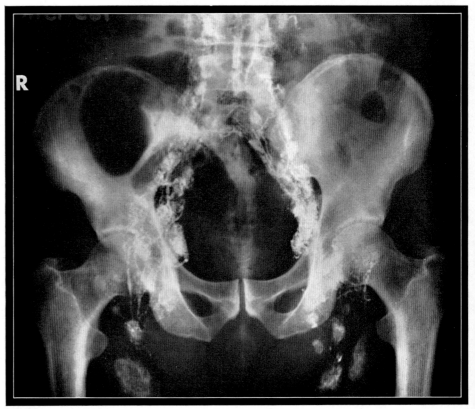

2074b

25

SOFT TISSUE

25 SECTION 25

SOFT TISSUE

As in many of the foregoing sections some reference is made to soft tissue technique, this section is intended to include only such conditions as have not been previously discussed.

Although 'soft tissue' could be applied to all body structures other than bone, the term, as generally understood, implies the superficial tissues of the limbs and trunk requiring differential exposure technique to enable these low density, low contrast tissues, with any changes therein, to be visualized. Included in this section is a review of Mammography Technique.

Sometimes, as shown on page 618, a contrast medium is used to indicate the direction of a fistulous tract (2123) or to outline a cavity in the soft tissues (2121,2122).

Mammary Glands

Mammography
The technique of recording maximum soft tissue differentiation within the mammary glands with the subsequent visualization of tumour tissue if present.

Shape, Size and Age
The profile of a breast lying against the pectoral muscle is shown in 2075. The ovoid shape of the breast provides an extensive range of densities from the base to the periphery.

There are also differences in size and density of the normal breast due to parity (the condition of a woman with respect to her having borne children).

Whereas parity and increasing age from 40 (2076b) years tends to promote changes in the glandular tissues and replacement by fat which requires less exposure, the breast tissue of a young person without children is denser and requires more exposure (2076a).

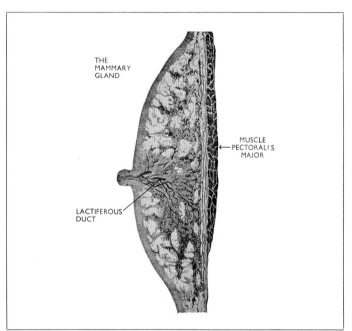

2075

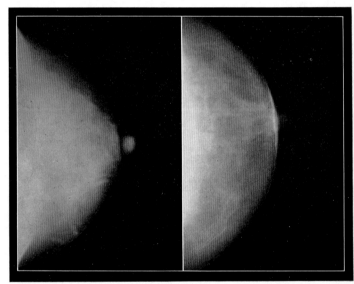

2076a   2076b

The situation arises therefore that due to shape and contour, we have a condition of steep overall subject contrast, with low inherent contrast of the internal soft tissue structures of the breast.

The need therefore to provide sufficient intimate contrast to record pathological changes in the internal soft tissue structures is extremely critical, coupled with the fact of recording the steep overall subject contrast at a suitable density.

Efforts to diagnose the conditions at a much earlier stage have led to limited mass X-ray examinations of the mammary glands in presumably normal subjects. Initially, it was essential to know how much could be shown of the changes taking place at various stages in abnormal conditions of the breast, and the earliest stage at which the conditions could be diagnosed by radiology.

From the evidence of intensive investigation a routine procedure of X-ray examination has been devised for positioning, exposure conditions and materials used, to provide the most satisfactory diagnostic evidence. Both breasts are X-rayed for comparison.

The right and left breasts are exposed in the lateral and craniocaudal (superior-inferior) positions (2077).

The result demonstrates normal breast tissue.

As the illustrated radiographs demonstrate, accurate marking of the result is imperative to determine side and site. As a check against movement blurr a lead pellet may be attached to the breast itself, and for an abnormal condition requiring further examination, small lead pellets may be placed on the skin surface in relation to the lesion to identify its position in each projection.

Radiographs (2078) compare normal and abnormal conditions respectively, (2079) being reported as a carcinoma.

It should be noted that although a condition related to women, occasionally male subjects develop carcinoma of the breast.

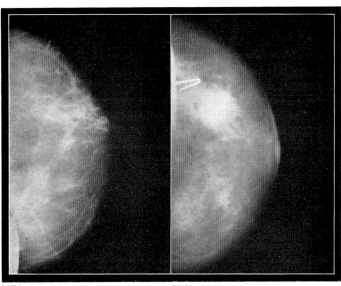

2078   2079

2077

Positioning

Routinely the most suitable projections are from the cranial caudal and medial lateral aspects, with follow up additional projections as necessary when an abnormal condition has been disclosed. Specialized isocentric movement X-ray units have been devised for convenience to the patient in obtaining the respective positions. These units also utilize an X-ray tube incorporating a molybdenum target, which at the low kV in use provides an emission most suited to provide soft tissue contrast and detail.

In the absence of such a specialized unit adaptations have to be provided. Although the lateral view can be taken in the seated erect position, it is the reclining posture that has been favoured and use is made of the full length couch (2082). A variable height platform is required to support the breast with the patient erect or sitting for the cranial caudal projection (2080a,b). A long localizing cone flattened on one side at the aperture enables the cone to be brought into contact with the breast with the flattened side against the chest wall.

It is important in placing the breast position to avoid puckering or creasing the skin surface which could appear as an added confusing density in the radiograph. In each position the nipple should be in profile.

Further information may be obtained with the patient in the prone position, from a radiograph taken with horizontal projection of the pendant breast, particularly when the breast is immersed in fluid, such as mineral oil, to obtain uniform density.

There appears to be difference in opinion as to whether or not compression of the breast should be advocated and the radiographer is advised to follow the radiologist's ruling with regard to this.

Superior-inferior

With the patient sitting or standing each breast in turn rests on the film placed on a table support which can be raised or lowered to suit each patient. The nipple is in profile. The patient presses forward against the film with the head turned away from the localizing cone. The cone is flattened on the lung aspect and is lead lined, thus serving to restrict the beam to the mammary area and protecting the near-by lung tissue (2080a,b, 2081).

A 14 inch—35 cm. focus–film distance is shown in (2080a), and 20 inches—50 cm. in (2080b).

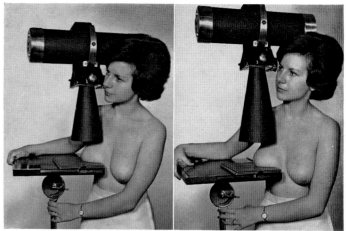

2080a   2080b

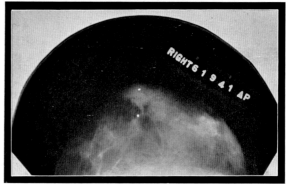

2081

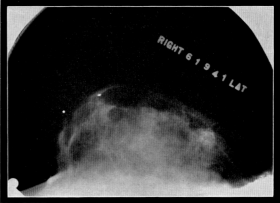

2083

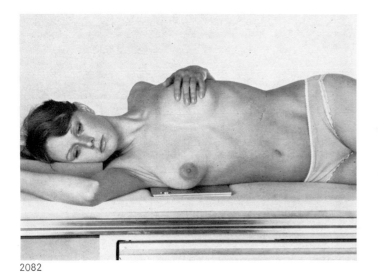

2082

Medio-lateral

With the patient lying on each side in turn, the hand on that side is abducted and placed under the head, the film is supported on a foam pad and placed under the breast. A slight backward tilt of the patient may be required to bring the breast into the lateral position with the nipple in profile, this also assists in separation of the breasts. With pendulous breast subject it may be necessary to ask the patient to withdraw the other breast from the vicinity of the cone (2082, 2083).

NOTE—On occasion the latero-medial projection may be preferred.

Axilla

This may be taken in the sitting, erect or horizontal position. The patient is rotated 30 degrees to the affected side to allow the breast to recline away from the chest wall, with the humerus abducted at least 90 degrees to avoid superimposition of the scapula over the axillary region. The film should include both the axilla and breast.

■ Centre 5 cm. below the axilla, both sides should be taken for comparison (2084, 2085).

NOTE—For the direct exposures to the breast the conventional 2 millimetre aluminium filter is removed, but replaced for the projection through the axilla.

On disclosing an abnormality at the initial survey, further investigation may include tangential projection (2086) from each aspect of the breast.

The site of the lesion is identified by small lead pellets attached to the skin surface (2086, 2087).

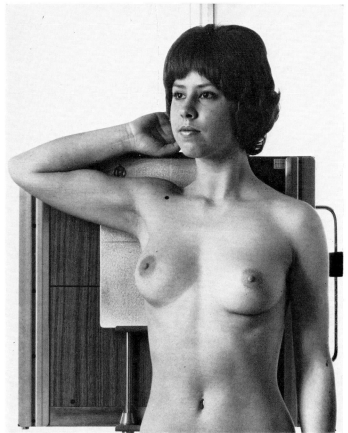
2084

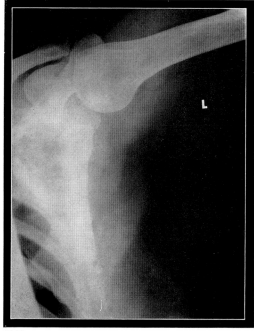
2085

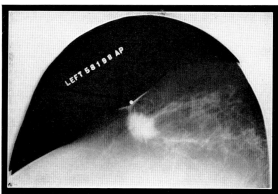
2086

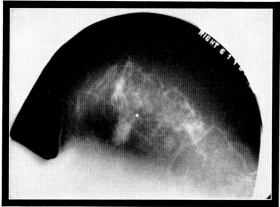
2087

Exposure technique

The recording technique to show minute detail in the soft tissue of the glands down to the dimension of pathological particle size in keeping with the smallest available foci spot has been a matter of considerable investigation. The system should provide—

(1) Minimal conditions of unsharpness.
(2) Suitable conditions of exposure.
(3) Low grain.
(4) High amplification of subject contrast.

An appreciation of the radiation hazards must also be taken into account.

Types of Film Available

An extensive range of non-screen film is available of increasing speed, with approximately a ×10 difference in speed between the slowest (in use for gamma radiography) and the conventional speed medical non-screen type of film.

The relative grain size of the faster material is approximately ×2 that of the slower film.

High gamma can be obtained with suitable development on all films, and the existing contrast difference within the range is marginal.

These films have a high DMAX and as a consequence their recording ability is compatible with reproducing the steepest subject differences with progressive contrast.

Relative Exposure Requirements:

Slow speed film: 2000 mAs:
Intermediate non-screen film: 500 mAs:
Conventional Medical non-screen film: 200 mAs.

Apparatus

Specially designed equipment and X-ray tubes are now available for this technique. Standard equipment however can be modified so that the transformer is regulated to provide low kilovoltage in the region of 20 to 40 kVp.

For direct exposure to the breast, only the inherent filtration of the tube is in use, all additional filtration being removed to improve contrast.

Technical Approach

The use of the finest focal spot size available is imperative, compatible with the loading required for the examination. Kilovoltage in the region of 20–40 kVp in conjunction with the high contrast film suitably processed provides the maximum soft tissue differentiation, choice of film speed is dependent on the available output and the consideration given to the patient dosage factor. Focus–film distances are in the region of 14–20 inches.

Immobilization

The posture of the patient should be as comfortable and relaxed as possible in view of the duration of exposure time, so that full co-operation in avoiding subject movement is obtained.

Radiation Protection

Protection of the gonads particularly in the cranial caudal projections is essential.

Single Film Technique

This should be backed with sheet lead or lead rubber during exposure. Adequate exposure should be given to ensure that the internal soft tissue structures are recorded where the film responds with progressive contrast. (An appropriate density range to ensure this is between D 0.7–D 1.4, the peripheral structures are then recorded at a density level between D 1.8–D 3.5.) Alternatively, automatic conditions of exposure control is now available to ensure this.

Conventional viewing conditions are suitable for viewing the lower subject density range but higher intensity (photoflood) viewing is essential to visualize the contrast change of the higher density range (2088).

Double or Tri-pack Film Units

Double Film Pack: An extension of the multiple radiography principle applied to the use of films of differing speeds. There should be approximately a 4:1 difference in speed between the two films and the faster film of the two should be placed in closest relationship to the tube (with the low kilovoltage, the top film absorbs at least 60% of the incident radiation). Consequently if the films are placed in reverse speed order to this recommendation, this adds considerably to the exposure required and also dosage to the patient (2089a,2089b).

Tri-Pack: There should be a 2:1 speed relationship between the three films with the fastest film in closest approximation to the tube and subsequent decreasing speed downwards.

Both the double and triple packs should be backed by sheet lead or alternatively placed on lead rubber during the exposure.

The above application of the multiple procedure provides for a suitable scale of densities on the alternate films to suit the respective differences in subject contrast.

Due to error in exposure, at least one of the films may contain the necessary information.

The method may also provide greater tolerance to variation from the normal in size, shape and density.

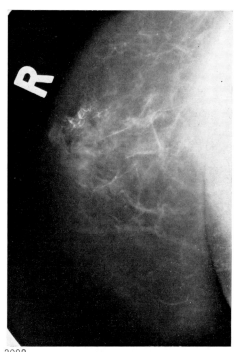

2088

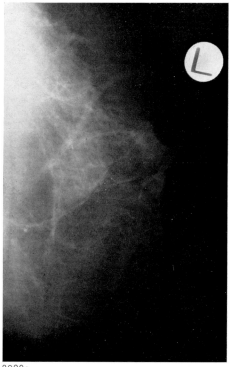

2089a

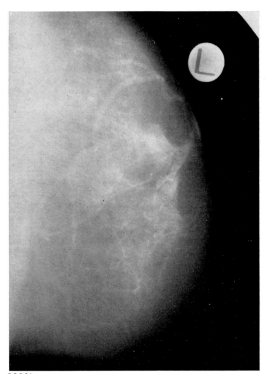

2089b

25 Soft Tissue

The radiographic examination of soft tissues involves the alternatives of demonstrating;

(a) maximum distinction between the low inherent contrast of the soft tissues themselves—or recording

(b) calcification, associated with the soft tissues, or tendons and arteries within the soft tissues, to

(c) where there is invagination of pathology either from the soft tissue to the adjoining bone structure or vice versa.

The study of appropriate kilovoltage, adequate exposure, effective collimation and suitable processing in Mammography technique, has tended to make us more critical in the choice of these features in general soft tissue radiography.

With regard to kilovoltage the choice should be flexible varying from low, to suit low inherent tissue contrast to higher where the inclusion of bone, gas or air extends the range of subject contrast.

Equally important is adequate exposure to ensure that the subject range is recorded with progressive contrast. In soft tissue radiography there is a tendency to underexpose, probably due to associating low tissue density with low film density. Processing should then ensure the clarity and density suited to this subject range. Where however, to obtain maximum emulsion speed, high activity and temperature chemical processing is in vogue, this may not be suited to recording the subtlety of minor changing contrast as would low temperature chemicalization.

Kilovoltage

We should endeavour to relate kilovoltage to the soft tissues themselves, appreciating that the density of these structures will require in the region of 15 kV less than that required for bone structure. However it should be fully appreciated that where the subject increases in its range of opacity a compromised quality may be necessary, in both the bone and associated soft tissue structures.

Kilovoltage should then be increased by approximately 20 kVp to that for the bone structure alone and exposure time reduced to record a density at which the bone and soft tissue structures can be viewed simultaneously.

In regions of greater thickness, e.g. shoulder and hip joint, spine and the soft tissue of the abdomen, multiple radiography adopting the two-film steep range technique (page 634) is an ideal method of demonstrating a suitable scale of densities for each area. With this method contrast in bone and soft tissue is superior, in that kilovoltage need not be increased beyond that required for bone structure.

Unusual Projections

It will be understood that there will be many diversions from routine projections for soft tissue work, considerable use being made of the profile view of the lesion. An example is shown for the post-traumatic calcification over the scapula in (2090), for which the patient was rotated to enable the protrusion to be shown in profile away from the posterior wall of the chest. In this instance, in showing the substance of the calcification, structural details in the adjacent tissues are not shown.

A further example, revealing the complete outline of the small lipoma on the inner thigh, is shown in (2091).

In profile or Skyline projections as above, a non-screen film placed on top of the cassette records complementary information to the screen film within the cassette.

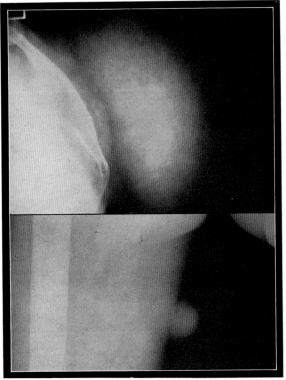

2090 (top)   2091 (above)

Conditions Pertaining to Soft Tissue
Adenoids

Two films exposed from the lateral aspect of the upper pharynx show (2092a) the soft tissue structure of enlarged adenoids encroaching upon the nasal pharynx, and after (2092b) an operation for removal of the adenoids. The lateral position of the head and neck is assumed with the chin slightly raised.

■ Centre 2 inches (5cm) above the angle of the jaw

Positive reproductions replace the negative illustrations generally shown.

Aneurysm, arteriovenous (2093) of hand showing soft structure swelling.

Cyst, a tumour containing fluid or solid substance, which in the latter state, depending on the region concerned, may be visible on a soft tissue radiograph. Calcification in the wall of a cyst renders it opaque to X-rays, presenting an annular appearance as shown in the two projections of the neck (2094).

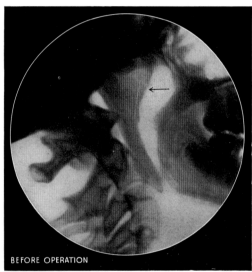

BEFORE OPERATION

2092a

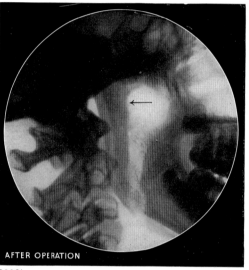

AFTER OPERATION

2092b

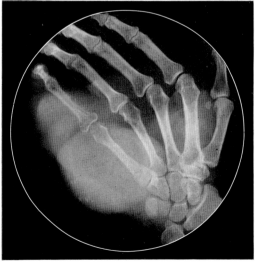

2093

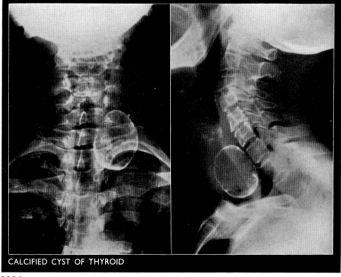

CALCIFIED CYST OF THYROID

2094

Emphysema, air in the tissues following an injection, and gas gangerene, a serious condition following a projectile wound, show as numerous dark striated shadows in the tissues. It is most important to include the whole outline of the region in the radiograph, as in (2095) of a child. An example of surgical emphysema of the chest wall is shown in (2096a) and of trauma (2096b). An example in the lower limb, query emphysema or gas gangrene is shown in (2097). Haematoma, which, if the blood is not absorbed, later calcifies and thus becomes visible in the tissues (2098).

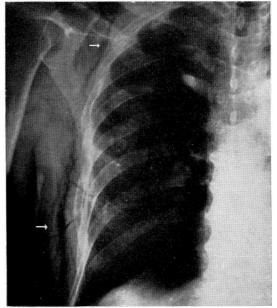

2096a

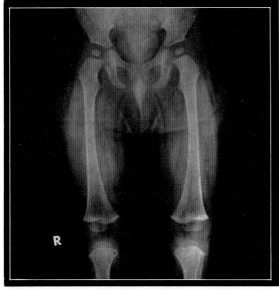

2095

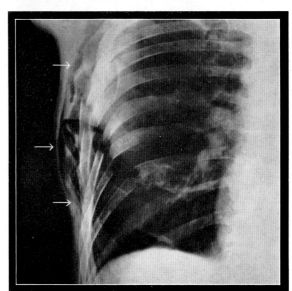

2096b

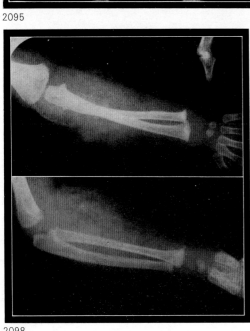

2098

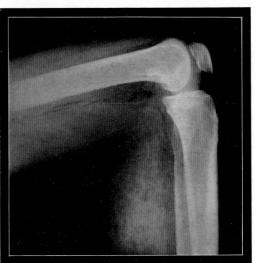

2097

Lipoma, a fatty tumour which is more transradiant than the other tissues and which appears, therefore, as a dark shadow on the radiograph as shown in the upper arm (2099). Shown in profile, the appearances are rather different in the protrusions from the lateral chest wall (2100), and scapula (2102) and on the inner thigh in (2103).

Loss of soft tissue mass in any appreciable degree appears as a darker shadow in the tissues, as shown in the lower arm (2101).

NOTE—In soft tissue X-ray examinations the presence of skin lesions such as warts, moles, cysts, etc., should be recorded for the information of the radiologist; as due to the lower range of kilovoltage in use these may be recorded and confuse the diagnosis.

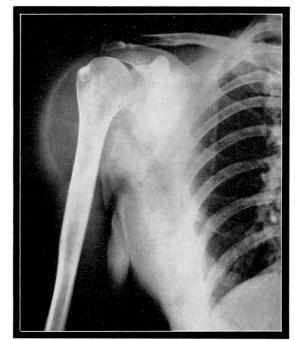

2099

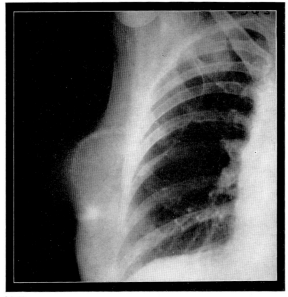

2100

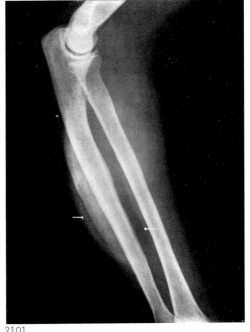

2101

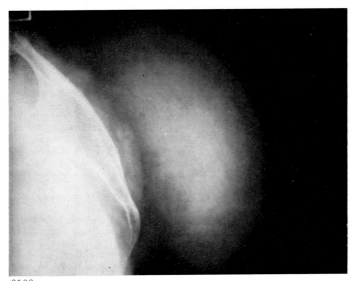

2102

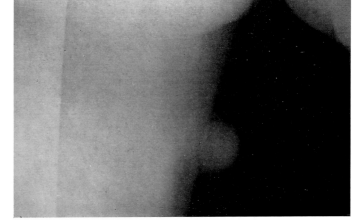

2103

Calcification in Soft Tissues
The Arteries

When the walls of the arteries become visible due to calcification, an examination of the limbs should include films to cover the course of the arteries concerned from their main trunk origin to distal extremity. A reduction in either kilovoltage or exposure time being made to obtain the required quality to show the calcification. The series should include:

(a) A general film of the pelvis using the grid.

(b) Right and left thigh and upper limb area taken with the grid.

Thereafter lateral projections generally suffice and are to be preferred.

(c) Right and left lateral lower limb to include the foot (taken without the grid).

Illustrations (2104, 2105, 2106) indicate the presence of calcified arteries in pelvis, leg and ankle.

Phleboliths, are clots or thrombi in the veins which have become calcified, forming small, round or oval shadows (2107).

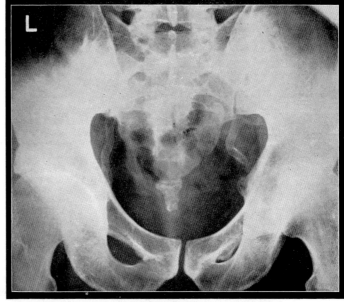

2104

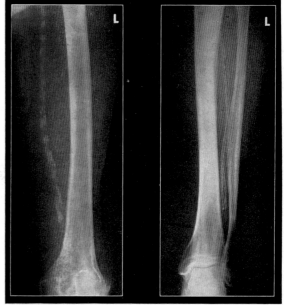

2105

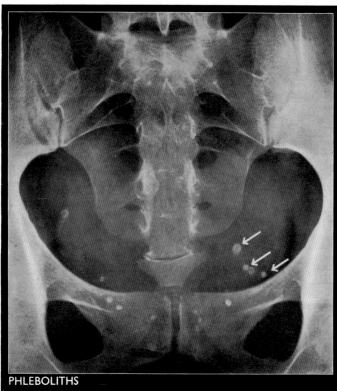

PHLEBOLITHS

2107

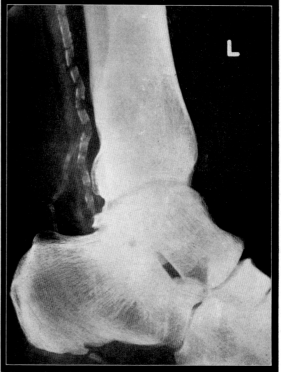

2106

Calcification in Soft Tissue
General Procedure

In a condition such as cysticercosis the patient is X-rayed extensively but only one projection each of limbs, trunk and head is included in the examination (2108, 2109, 2110).

Where the patient is examined at intervals throughout the period of treatment or observation there should be no variation whatsoever in exposure and processing, in order that true comparison may be possible from one examination to another.

Calcification due to trauma (2111) in relation to a shoulder joint dislocation. Calcification of tendon to bone attachments.

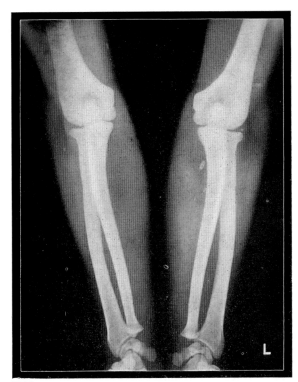

2108

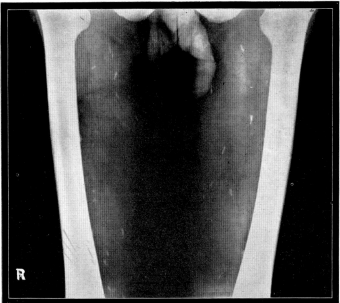

2109

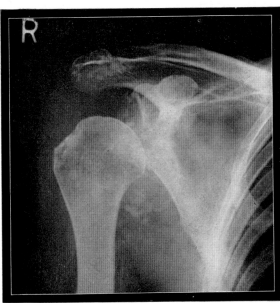

2111

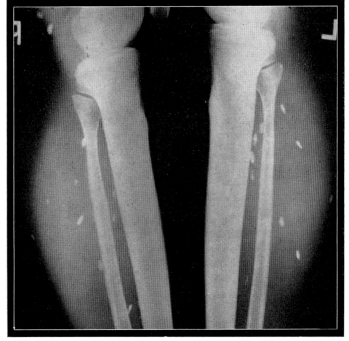

2110

Myositis ossificans, the formation of bone in the muscles as shown in the upper arm (2114) and in the shoulder (2112); as a local condition it occurs at the site of pressure or repeated trauma (2113) and in the region of fractures and dislocations. There is also a generalized condition, but this is very rare. Bone may also be formed in operation scars, especially of the abdominal walls. Neurofibromas and other soft tissue tumours may cast a shadow, or reveal their presence by the deformity of the skin surface outline, or by the displacement or deformity of adjacent normal soft tissue structures.

For a plastic replacement of bone as shown in the upper arm in (2115), soft tissue technique is again essential to give all possible information to the surgeon.

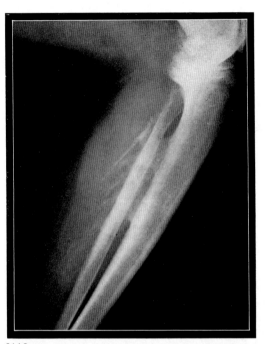

2113

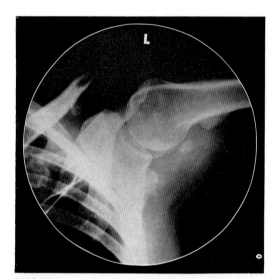

2112

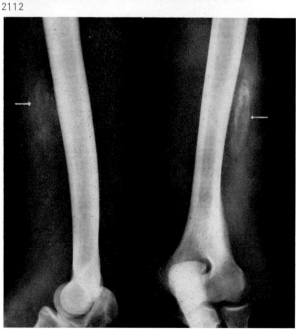

2114

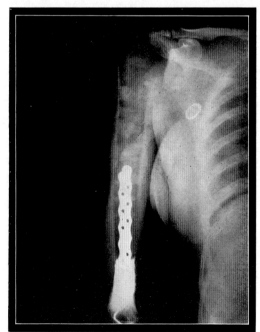

2115

Bone and Soft Tissue Involvement

Rheumatoid arthritis (2116) and gout (2117,2118), in which there is considerable involvement of the soft tissues around the joints, are examples of the essential demonstration of both bone and soft structures. An enlargement of an interphalangeal joint shows in detail the structures involved (2118).

Sequestrum (2119), detachment of a small fragment of bone due to pathological conditions, the position of which must be identified.

Ulcer, tropical, a disease of the tropics occurring in the native population and affecting bone and soft tissues, chiefly of the lower limb.

Yaws (2120), also a disease of the tropics occurring in the native population, affecting the hands and feet, long bones and adjacent soft tissues to skin surface.

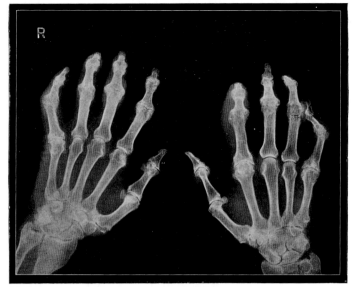

2116

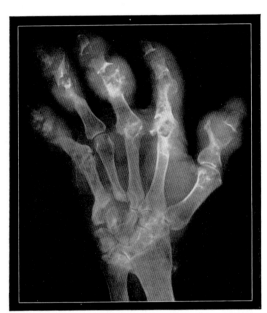

2117

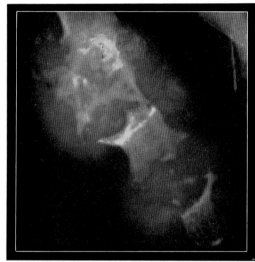

2118

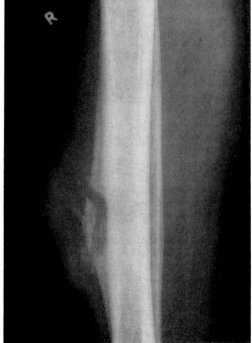

2119

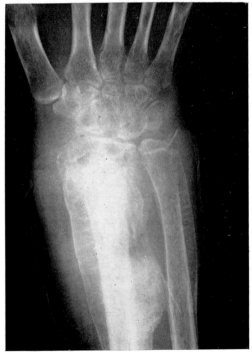

2120

Injection of Iodized Oil

It is sometimes necessary to make radiographic examination following an injection of iodized oil into sinuses and fistulous tracts in the soft tissues leading to cavities or bone lesions. As previously discussed, the success of these examinations depends on the technique of injection, it being essential that the films should be exposed while pressure on the syringe is maintained (2121).

When conditions are suitable, exposures are made from both antero-posterior and lateral aspects of the limb and may sometimes be stereoscopic. The position of the skin exits of such sinuses may be shown on the films by small metal rings placed on the skin surface. A radiograph of the hip joint shows the appearance after injection of iodized oil with sinus exit rings in position (2122), stereographs in this case being of considerable value.

Thyro-Glossal Fistula

A cannula is inserted into the tract at the skin opening of the fistula which, in the case illustrated (2123), is at the crico-thyroid level. 3 to 7 millilitres of iodized oil are injected at blood heat, pressure being maintained on the syringe during the exposure, which is made from the lateral aspect of the neck. The arrow indicates the position of the fistulous tract. Soft tissue technique is employed.

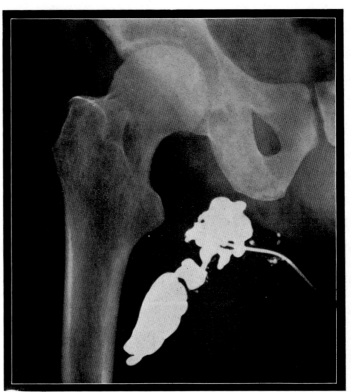

2121

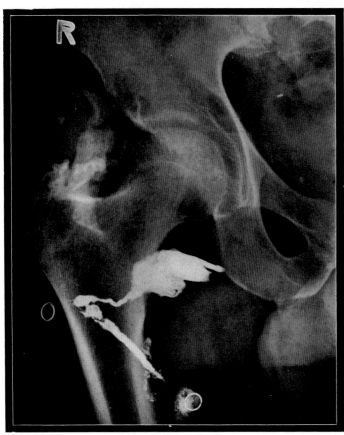

2122

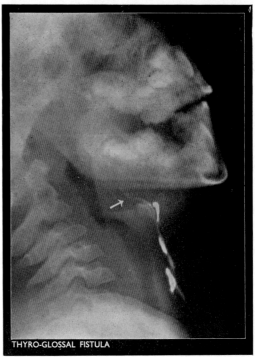

THYRO-GLOSSAL FISTULA

2123

26

MACRORADIOGRAPHY

MACRORADIOGRAPHY

Macroradiography is a method whereby direct enlargement of the image is obtained by interposing the subject between the X-ray tube and film at such a distance that the continued divergence of the beam produces the required degree of magnification. The relationship of the focus–film distance to the focus–object distance determines the magnification factor, and can be obtained if necessary by the simple geometric formula:

$$M = \frac{D}{d} = \frac{\text{focus–film distance}}{\text{focus–object distance}}$$

Alternatively knowing the desired magnification the focus–object distance is acquired from the following:

$$\text{Focus–object distance} = \frac{\text{FFD} \times 1}{M} = \frac{36 \times 1}{1 \cdot 5} = 24''$$

Subject–film displacement = 12″.

In estimating distance relationship between subject, tube and film the level of a known lesion or the mid-thickness level of the subject should be the reference plane rather than the table-top, or vertical chest support in the erect position.

The procedure is advantageous in resolving fine particle detail of bone structure and minimal lesions and subsequently projecting them up to a size they can be more readily perceived.

With the subject displacement involved it is essential that small foci in the region of 0·3 mm² or 0·6 mm² are available to offset the increasing geometric unsharpness. With the 0·6 mm², enlargement with acceptable definition can be obtained up to ×1·5; with the 0·3 mm² dimension ×2 enlargement is practical, beyond this the unsharpness of the image becomes progressively unacceptable.

For the smaller regions non-screen film is recommended and enlargement up to ×2 with acceptable definition is practical. As the subject thickness increases the use of intensifying screens will be necessary and the type used will also influence optimum enlargement. With High Definition screens this will be ×1·5, and Fast Tungstate screens ×2.

The feature that screen grain is a constant factor irrespective of the degree of enlargement permits extensive use of the fast type screen to complement the restricted rating of the small foci.

With a focal spot as small as 0·3 mm output is obviously restricted and the tube rating chart should be carefully examined to appreciate the limitation and duration of exposure time thus imposed. The greater loading opacity of the 0·6 mm² foci is an obvious advantage particularly for the extension of this technique into heavier regions (e.g. angiography) provided the enlargement is restricted to ×1·5 times.

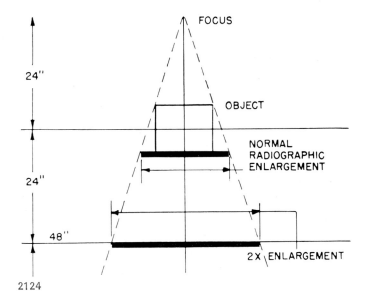

2124

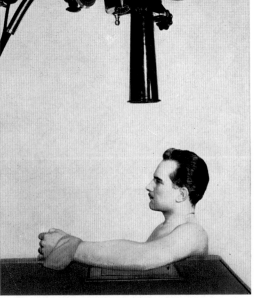

2125

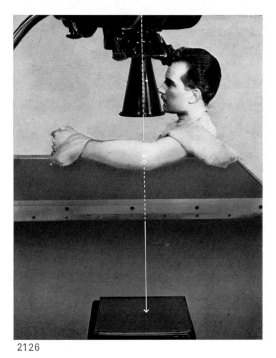

2126

Complete immobilization with precise collimation of the part is essential, as is accuracy in centring, and alignment of focus, subject and film. Specialized equipment is available but adaptation to existing circumstances to provide for subject–film alignment; (transparent window) and platform cassette support, at the required under-table distance for the usual ×1½ and ×2 enlargement is well within the ingenuity of the radiographer.

The use of the grid and the added exposure required may make its use prohibitive in macroradiography, and contrast is maintained by precise collimation of the beam, and the fact that within the air-gap distance between subject and film the obliquity of a high proportion of the emerging subject scatter extends outwith the area of the film. With the non-screen subject, contrast is thus higher in the enlargement and increased kilovoltage can be used to reduce exposure time. With non-grid procedure however the selection of kilovoltage should be with a view to providing acceptable contrast within the capability of the air-gap, to limit the effect of scattered radiation (2127).

In macroradiography of the extremities generally the original contact FFD is maintained, for example 30″, and the film is then displaced the necessary distance for the enlargement, below the table. For macroradiography of the skull, vertebral column, abdominal content (angiography) the enlargement may be encompassed within the normal FFD, eg 36″ Focus–film distance × 2 enlargement—subject 18″ from film, × 1·5 enlargement—subject 12″ from film.

With this procedure focus–skin distances are much reduced, as the possibility of excessive radiation to the near skin surface must be constantly in mind, avoiding repeat exposures and ensuring that the conventional 2 mm aluminium filter is at the tube aperture.

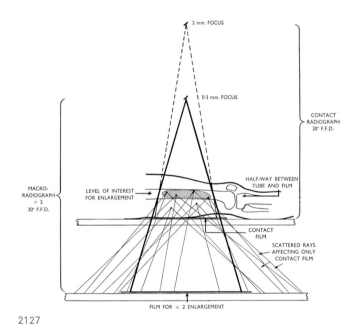

2127

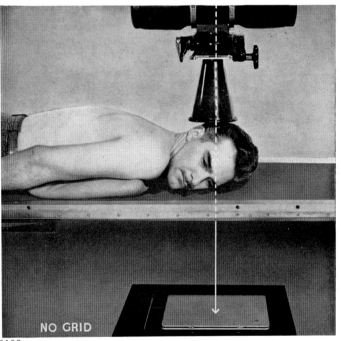

2128

(2129,2130) show a comparison between the conventional contact radiograph of the elbow joint and a ×2 enlargement of the elbow joint. The fine detail and contrast in the bone around the upper part of the screw can be clearly seen in the enlargement.

A selection of various degrees of enlargement of the wrist joint is shown in

Wrist	Elbow
(2131) in contact with the film	(2135a) ×1$\frac{1}{2}$ enlargement
(2132) ×2 enlargement	(2135b) ×1$\frac{1}{2}$ enlargement
(2133) ×1$\frac{1}{2}$ enlargement	
(2134) ×1$\frac{2}{3}$ enlargement	

These radiographs are produced in actual size.

Fifty per cent increase in exposure is required for the enlargement due to the loss of total intensity within the intervening airgap.

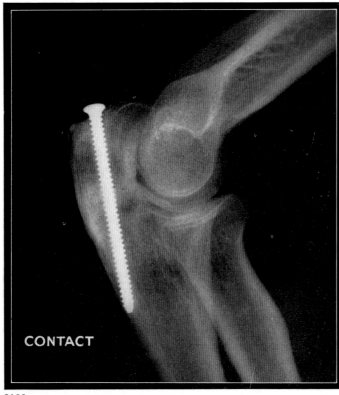

CONTACT

2129

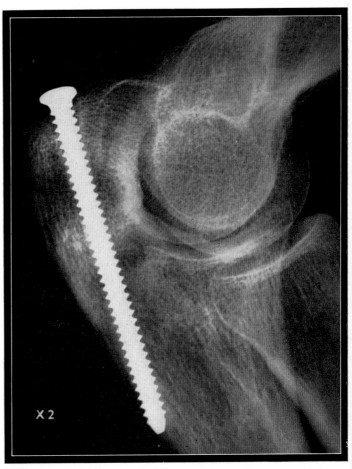

×2

2130

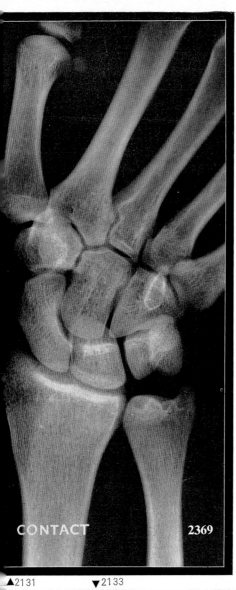

CONTACT   2369

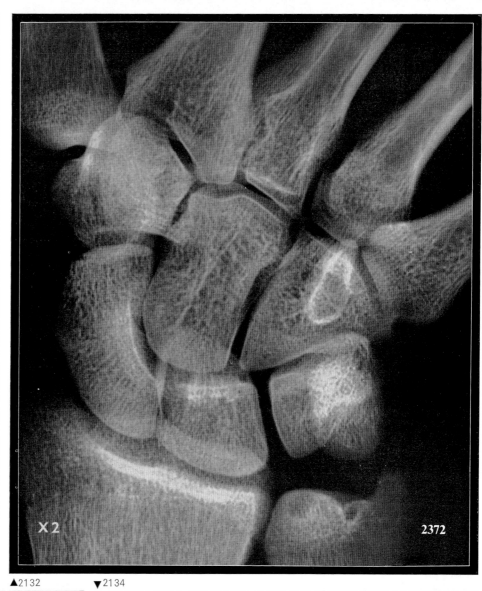

X 2   2372

▲2131   ▼2133   ▲2132   ▼2134

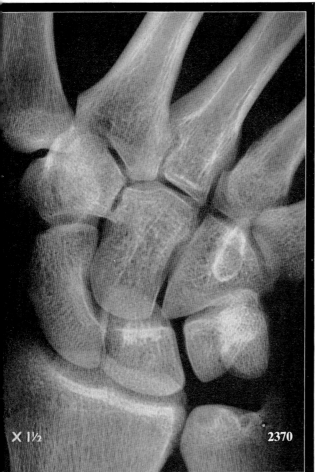

X 1½   2370

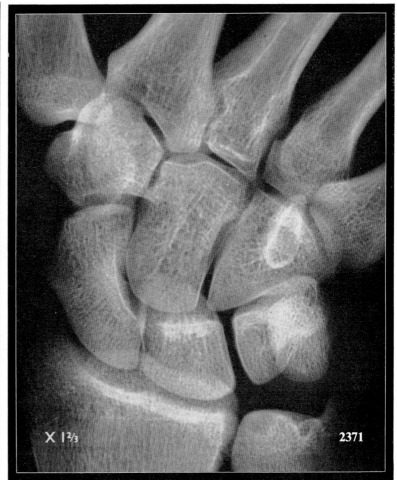

X 1⅔   2371

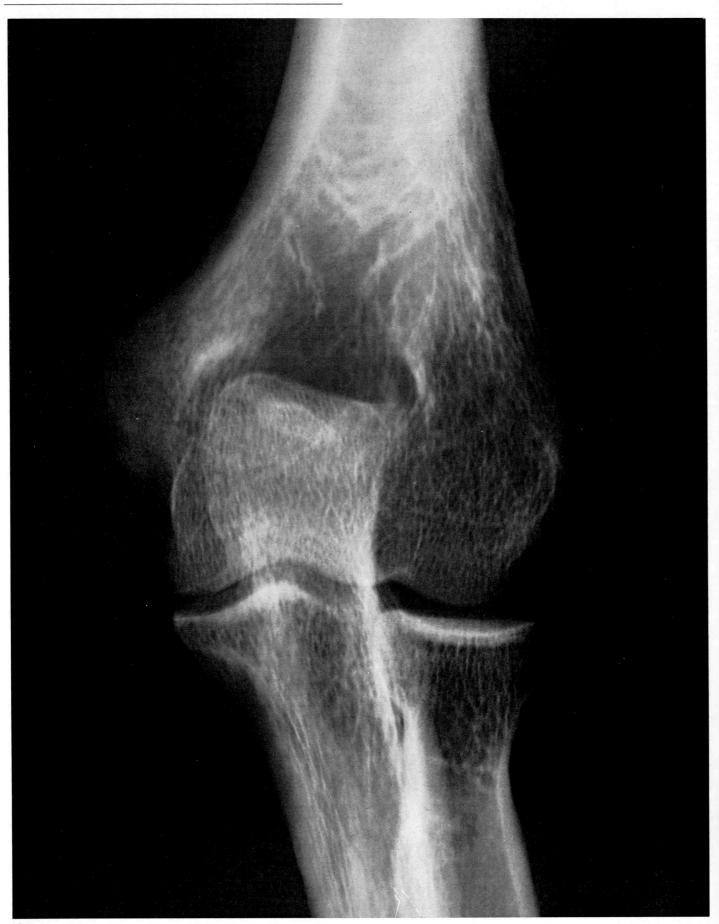

2135a

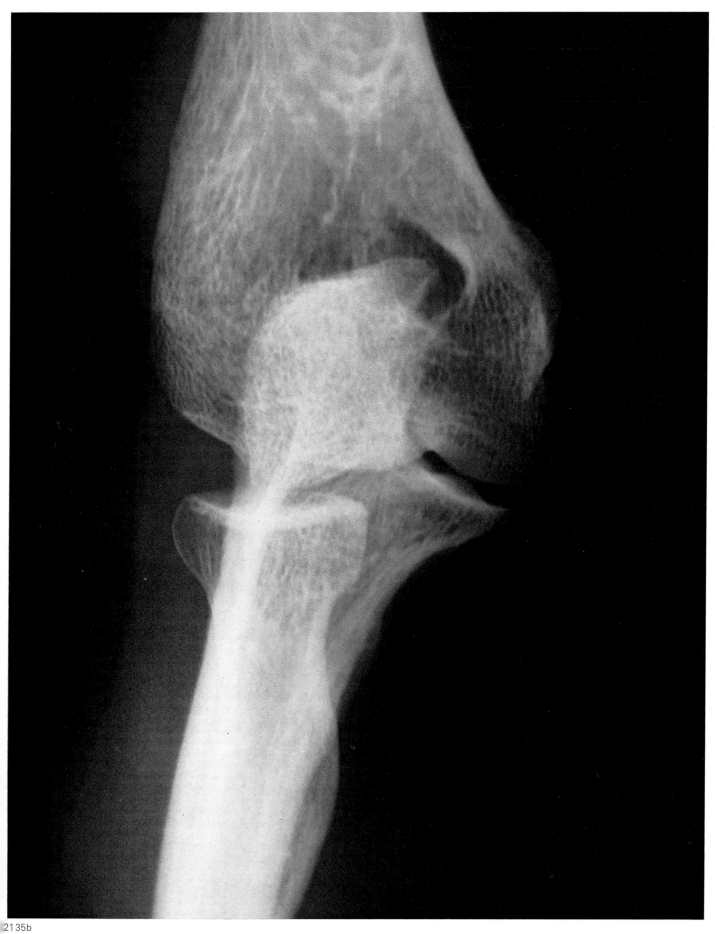

2135b

Petrous Temporal

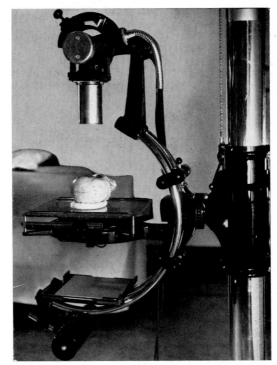

2136

The skull unit with the appropriate focal spot size, the grid removed and film positioned on the lower aspect of the counter-balancing arm provides an ideal set-up for macroradiography.

Macrographs, together with comparative conventional contact radiographs of the petrous part of the temporal, are shown in the series (2137a and b).

Using the 0·3 millimetre tube focus for the ×2 enlargements the following technique was employed:

(2137b) macrograph and (2137a) contact radiograph lateral, with 25 degree caudal tube angulation.

(2138,2140) fronto-occipital projection, patient supine. OMBL at 90 degrees, centre in the mid-line at the level of the lower border of the superior orbital ridge. Clearly defined details of the semi-circular canals, the cochleae and adjacent structures are shown within the orbital margins in macrograph (2140).

(2139,2141) for the half-axial projection the tube was angled caudally 25 degrees for the macrograph (2141) and 35 degrees for the conventional contact radiograph (2139).

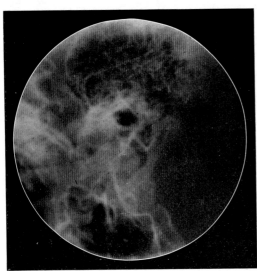

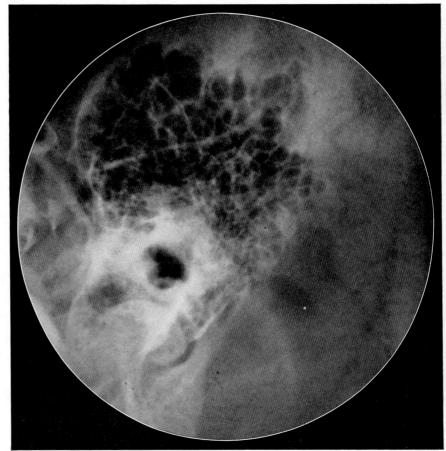

2137a

2137b

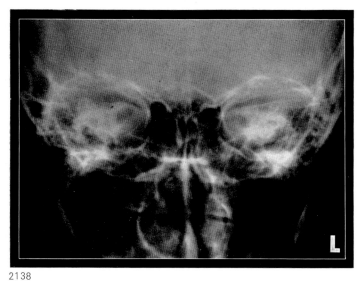

2138

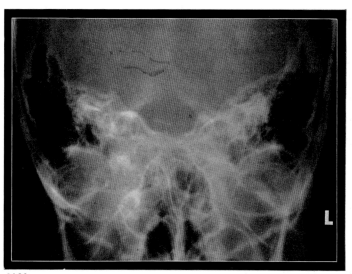

2139

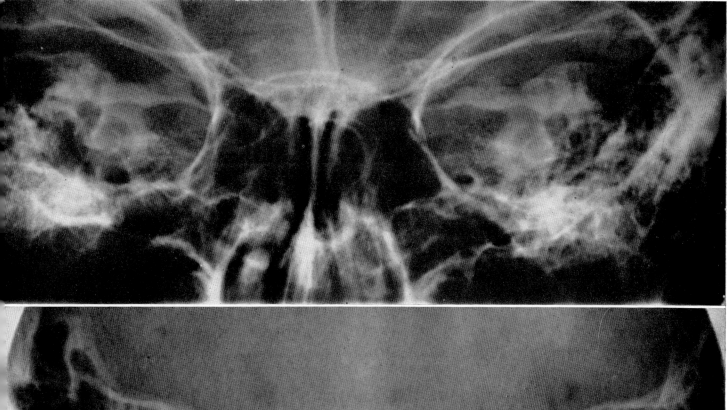

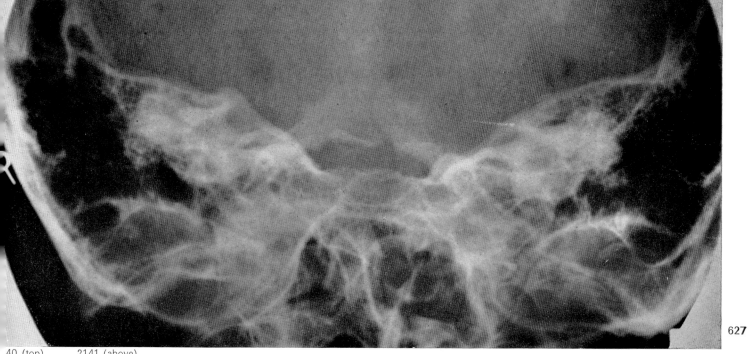

40 (top)   2141 (above)

Lungs

For routine macroradiography of the lungs, the chest surface area is divided into four parts to enable a full size ×2 macrograph to be taken of each section on a 14 × 17 inch film. The preliminary contact radiograph (2142) is lettered to show the four divisions. The upper zones (1) and (2) at the level of the spine of the scapula and the lower zones (3) and (4) at the level of the inferior angle of the scapula, are centred each in turn 3 to 3½ inches from the mid-line and the skin surface is marked accordingly for guidance in centring for the macrographs.

A sectional macrograph is included, section (3) the right lower zone. This macrograph has been trimmed down from the original 14 × 17 inch film to enable full size enlargement of the actual lung tissue to be included.

Note—The preliminary film (2142) was taken with High Definition intensifying screens and the macrograph with standard speed screens and fast film.

Exposure factors:

Upper zones 110 kVp, 1·6 mAS at 25 mA.
Lower zones 120 kVp, 2·0 mAS at 26 mA.

The chest support shown in the (2144) is adjustable to any selectable degree of enlargement up to ×2. The patient is positioned against the ¼″ perspex sheet. (2143) depicts the set-up for routine contact radiography at 60″.

(2145) The macroradiograph ×2 at 60″.

Because of the reduction in the effect of scatter in the intervening air-gap, high kilovoltage can be used with advantage in conjunction with the small foci to reduce exposure time.

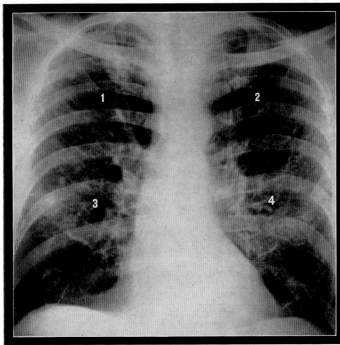

2142

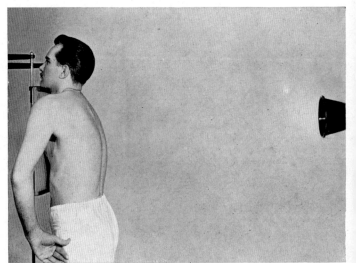

2143

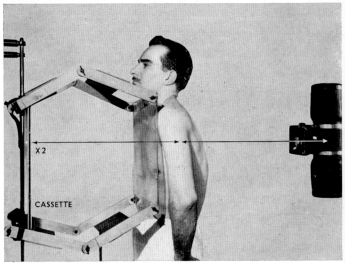

2144

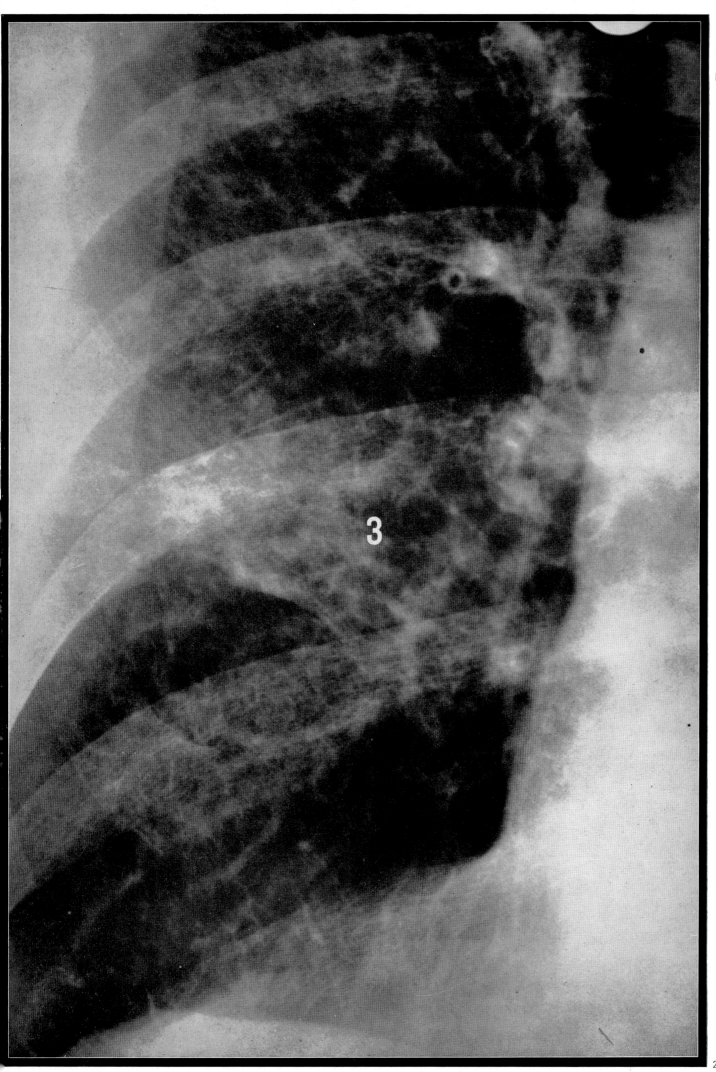

3

The Lacrimal System

The main description for the lacrimal system with the injection procedure is given in Section 20 page 505, but only a brief reference is made to macroradiography.

The specially designed macroradiography table used for skull work is shown in (2146). For the lacrimal system a magnification of $\times 2\frac{1}{2}$ is used and the photograph shows the relative positions of tube, head and film, the greater than $\times 2$ enlargement having been obtained by displacing the film at a greater distance from the head than that of the head to the tube focus.

Using the occipito-mental position, OMBL angle 40 degrees, and the lateral position, one pair of macrographs and one pair of conventional contact radiographs are shown.

Only the essential part of each macrograph is included. For the macrographs the exposure technique was: occipito-mental 1·5 seconds and lateral 0·15 second at 125 kVp, 10 mA, using Standard intensifying screens and fast film without a grid.

The radiological report is as follows:

(2147) An incomplete low level obstruction of the naso-lacrimal duct with slight distension of the duct.

(2148,2149) Incomplete obstruction of the lacrimal passages above the bony canal with dilatation of the lacrimal sac. The opaque medium is retained in the canaliculi, with a residue on the floor of the nose.

(2150a,2150b) Conventional contact radiographs. This technique for the lacrimal system is referred to as macro-dacryocystography.

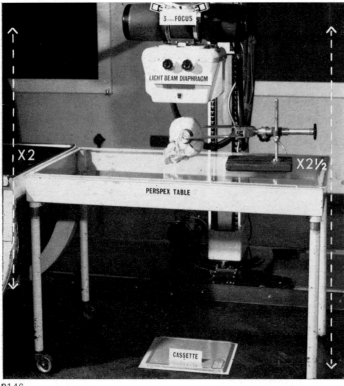

2146

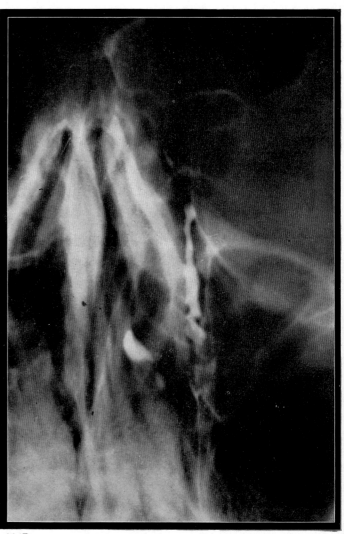

2147

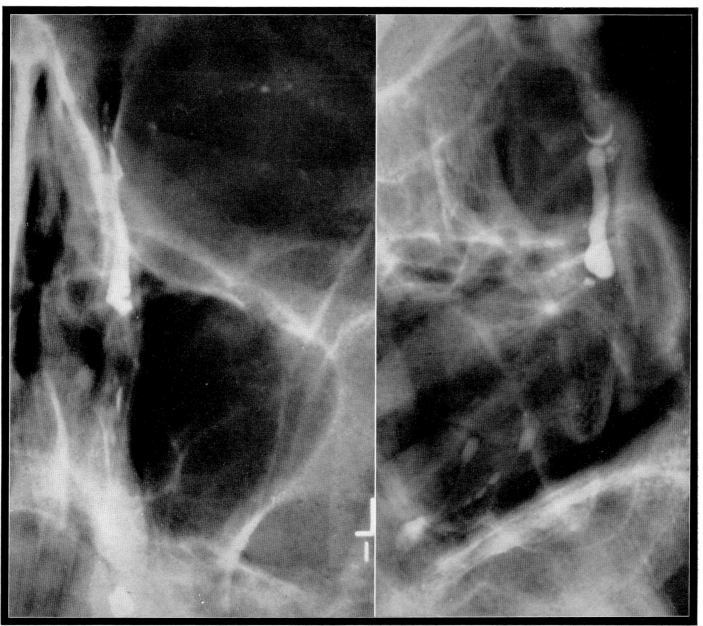

2148

2149

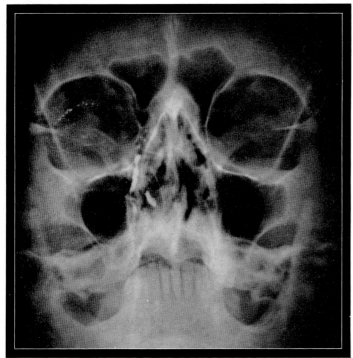

2150a

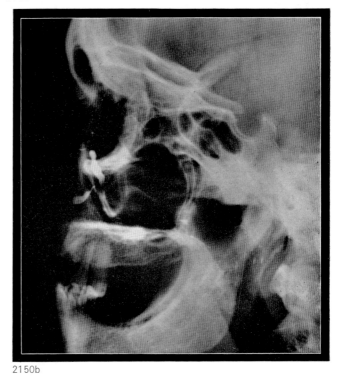

2150b

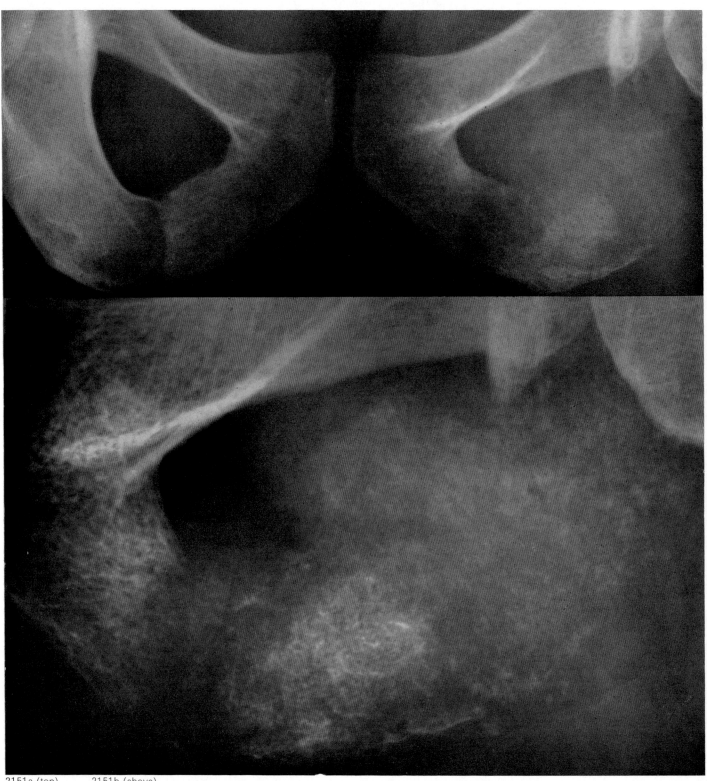

2151a (top)   2151b (above)

27

MULTIPLE
RADIOGRAPHY

SECTION 27

MULTIPLE RADIOGRAPHY

This technique with its many potential applications is designed to permit the exposure of two films simultaneously. The method makes use of appropriate selection of two pairs of conventional type screens from the currently available range of High definition, Standard and Fast Tungstate routine intensifying screens. Choice of two pairs from the above range, placed within a single cassette and loaded with an X-ray film in each screen position, allows the two films to be exposed simultaneously. Positioning the faster pair of screens in the cassette in closest relation to the tube, with the slower pair to the rear, result in the two films receiving different exposure to the extent that a distinct difference in subject is recorded on each film.

No. 1. film emphasizing the greater opacity range of the subject including bone structure.

No. 2. film—the lower opacity range of the subject including soft tissue.

Vice versa, if the screens are arranged in progressive speed within the cassette, the faster rear screen compensates for loss in exposure due to absorption of the beam in the front pair of screens and consequently density on each film is similar.

Irrespective of the arrangement of the screens within the cassette, the exposure requirement for the region examined is in accordance with the speed of the pair in closest approximation to the tube.

Wide Range Radiography

Where it is necessary to reproduce a considerable variation of subject opacity within a region being examined the multiple method is used with the screens placed within the cassette in descending speed order from the Tube.

In subject of the type (2153a,2153b) (2154a, 2154b) ×2 drop in exposure between the two films is suitable to record the bone structure on film No. 1 and soft tissue structure film No. 2 at correct density level for each.

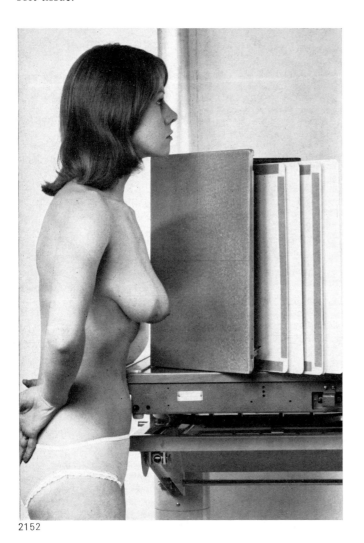

2152

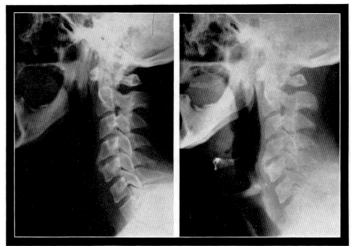

2153a   2153b

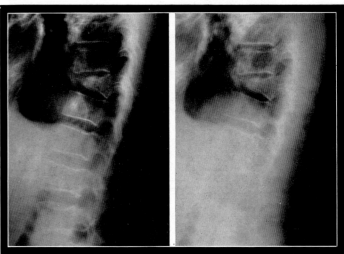

2154a   2154b

Recommended combination

Fast Tungstate (pair) nearest the tube.
Standard screens (pair) at the rear.

Where the variation in subject opacity is marked, the difference in exposure received by the two films has to be extended and in such an instance the combination of, Fast Tungstate (pair) nearest the tube, High Definition (pair) to the rear is more appropriate (2155a, 2155b).

The gain in information due to this method is particularly exemplified in the two appropriately simultaneously exposed films for Placenta Praevia.

Film No. 1 (2156a) is of sufficient density to show the relationship of the foetal head with the maternal vertebrae and pelvis.

Film No. 2 (2156b) shows the contents of the maternal abdomen right out to the anterior abdominal wall.

Advantages of the above method

(1) Its convenience in simplifying the technical difficulty associated in the above subjects.
(2) The single exposure is suited to the fast pair of screens minimizing patient dosage.
(3) The general quality of both films is decidedly superior with respect to definition (sharpness and contrast) compared with the result obtained when High Kilovoltage is applied to reduce the scale of subject contrast.
(4) As a safety factor in obtaining a suitable exposure in a less familiar examination.

Wide range technique may be applied, of course, to many of the regions discussed in the various sections of this book, in every case bringing with it the advantage that only a single normal exposure is required to produce the necessary related densities.

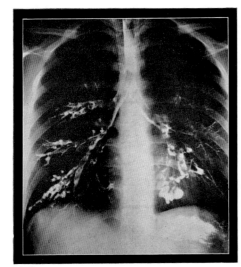 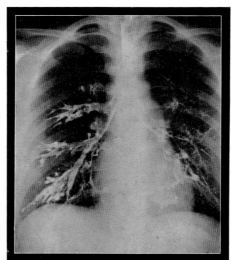

2155a   2155b

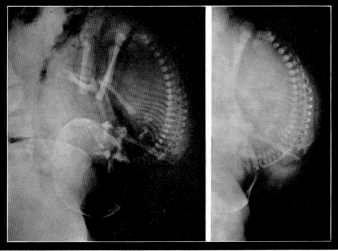

2156a   2156b

Duplication

Placing two pairs of screens in the cassette in progressive speed order eg: No. 1. Standard pair; No. 2. Fast Tungstate pair, and with an X-ray film in each screen position, produces two similar density films with one exposure. The faster screen at the rear balancing the absorption of the radiation passing through the first pair of screens. The potential of this application is perhaps less striking than its wide range application, nevertheless it gives (a) an authenticity of duplication that may be absent with two separate exposures. (b) Reduction in dosage and convenience to the patient.

Situations where for instructional purposes additional radiographs are required in building up a radiological library, or in providing a series of radiographs for instruction in radiographic positioning, are suited by this technique.

Cassette

The added well depth of the grid cassette, with the thickness of the second pair of screens replacing the grid, permits the ready application of either forms of this method. An alternative to this is to single out a cassette where the contact is suspect with a single pair of screens, the deficiency being rectified by the added thickness of a second pair of screens.

It must be emphasized, however, that in both procedures a conclusive test for contact with the two pairs of screens in situ must be confirmed.

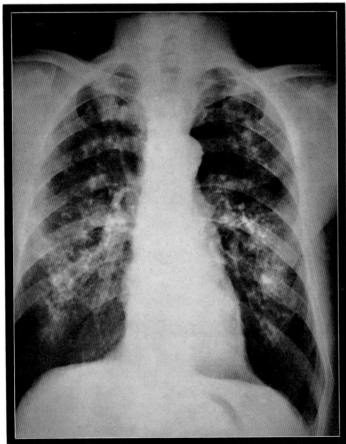

2157a

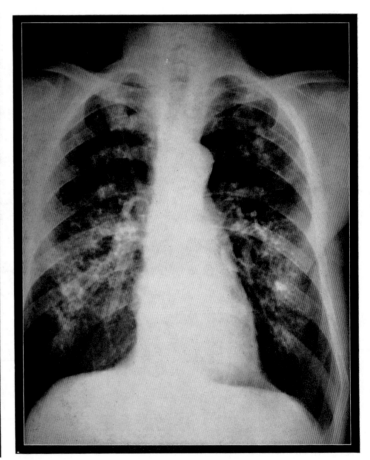

2157b

Simultaneous Contact Radiography and Macroradiography

A further form of multiple radiography is in the link-up with enlargement technique, making it possible to combine the production of the contact radiograph with that of the macrograph at a single exposure. For the smaller regions a non-screen film is used for the contact radiograph and a pair of high definition screens with the appropriate film for the ×2 macrograph. The contact and enlargement are taken simultaneously. The speed of the screen combination ensures that the macrograph is comparable in density to the contact film with simultaneous exposure.

In heavier regions where the use of intensifying screens is required for the contact radiograph, the cassette should be minus the lead protective backing to allow the remaining emerging rays to reach the displaced cassette and film for the enlarged radiograph.

The respective screen speed should be high definition for the contact radiograph and fast tungstate for the enlargement. With the grid removed the skull unit, as demonstrated (2135) provides an ideal setting for simultaneous contact and enlargement particularly for such techniques as macrodachryocystography.

Employing the multiple cassette for the enlargement allows the full facilities of multiple radiography to be obtained, either wide range technique or producing a duplication of the result.

Additional advantages of this approach to macroradiography are the:

(a) Reduction in exposure by exposing the contact and enlargement simultaneously.

(b) The subject position is an exact duplication where, as with separate exposures the possibility always exists that there can be a shift in the subject position.

Contact radiographs (2158a, 2159a) and macrographs (2158b, 2159b) were exposed simultaneously.

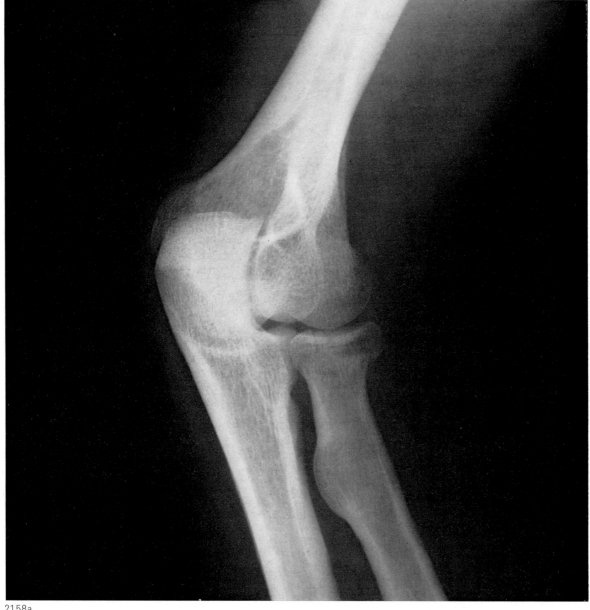

2158a

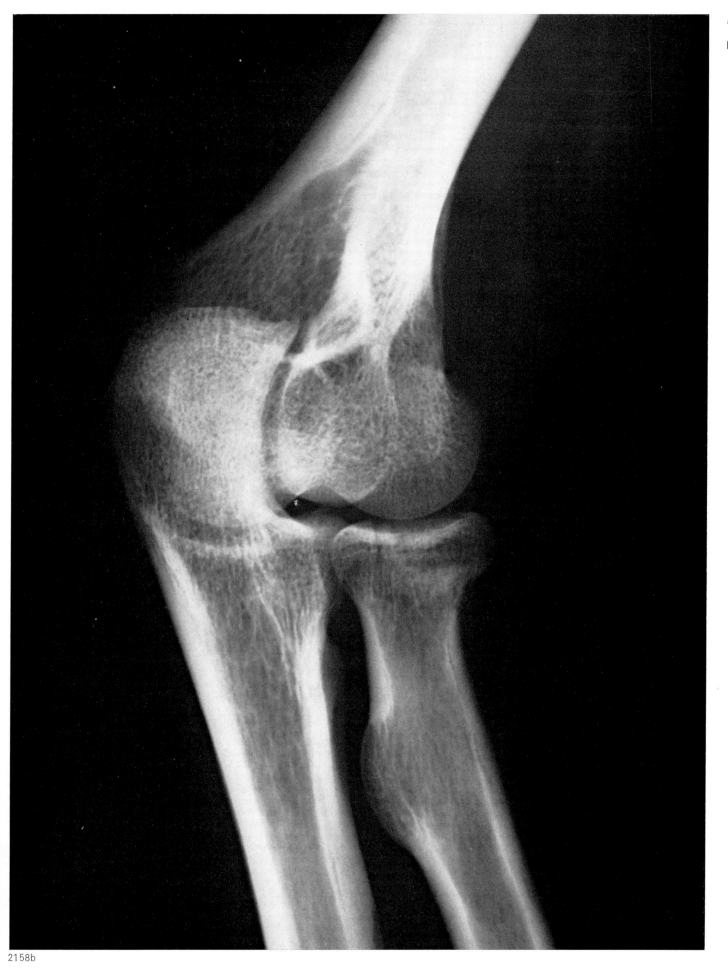

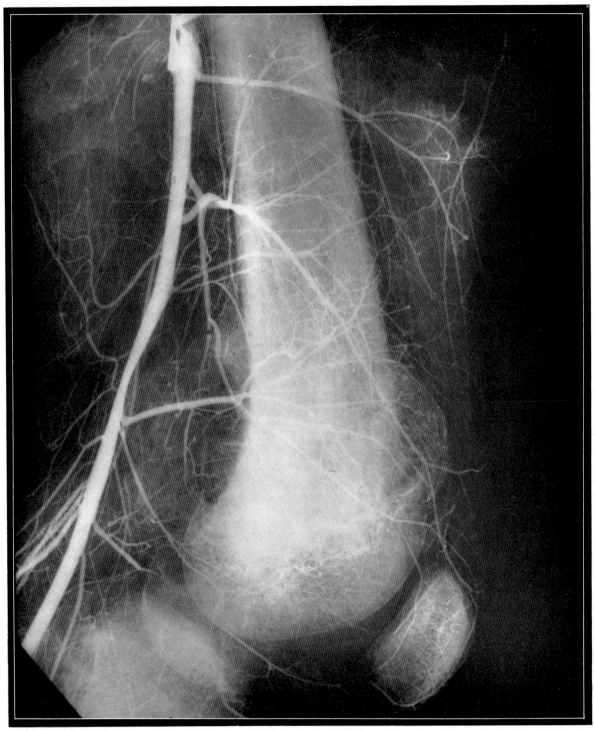

2159a

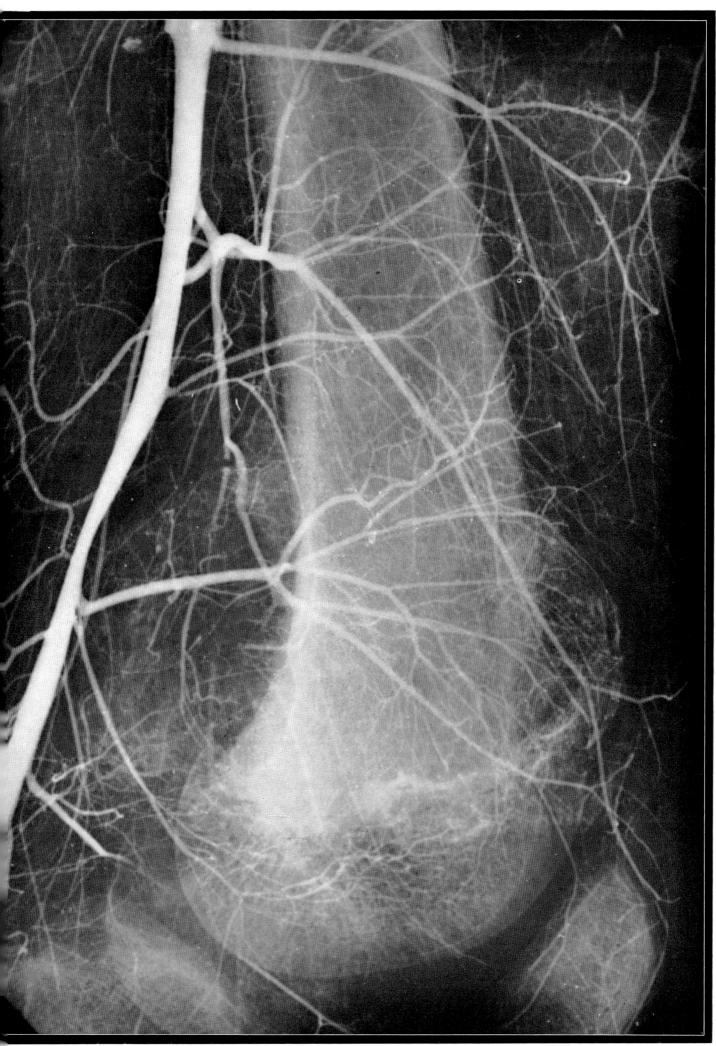

2159b

28

TOMOGRAPHY

TOMOGRAPHY

The method for taking radiographs of individual layers of the body has been known under various names chiefly to define the type of apparatus used. Of these, tomography has been officially adopted for all systems producing body-section radiographs which are called tomograms.

Principles

The conventional radiograph produces a two dimensional image of all structures within the total depth of the subject between the X-ray tube and the film. As a consequence of this all structures in a direction at right angles to the plane of the film are superimposed. Due to this superimposition the clarity with which image detail can be seen at various levels of the body, at times is not distinct.

The elimination of unwanted shadows by diffusion has long been practised for specified regions by the controlled use of respiratory movement and short distance technique. Tomography is a further means, whereby selected levels within the body can be isolated and freed from superimposition of images above and below this level.

In tomography the isolation of a particular level is achieved by relating the movement of any two of three components (namely the tube, the patient and the film) the third component remaining stationary. Conventionally it is generally the tube and film that are moved and the patient remains stationary.

Objective Plane. This represents the level in the patient through which the opposing tube and film movement is taking place.

An invariable principle of tomography is that the objective plane is always parallel to the film. Where the lie of the structure is oblique, the patient's position can be suited to bring it parallel, or alternatively the film can be tilted from the usual position, eg trachea and main bronchus, sacro-iliac joints, etc.

Apparatus. Basically the apparatus consists of a pivoted metal bar joining the tube and potter-bucky diaphragm by means of which they are given opposed movement about an adjustable axis (the fulcrum or patient axis).

Constant tube centring is maintained due to the rotation of the tube through the axis of the focus.

(2160) The position of the fulcrum can be adjusted to the height of any layer required, on a graduated cm scale indicating the height of the layer above the couch top. To ensure that this particular level is recorded it is essential for the film-driving pin (film axis) to be positioned in line with the level of the film in the potter-bucky tray.

A constant focus–table-top distance is generally adhered to, the tomographic movement being variable, a total angle from 20 to 60 degrees is generally possible. The exposure angle is varied in accordance with the linear distance travelled by the tube column, but the angle rather than the distance factor is generally quoted.

The chosen exposure angle can be preset by means of adjusting the position of 'on and off' switches (2161) tomographic switches actuated by the lever on setting the required angle.

Generally the exposure angle is equidistant on either side of the tube centring position (symmetrical). On occasion however the exposure angle may be confined to one side of the tube centring position (unsymmetrical exposure angle). For consistency the exposure should be controlled by the tomographic switches, the bucky contacts operating before and after. They should also be independently adjustable, so as to produce either a symmetrical or unsymmetrical movement.

Power for the motivation is either by traction spring or motorized electrically, and should preferably be from table top height to improve the possibility of smooth movement.

Generally a moving grid is used for all exposure, this should be efficient at the kilovoltages in use.

Equally important to the grid in the control of scatter, is close collimation of the beam and carelessness in this respect is decidedly detrimental to quality.

Essential Requirements. A smooth stable movement is essential with total absence of vibratory movement. There should be constant tube centring with avoidance of any slack in the reciprocal tube and film movement.

Exposure for a tomogram is increased by 30 per cent as compared with the standard radiograph.

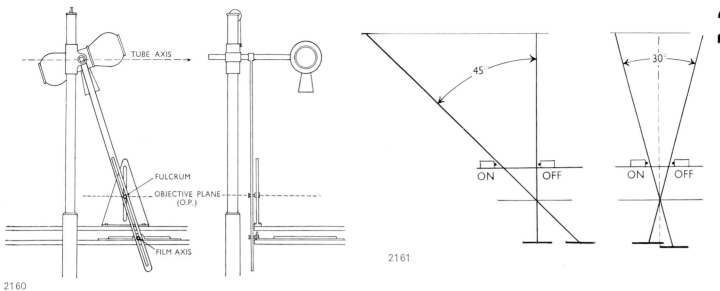

TUBE AXIS

FULCRUM

OBJECTIVE PLANE
(O.P.)

FILM AXIS

2160

45

30°

ON | OFF

ON | OFF

2161

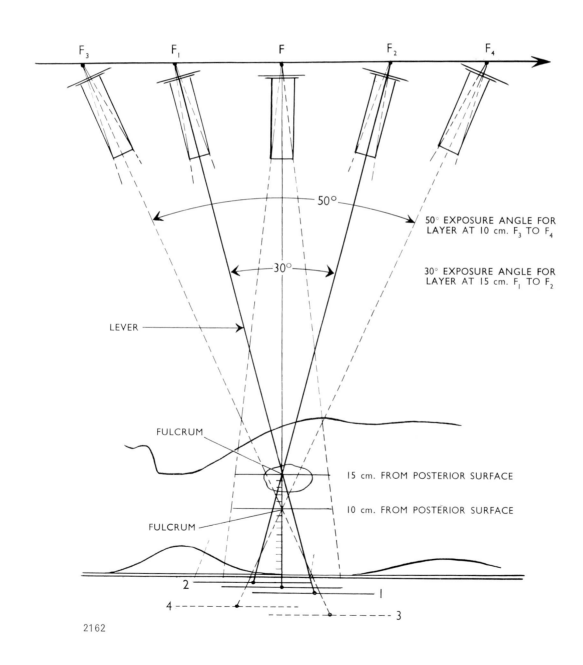

F_3 F_1 F F_2 F_4

50°

50° EXPOSURE ANGLE FOR
LAYER AT 10 cm. F_3 TO F_4

30° EXPOSURE ANGLE FOR
LAYER AT 15 cm. F_1 TO F_2

30°

LEVER

FULCRUM

15 cm. FROM POSTERIOR SURFACE

10 cm. FROM POSTERIOR SURFACE

FULCRUM

2   1

4   3

2162

Line to Line Movement (Plane Parallel)

This embraces an opposing straight-line parallel movement of the tube and film, ensuring constant focus–object object–film ratio throughout the movement. As a consequence of this, the objective plane, parallel with the tube and film movement at the fulcrum level is constantly selected.

Constant centring is obtained with rotation of the tube through the focal axis.

As can be seen however in (2163) the focus–film distance, and absorption of the beam in an increased thickness of the body, is greater at the start and finish, than at the centre of the movement, therefore theoretically, movement should accelerate and decelerate throughout, in order that the exposure is uniform at all angular positions.

This discrepancy in exposure at the peripheries can be accepted in thin type subjects but with heavy subjects and increasing operating angle a stage may be reached where there is deficiency in exposure and in consequence, a disparity between the recorded angle and the operating angle.

Recently automatic exposure control has been incorporated which in addition to arranging the exposure, controls uniformity, and the effective angle.

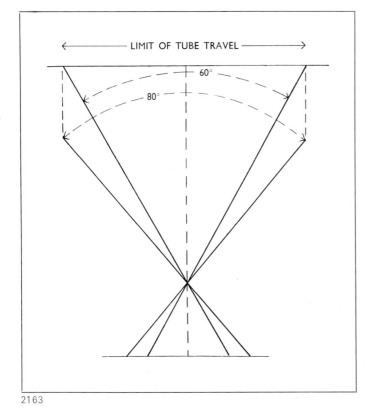

2163

Arc to Arc Movement (2164)

This comprises an opposing synchronized arcuate movement between the tube and the film. The arcs of the circles centred about the pivoting point. The film is maintained parallel to the objective-plane, although its centre follows the arcuate movement. Both the focus–film distance and the focus–object, object–film ratio are constant and consequently the objective plane parallel with the film at the fulcrum level is constantly selected.

Arc to Line Movement (2165)

This comprises an opposing synchronized arcuate movement of the tube with a straight line movement of the film. Although this system does not ensure a constant magnification the error can be tolerated in view of the closer subject–film relationship compared with the arc to arc movement.

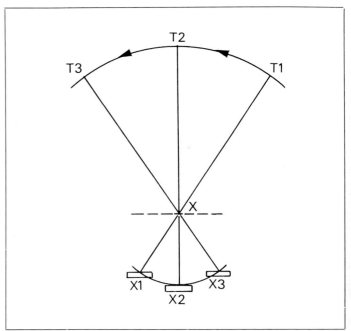

2164

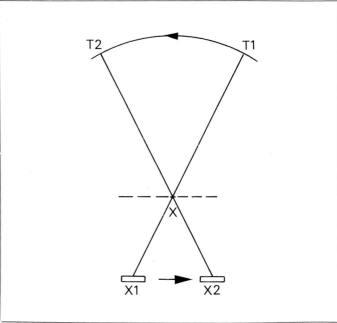

2165

Confirmation of Depth and Exposure Angle. To correlate the scale of readings for the objective plane with the actual subject depths recorded in the radiograph, a standard test object is used such as those shown in (2166, 2169). The scale is marked from 0 to 21 centimetres, increasing by 0·25 centimetres by means of lead wires placed transversely; there is also a single wire placed longitudinally. A tomogram of this test object, with the movement at right angles to the longitudinal wire, will be similar to that in (2167, 2170). The actual height of the objective plane is at the sharpest point on the longitudinal wire image (2170). For consistency the test exposure should be duplicated. Any discrepancy between the scale setting and the test tomogram, means that the scale pointer needs adjusting, or that the film axis is above or below the film; more likely it is the latter. The scale pointer can be checked against the measured height of the fulcrum above the table. In doing this it should be appreciated that a scale is often placed in a convenient position and not necessarily with the zero at table top level. If the scale pointer is correct then the discrepancy is due to the film axis being either above or below the film; above, when the test indicates a lower level than the scale, and below, when the test indicates a higher level. Small errors can be due to the various thicknesses of cassettes, therefore the same type of cassette should always be used, if absolute accuracy is desirable.

It may again be emphasized that errors in localization of the objective plane make no difference to the quality of a tomogram.

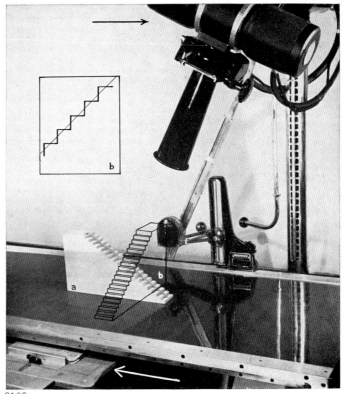

2166

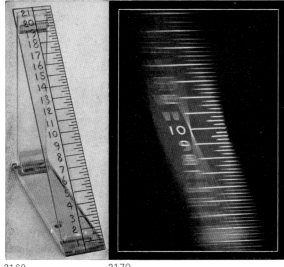

2169   2170

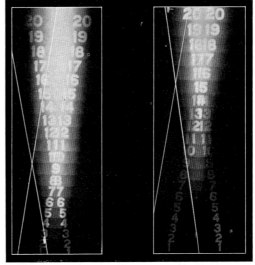

2167

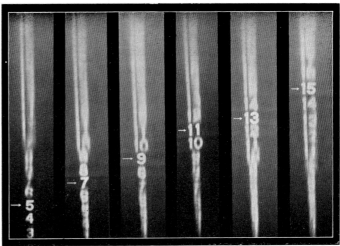

2168

Section Intervals

The intervals in a series at which tomograms should be taken depends principally on the exposure angle.

Tomograms must be taken at closer intervals as the exposure angle is increased.

The greater the exposure angle the thinner the section interval, and conversely.

The smaller the exposure angle the thicker the section thickness isolated with acceptable sharpness (2171, 2172).

Selection of the section interval depends on the condition investigated. For an image pattern of 3 millimetres diameter size the section interval must be less than when diameters of not less than 10 millimetres are anticipated, for instance, bronchioles as compared with the larger bronchi, bone trabeculation as compared with cavitation, or alternatively the minute bony labyrinth within the petrous compared with its total thickness.

As already stated only an approximation of the thickness of the section interval relative to the exposure angle can be given, and the method adopted to ascertain this should utilize similarity of Phantom material to body substance to produce the closest approximation. As a consequence the following estimation can only be quoted as a guide.

Linear Movement

10 degree arc	+2 cm section thickness
20 degree arc	1 cm section thickness
30 degree arc	0·5 cm section thickness
50 degree arc	2·4 mm section thickness

As a general rule a 30 degree arc is suited to chest tomography.

Initial exploratory spine tomography and general skull, 1 cm section (20 degree arc), thereafter on localization it may be necessary to do more intimate sections using a 50 degree angle.

For petrous, sinus, optic foramina, etc., it is essential to the use the maximum angle.

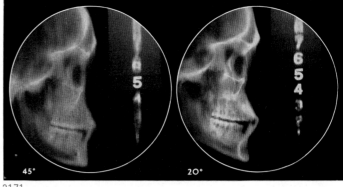

2171

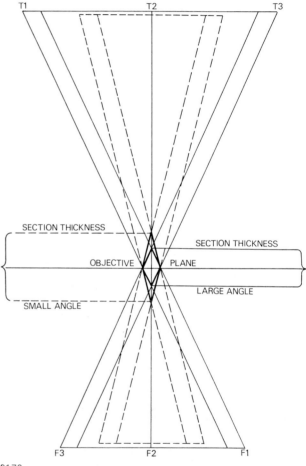

2172

The Tomographic Image

Sharpness

The quality of the tomographic image depends on the precision and accuracy with which the image pattern within the interval in focus is recorded. Within this interval the total accepted unsharpness is greater than that would be accepted in routine radiography, due to the moving system, and the progressive unsharpness from the vicinity of the sharp objective plane.

Subject contrast may also be lower because of the thinner section, and the approach necessitates critical appreciation of the section interval required, relative to the initial subject contrast, to obtain the best balance between objective contrast and sharpness.

The situation depends on:

(a) How well defined the image pattern is in itself.
(b) Accurate localization and efficient blurring.
(c) Choice of the most suitable angle.
(d) Minimum routine unsharpness.
(e) Suitable and accurate movement.

Precision engineering and efficient installation play a major part in reducing unsharpness, due to any non-synchronous movement in the tomographic travel.

It should also be appreciated that the possibility of vibration increases with increasing angle.

Sharpness of the Image. A major feature in determining the definition of the tomographic section interval, is the most appropriate choice of the factors concerned in the formation and sharpness of the routine image.

Exposure Time. In tomography, the film density depends on a factor of time during which the objective image accumulates, therefore the process cannot be instantaneous, the briefest exposure, tends to be limited to the region of 0·25 second, suitable mechanical movement to give adequate tomography below this exposure value being difficult to achieve, due to the travel time required for the various angles. As a result of this we do not have the same possibility of controlling, particularly involuntary movement as we have when taking the routine film.

In addition to this, exposure time will vary in accordance with the necessary travel time to complete the differing angles, and path of movement.

Immobilization. From the above it will be seen that it is imperative to ensure that there is no patient movement during both the single exposure and throughout the whole examination. Steps to assist in this take the form of clearly understood instructions to the patient and attention to the patient's comfort. When appropriate the use of compression bands and head clamps may afford further assistance. Patient positional movement is most likely to occur if they are left unattended, in this respect sequence exposures such as for the Petrous should be completed consecutively.

Geometrical Unsharpness. Minimizing unsharpness in the isolated interval is all important in view of the fact that contrast is lower in the tomograph than in a routine film, added to this our assessment of the image pattern is more critical when we remove all other extraneous detail. It is recommended therefore that to limit the magnification unsharpness in the line to line movement a focal spot no greater than 1 mm should be used.

In arc to arc travel, where to accommodate this movement we have an additional design magnification of × 1·3, a 0·6 mm focal spot should be used.

With hypocycloidal movement (to be explained later) the system produces a × 1·6 subject magnification and the use of a 0·3 mm focal spot is essential.

Screen and Film Combination. During the tomographic movement, image points resolved by the screen tend to be elongated in the direction of the movement. The greater the angle and the more continuous the angle the greater the screen unsharpness and the possibility of parallax between the two emulsion images. This is particularly detrimental to the image where the diameter of the detail to be recorded is small. Where other factors do not exclude their advantage, the use of high definition screens is advocated. Alternatively the use of a single screen of suitable choice in speed to compensate for exposure and used as a backscreen could be used. Other than in the above instance, choice of appropriate screen speed is generally associated with appropriate exposure time, and with a view to reduced dosage.

Border or Marginal Sharpness. The greater the opacity of the object border to the adjacent area the better the distinction due to greater differential contrast. Conversely with minor opacity change the lower the distinction. To obtain maximum distinction, however, in either instance, the object border should assume a close parallel relationship to the beam.

In tomography the probability of attaining a suited tangential angle to the border segment at the objective plane is greater with linear movement than with more complex movement.

With linear movement due to the constant changing viewpoint of the focus within the movement from zero to maximum angle, a greater compromise to variation in marginal orientation is thus presented, than with complex movement operating at maximum angle throughout. Edge distinction of the interval selected will also be accentuated due to the closer association of the total movement with this suited orientation of the beam.

Efficient Blurring. This is achieved where there is efficient removal of all images other than the detail required in the isolated structure. (Thus allowing this detail to be seen with complete clarity.) To achieve this efficiency in blurring, consideration must be given to a number of factors.

(a) *The relationship of unwanted shadows to the required level.*
The greater the angle of movement the more effective the dispersal or blurring of unwanted images. Their proximity to the subject level will necessitate a larger movement angle to produce sufficient blurring to be out with the accepted sharpness of the subject interval. When the position is remote from the required structure level a smaller angle of movement will produce the necessary effective blurring.

(b) *The direction of the long axis of the object relative to the tube movement.*
Maximum blurring will be obtained when the direction of the long axis of the object is at right angles to the direction of the movement. As a result of this linear movement produces effective blurring in one direction only, and images or a superimposition of images lying in a plane parallel to the movement are not effectively blurred. Where their opacity is sufficiently great they produce the characteristic blurring shadow defect (tomographic lines) which may intrude upon the clarity of the true image.

(c) *Whether they lie above or below the objective plane*
The blurring of unwanted shadows below the objective plane level is less than the blurring of unwanted shadow detail at the same distance above. As a consequence of this, where the intruding shadow detail lies below, a greater angle of movement is necessary to effectively remove it.

(d) *The opacity of the unwanted shadows*
The greater the degree of opacity of the unwanted shadow detail the more effective the degree of blurring necessary to remove it. A major problem exists where this is in close proximity to the required level and its opacity is greater than that of the required structure itself. In such an instance a more complex movement than linear may be required to effectively diffuse its pattern in more than one direction.

Tomographic Contrast
In general this is lower than the routine radiograph.
(a) The smaller the angle and as a consequence the greater the number of planes that are superimposed with suitable sharpness, the better the image contrast.
(b) It should be appreciated that only a portion of the total exposure contributes to the formation of the isolated image, the remainder is efficacious in blurring out unwanted shadow detail. This blur density produces a screening effect on the contrast of the true image.

Scatter also produces a veiling effect on the true image, consequently the use of the lowest kilovoltage giving adequate penetration is essential to minimize the effect of scatter.

Subject Contrast. The initial subject contrast limits the intimacy of the intervals that can be obtained. Bone structure (eg the Petrous) maintains sufficient contrast down to 2 mm–1 mm intervals, on the other hand soft tissue subjects such as the Kidney, Gallbladder, etc., are dependent on the contrast of a thick section to retain definition.

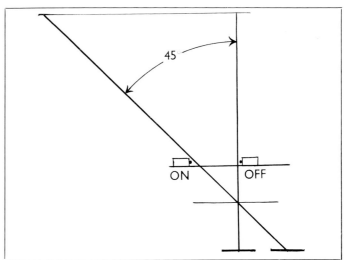

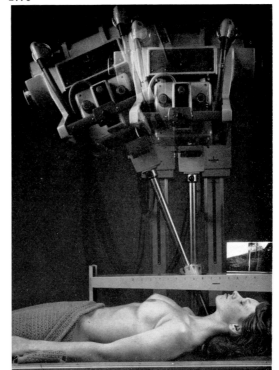

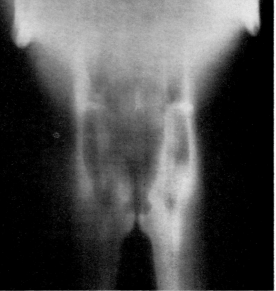

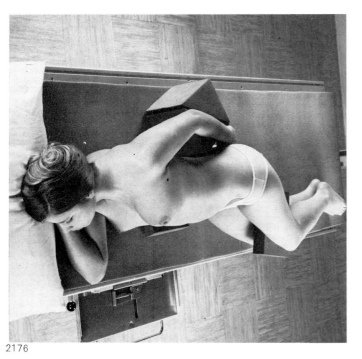

Symmetrical–Unsymmetrical Movement

Generally the total angle of movement is uniformly distributed on either side of a perpendicular centring point, in a number of instances, however, confining the exposure angle to one or other side of this perpendicular centring point is advantageous.

The method is useful:

(a) In circumventing two adjoining areas of steep differences in opacity.

(b) Assisting the tomographic movement by projecting remote dense structures clear of the centred area.

(c) Exposure and radiation absorption are reduced (2173, 2174, 2176).

For example:

(1) Using a caudal unsymmetrical angle a tomogram can be taken of the base of the lungs with minimum radiation to the abdomen.

(2) *Larynx* (*supine*) 2174.

With a cephalic unsymmetrical angle, the superimposing lower jaw is projected to a higher film level and heavy absorption through this area is avoided.

As stated previously the facility to adjust the position of the contactor switches should be available where this is not present, the *total* angle should be set for one side and the control table timer set at a travel time to terminate the exposure just prior to the perpendicular tube position.

(3) *Cervical-Thoracic Region* (*lateral*) 2176.

If a caudal unsymmetrical movement is used, heavy absorption of the exposure through the dense superimposed shoulders is avoided.

2173

2174

2176

2175

28 Tomography

Zonography

This tomographic approach is primarily associated with producing what is virtually a stationary radiograph of an isolated structural section in the region of 2–3 cm in thickness, with blurring of underlying and overlying obtruding shadows at a considerable distance from the objective plane. Tomographic angles of 3°–5° and 10° are generally used.

Because of this remoteness from the objective plane the small angles in use introduce the necessary blurring of the remote shadows and produce a section of acceptable sharpness in keeping with the structure thickness. A situation exists where the ideal is to produce the maximum efficiency of blurring at the small angle with the endeavour to form the stationary sharp image with minimum added tomographic unsharpness. With respect to efficiency in blurring at these small angles the circular path tends to be favoured. It is imperative that the maximum in true image sharpness is maintained by judicious selection of the most appropriate image formation factors in terms of small foci and high definition screens in order that the maximum differentiation between the sharpness of the true image and the blurring of unwanted detail can be readily perceived.

The technique is also useful as a preliminary localizing procedure and in the form of a general survey of joint spaces (Shoulder and Hip) and the spine (Lumbo-Sacral). It tends to be applied particularly to low opacity structures, eg Kidneys and Gallbladder where the amplification of contrast due to the thick section improves definition.

Precise positioning in zonography is important to ensure that the structure is orientated in profile to the minor changing beam direction.

The border segment to which the beam forms a suitable tangent is generally remote from the objective plane. Multi-section technique with two films interspaced +1 cm apart demonstrates the complimentary information that can be obtained on two films due to their difference in area sharpness.

Linear Movement

Although the maximum angle through which the tube and film move is generally quoted, it should be appreciated that this is attained only during a brief interval of the total exposure angle and the image is really a summation of the recorded exposure from zero to the maximum angle. This feature produces a more stabilized image, and is a factor in favour of linear movement.

Multidirectional Movement

Demonstrated in (2178) are various forms of more complex tomographic movement available particularly in circular, elliptical and hypocycloidal form.

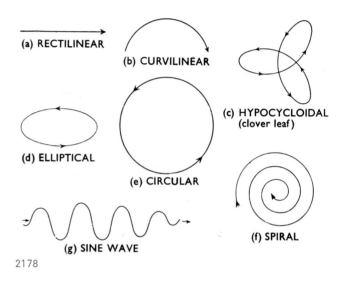

(a) RECTILINEAR
(b) CURVILINEAR
(c) HYPOCYCLOIDAL (clover leaf)
(d) ELLIPTICAL
(e) CIRCULAR
(f) SPIRAL
(g) SINE WAVE

2178

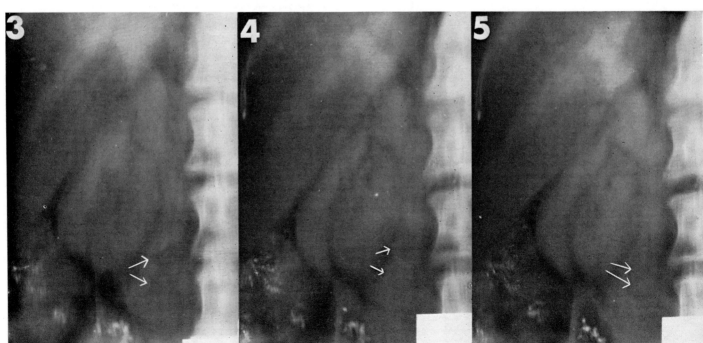

2177

Circular Movement

As we have seen two factors predominate in the effective blurring of unwanted image detail.

(a) The direction of the structure relative to the movement.

(b) The length of travel (the operating angle) and as a consequence the length of travel of the unwanted image points relative to the film.

More complex movement therefore in the form of circular movement will increase the effective blurring for the following reasons.

(c) Due to the greater travel distance of the circular path at constant maximum angle the blurring effect will be greater.

(d) A truer cross-section will be obtained from all aspects.

(e) There is a greater probability of multidirectional shadows being orientated in a suitable direction across the movement, maximum blurring of curved structures occurring when the movement is along a path opposing the main curvature of the object outline.

This is a pointer to the reason why the circular movement gives greater selectivity in bone tomography compared with the linear, and also why the spine is blurred out more effectively when tomographing the hilar region in the prone position. However when the main arc of the object (eg the cochlea) takes the same circular path, inefficient blurring results and the blurred shape is continued and not effectively eliminated (Circular Striation).

Circular movements of various radii are provided and the greater efficiency of this movement is amply demonstrated in many aspects of bone and soft tissue tomography.

A tomogram with circular movement is often taken to compliment a linear result. If both are taken with the same operating angle the result with the circular movement may be disappointing in comparison due to lower contrast because of the more effective blurring.

If however a circular angle is chosen with a travel distance similar to the linear traverse, the advantages of the circular path movement will be apparent because of the improved contrast compared with that obtained with the previous circular angle.

28

Circular

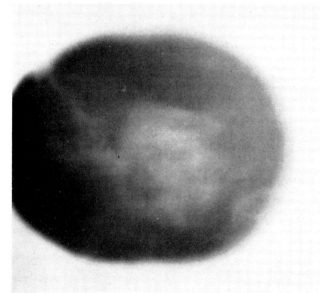

2179a

Linear

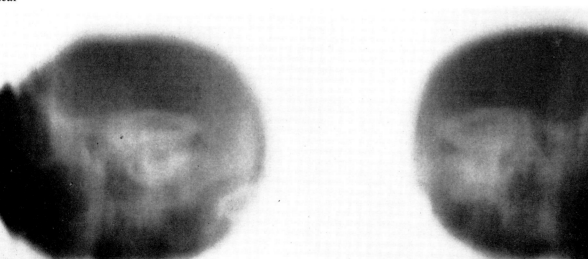

2179b

Hypocycloidal Movement (Clover Leaf)

A more tortuous movement such as the above increases still further.

(a) The homogeneous distribution of unwanted shadows in all directions, due to the further increase in travel distance required for the hypocycloidal path.

(b) A truer all-round cross-section is obtained.

At a 48° angle the above moment is effective to the extent of providing 1 mm, subject intervals.

Disadvantages. The cross-over pattern of the hypocycloidal movement however creates the possibility of pseudo-density blurring to the extent that extraneous shadows may be introduced producing confusion as to their authenticity.

It must also be realized however that the increase in travel distance, necessitates for the circular path a 3 second duration and for the hypocycloidal path a 6 seconds duration of movement, and as a consequence are unsuited for subjects with associated involuntary movement.

Precautions to avoid voluntary subject movement have also to be more stringent. With the increased selectivity, initial subject contrast limits unwarranted application.

The total absence of a retained routine image impression as is present with the linear method, adds to the difficulty of associated anatomical appreciation.

Petrous Technique with Hypocycloidal Movement

Due to the subject displacement factor it is essential to use the 0·3 mm focus to maintain acceptable definition. Close collimation of the beam to subject area in the form of an aperture or apertures 15 mm diameter reduces subject scatter. Recently the Air-Gap technique has tended to replace the Synchronous grid in removing subject scatter. The Air-Gap technique can be further complemented with the use of selective filtration.

To maintain subject contrast at the optimum level, kilovoltages in the 70–75 kVp region are preferred using the Air-Gap technique to the 120 kVp level with grid technique.

The speed of standard screens can be utilized to reduce dosage, their unsharpness factor being in keeping with the 'geometry of the system'.

Hypocycloidal

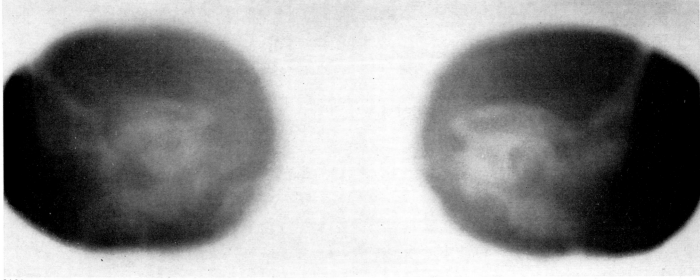

2180a

Linear

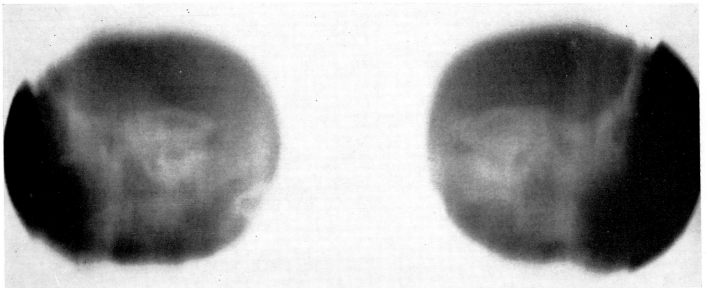

2180b

Localization

The preliminary views taken should have two objectives in view—either:

(1) To obviate the necessity of tomographic examination altogether.

In this connection the value of grid technique with adequate penetration of the opacity, and oblique views are valuable.

(2) If it is decided tomography is necessary, the preliminary views should provide the maximum amount of information as to the approximate depth and anatomical localization so that the extent of the tomographic examination and dosage to the patient is minimized.

In the upper lobe region where the lesion is of low opacity and would be difficult to determine in the lateral view, with a comparison of antero-posterior and postero-anterior positions the excursions of the lesion in relation to the anterior and posterior ribs will be indicated. The forward flexion in the A.P. view will produce an upward excursion of the lesion if posterior, and a downward excursion if anterior (2181a) (2181b).

If pertaining to the midlobe region on viewing postero-anterior and antero-posterior radiographs, the difference in the size and definition of the lesion is an indication of its anterior or posterior near film situation.

**28**

To accentuate this difference the two views should be taken at a reduced F.F.D. in the region of 36 in. This comparison is particularly useful when dealing with discreet opacity lesions in the midlobe region of the chest.

When the combination is of the lateral and postero-anterior projections, it is usually possible to estimate the position of the lesion fairly accurately (2181a, 2182).

Many structures can be measured directly from table-top height with the patient postured in the position ascertained for the preliminary views for tomography.

Where it is not possible to measure directly on radiographs or the patient, wall-charts should be provided to give approximate depth of organs in the average patient.

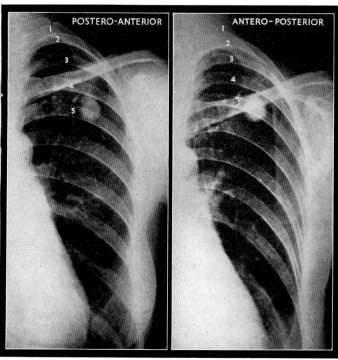

2181a   2181b

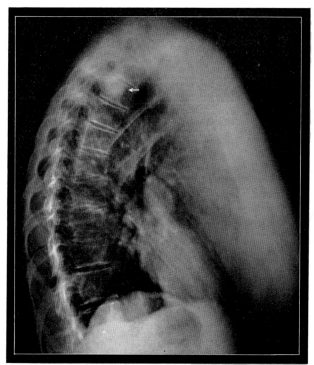

2182

28 Tomography

Procedure

Having ascertained the approximate position of the lesion in the three dimensions, the extent of the lesion is considered to enable a decision to be reached on the size and number of films required, also the measured intervals between the films.

Tomographic coverage necessitates the localized level and levels indicating its disappearance on either side. A discreet lesion may necessitate intervals of 0·5 cm and requires a coverage of at least four films. A lesion occupying a large area of lung from anterior to posterior would be exposed through the lung at approximately 2 cm intervals.

Where it has not been possible to predetermine the pathological level it is advisable to take three initial films at a suspected level using a small angle no greater than 20 degrees.

Photograph 2183 shows the relationship of patient, tube and film in two dimensions during the taking of a chest tomogram by the sequential method.

Positioning of the Patient

Generally the patient is positioned so that the half-section of the body within which the lesion or structure lies, is nearest the film in order to obtain maximum definition. Tomographic coverage is confined to this half-section. By restricting the underlying depth below the objective plane, effective blurring is obtained with a smaller tomographic angle.

Figure 2184 demonstrates the improved definition obtained with close subject–film relationship at 4 cm compared with a subject displacement of 8 cm. However, in order to achieve sufficient tube and film reciprocal movement to achieve the necessary tomographic effect the minimum pivoting level should be at least 4 cm from the table top level.

It may also be necessary to adjust the patient to bring the plane of the structure or lesion parallel with the film.

As stated, efficient blurring is obtained when the direction of the movement is at right angles to the plane of the structure. With linear movement therefore effective blurring tends to be limited.

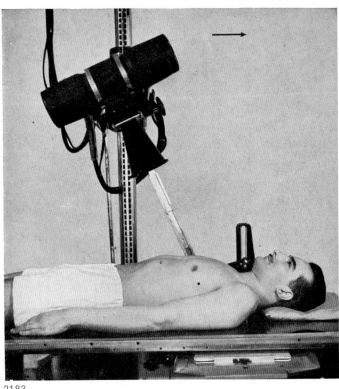

2183

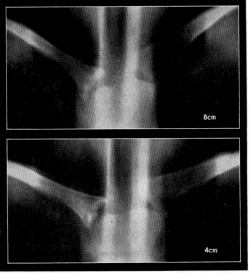

2184

In certain instances, orientation of the patient to offset two superimposed structures and to bring the required structure into a more suitable direction is useful and is demonstrated in two positions of the Sternum.

(a) R. anterior oblique with a slight cuddle curvature of the thoracic spine.

(b) Prone with the upper thoracic area offset from the midline position.

(2185,2186)

The above positions orientate the sternum oblique to the direction of the tube movement reducing the trailing shadow effect, with little alteration in the transverse rib right angled direction to the movement.

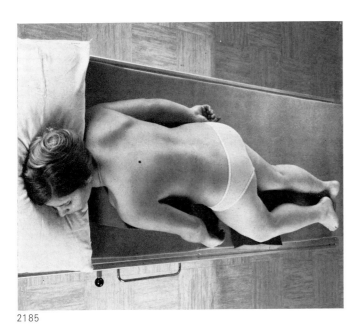

2185

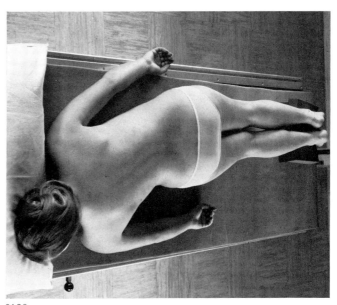

2186

Respiratory Tract

A study of a lateral chest radiograph will disclose the oblique direction of the trachea in its relationship to the bifurcation into the two main bronchi. To ensure that a single tomogram will encompass both areas it is necessary that the lie of the trachea, the bifurcation and main bronchi assume a line parallel with the film. Photographs (2187,2188) demonstrate how this can be achieved in both the prone and supine position.

Oblique

In the posterior oblique position centring is to the side nearest the film and in the anterior oblique position centring is to the raised side. The oblique position is of particular value for mediastinal and hilar lesions. A slightly oblique projection shows bifurcation of the traches very clearly in 2189.

In using the sequential method for the lungs every effort should be made to expose each film at the same stage of respiration and, instruction to the patient regarding this is time well spent.

When tomographing the chest in the antero-posterior position for lesions associated with the lower chest and diaphragm, it is helpful to have a slightly oblique presentation of the trunk, by raising the lower aspect of the patient (2190). A caudal unsymmetrical exposure movement should be used, to circumvent unnecessary abdominal exposure.

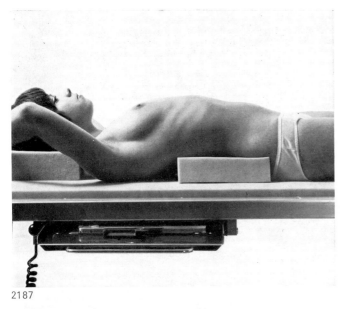

2187

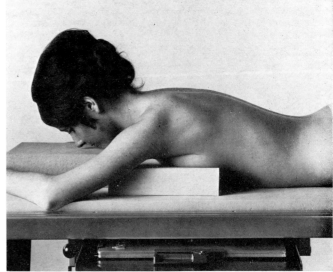

2188

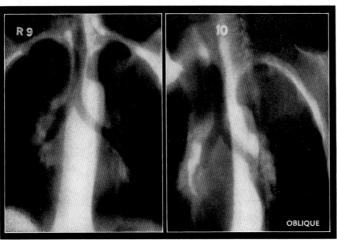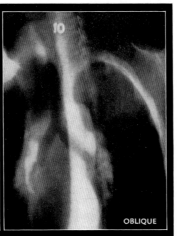

OBLIQUE

2189

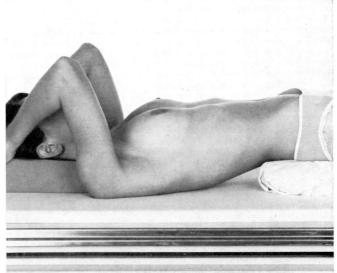

2190

Lateral

In taking lateral tomograms of the chest the patient is turned on to the affected side with the lesion in the near film position in order to obtain maximum definition. Exception to this procedure may occur when it is necessary to avoid compression of the lesion, in such a case the patient is placed with the diseased lung uppermost. In either instance tomography is restricted to the one half section. An unsymmetrical cephalic movement is recommended for upper lobe lesions with symmetrical movement over midlobe location. A.P. and lateral tomograms are (shown in 2196,2197) of enlarged vessels.

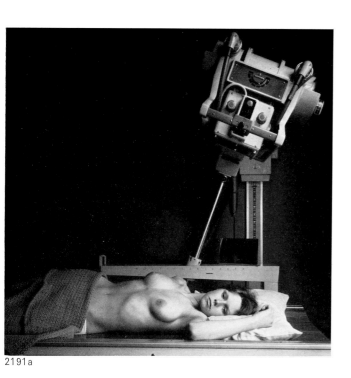

2191a

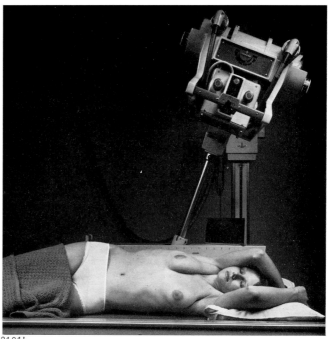

2191b

35° **Posterior Oblique** (Bifurcation of Main Bronchus into upper and lower bronchi).

With the side to be examined in contact with the table the opposite side is raised until the posterior surface is inclined at 35° to the film. This ensure that the bifurcation of the main bronchus on the side examined assumes a similarity in level, thus ensuring extensive information on the tomogram recording this level.

55° **Posterior Oblique.** From the lateral aspect with the side to be examined in contact with the table, the trunk is rotated backwards until the posterior aspect is inclined at 55° to the film.

This position is of particular value in the extensive survey it provides, of the upper lobe, the transverse fissure, pulmonary vessels, middle lobe bronchus and the apex of the lower lobe.

Planned Procedure

Work to a planned procedure whereby its familiarity eliminates the possibility of error. Reassure patient by giving explanation of procedure.

Read the request and appreciate what is required.
If it is a case which has been previously tomographed the new set of films should correspond to the previous set as closely as possible in both quality and levels.

If it is a new case the following information should be assessed.

(1) From which patient aspect and consequently the position of the patient. Approximate depth (from preliminary films measurement, or wall chart).
(2) Selectivity required relative to structure or pathological depth.
(3) Adjudge which operating angle will correspond to number 2.

Arrange the obtaining and disposing of unexposed and exposed cassettes in such a fashion that it avoids the possibility of double exposure.

Have available taped lead numerals over the approximated range of levels.

Procedure: Position patient to ensure site of pathology at its closest approximation to the film.

Set exposure angle
Set Pivoting height
Insert cassette
Position numeral

Three exploratory films should be taken initially.

(No 1) At the level approximated.
(No 2) At 2 cm or 1 cm intervals below the initial level.

(The film separation distance will depend on the subject depth and the intimacy of the levels required within the subject.)

(No 3) At a distance corresponding to the above, but above the initial level.

The result at the initial level will confirm the accuracy or otherwise of the approximation of level.

If an error is present the two additional films should confirm in which direction up or down in level the error lies, and where further intervening levels are necessary.

With practice it is surprising how accurate provisional localization can be, if care is taken.

Sufficient cuts should be taken to ensure full coverage of the subject and its disappearance on either side.

Processing: Half-cycle and particularly 90 second processing is a great asset in convenience to the patient and operator in a procedure such as Tomography which is time consuming.

Because of the rapidity at which results can be viewed, ultra-rapid processing has been responsible for a more exacting and increased use of the procedure. The steeper foot contrast on film suited to the above processing is useful in Tomography if minimizing the effect of scattered radiation.

The temperature and chemicalization of the above processing however is generally with a view to obtaining maximum emulsion speed, which unfortunately does not always result in the best quality in the shorter scale tomographic image. Where there is a prevalence to clogging of top densities in the image, improvement can be obtained by dropping the initial temperature to a level at which this is corrected. The alternative to this is the use of the more recently introduced low temperature chemicals.

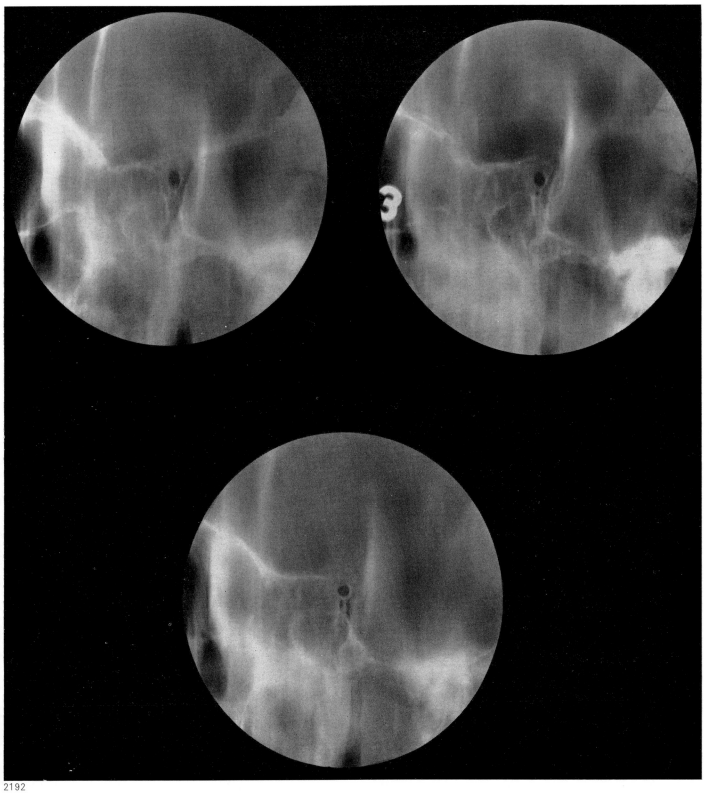

2192

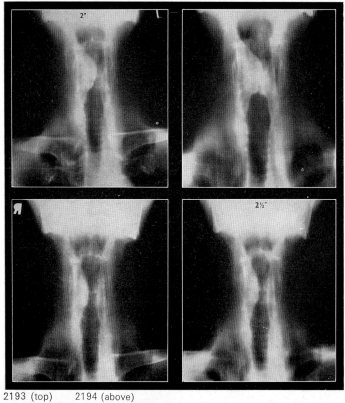

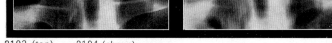

2193 (top)   2194 (above)

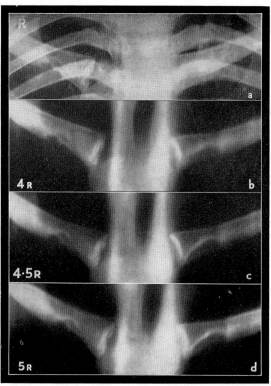

2195

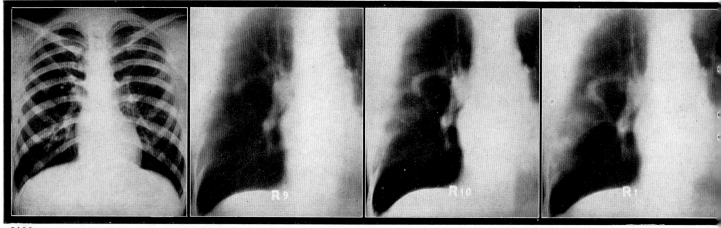

2196

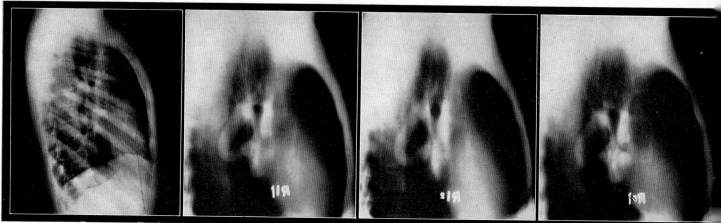

2197

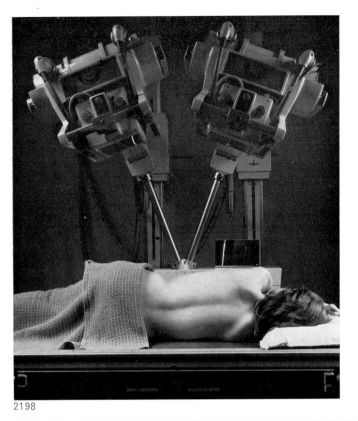

2198

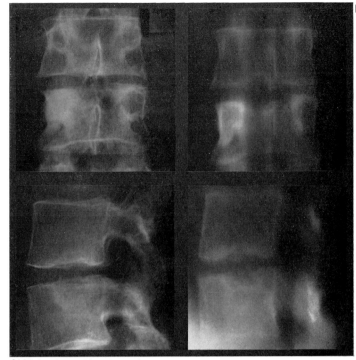

2199 (top)　　2200 (above)

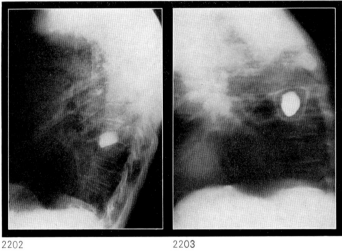

2202　　　　　2203

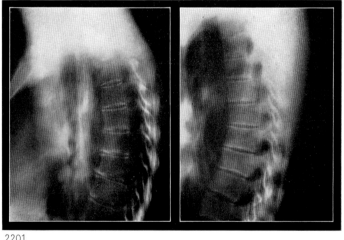

2201

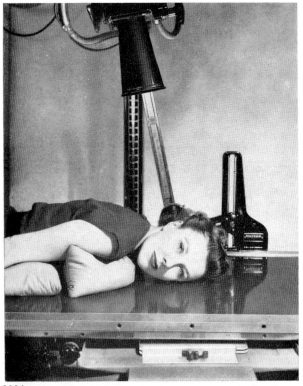

2204

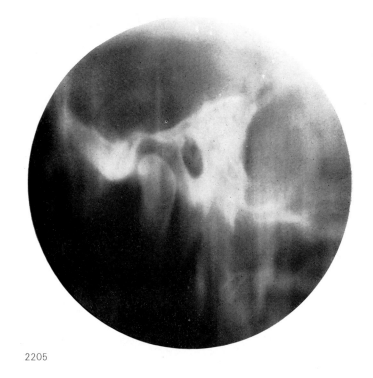

2205

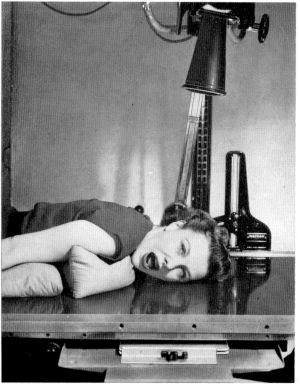

2206

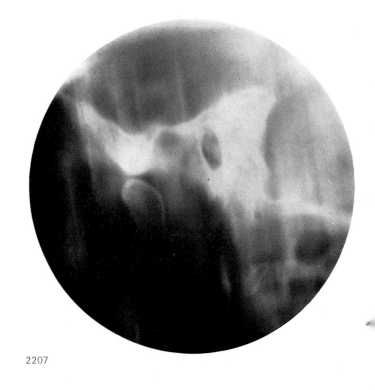

2207

Simultaneous Multisection Method, Multitomography

Multisection is a system which permits the taking of more than one body level simultaneously. The advantage of such a system is the time saving factor, both to the convenience of the patient and the department. Secondly, it is a method whereby all layers are recorded within the same phase of respiration, and as a consequence each level is separated by a more constant magnification factor than is the case with the sequential method.

Magazines are made to accommodate 3, 5, or 7 screen pairs with spacing provision for 0·5cm to 1 cm separation or more. The magazine is a light-tight box within which the screens are separated by transradiant polyester foam material. A compression block completes the anterior of the magazine to maintain the necessary screen contact throughought the unit. Supports are provided to maintain the magazine in position under the cut out aperture in the base of the bucky diaphragm. The film tray being removed to allow the top film level within the magazine to occupy the normal film position.

Uniformity of Exposure:
In order to compensate for the reduced beam intensity due to both the successive screen filtration and to a lesser degree the inverse square law factor, the screens are graduated in progressive speed from above down. The recommended screen combination for a tri-screen unit would be:
(1) A single standard and high definition screen combination.
(2) One standard and one fast tungstate screen combination.
(3) Fast tungstate pair of screens.

Five Screen Unit
(1) High definition pair of screens.
(2) High definition and standard single screen combination.
(3) Standard pair of screens.
(4) A single standard and fast tungstate screen combination.
(5) A fast tungstate pair of screens.

The progressive centimetre wedge scale placed alongside the phantom skull demonstrates that the film separation is sufficient to provide 1 cm subject intervals in simultaneous multisection procedure (2209).

Note: It is essential that the screens are maintained in the recommended sequence order.

Spacing Intervals: Due to the existing magnification the spacing between the film is greater than the distance between the body intervals.

The film spacing necessary to give the required body intervals can be calculated from the equation:

$$Fl = Bl \left(1 + \frac{d}{D}\right)$$

Bl = separation of body intervals
Fl = film spacing in magazine
D = focus to fulcrum distance
d = distance of fulcrum to top film

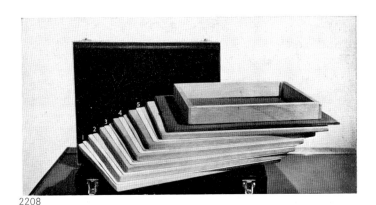
2208

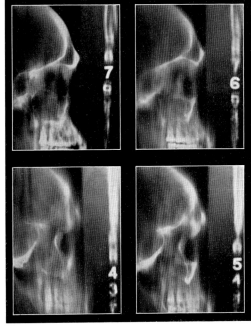
2209

Multisection Quality: The majority of criticism regarding the quality obtained with multisection compared with sequential tends to be too severe, in that it is doubtful that the films compared were identical in their similarity in level.

Recommendations: It is unwise to attempt too many film levels simultaneously.

The quality of the results from two separate sets of three screen units is decidedly superior to six taken simultaneously.

It is essential to ensure that there is good film and screen contact throughout the unit.

The magazine should be held rigid in position under the table, during excursion.

Strict columnation of the beam is essential.

Operating Angle Relative to Body Intervals
Quoting the section thickness approximated for each operating angle mentioned in the sequential section.

10 degree arc +2 cm section thickness
20 degree arc 1 cm section thickness
30 degree arc 0·5 cm section thickness
50 degree arc 2·5 mm section thickness

If we take a situation where we are employing 0·5 cm spacing intervals within the magazine irrespective of the angle chosen the objective level difference of each film will still be apparent.

Choosing a 30 degree angle giving 0·5 cm subject intervals will give distinction to the difference in localized levels beween each film.

On the other hand, we may wish to continue information from one film to the other, the choice of a 20 degree angle would result in part of the preceding and succeeding film information being retained on each film.

In the latter respect where zonography angles are being used, for example in kidney and gall-bladder tomography, such small angles do not produce a suitable tangent at the objective plane level. Subsequently using 2 or 3 suitably spaced films within the thick isolated section can give useful complementary information.

Exposure: This is dictated by the speed of the top pair of screens in the unit and dosage comparison to sequential is dependent on the speed of the screens used for the single film examination. In general the claim made for reduced dosage to the patient with this method is exaggerated being approximately the saving of one exposure irrespective of the number taken simultaneously.

Kilovoltage: To maintain good contrast with this method a good plan to work to, is to use the routine kilovoltage for the thickness of the part, adding 5 kilovolts for a 3 screen unit and 7 kilovolts for a 5 screen unit. The additional kilovoltage ensures adequate penetration of each screen ensemble.

The range of kilovoltage within the films are of comparible density is limited to between 70–90 kVp—where the kV is too low, the top film will be greater in density than at the bottom and vice-versa.

Operating Angle: With spacing in the order of 0·5 cm–1 cm the maximum operating angle should be restricted to 30 degrees in order to maintain uniformity of exposure, on each film.

Sequence of Body Intervals: Generally the top film records the fulcrum level, the lower films will then record levels successively below this. Where the pathological level can be measured or approximated however the fulcrum height can be set at a higher position so that levels are recorded above and below the localized position.

Note: It should be remembered both from the accuracy of level identification and the using of the screens in the correct sequence, that where the cassette loads from its lower aspect the film at the fulcrum level will be the last extracted. A check on possible error in marking and loading is to have the screens numbered to record their position in the magazine on the film.

Methods of Identification
Phantom Scale
With this method each successive film will record its own marker level. The method has the further advantage in that it provides a constant check on the accuracy of the fulcrum relative to the top film position in the magazine. It will also confirm error in the setting of the fulcrum height.

Disadvantages are however:
(a) It is not always possible to place it in close association with the subject.
(b) Where possible, it necessitates an increase in the opening in the diaphragm area.

Printed Height Identification
(a) This necessitates a printed numerical strip (1 to 15 cm) and the appropriate height number, for each film printed adjoining the typed name identification.
(b) An appropriate level number written on each film with a Tempo type marker pen.

Deep Cassette Multisection Radiography
This has the advantage that it can be placed, and held rigidly in the normal cassette position. The internal depth within the cassette provides for the spacing of two films 1·5 cm apart, a 4 film-screen combination spaced 0·25 cm down to film spacing the thickness of two screen apart (2212).

This provides an ideal system to record the intimate levels required in the Petrous examination, (2214) and in shallow structures such as the Optic foramen, sinuses, etc. The 1·5 cm spacing of 2 films is suited to producing complementary information in examinations such as the kidney gallbladder, etc., using small angles.

With maximum linear and circular angles, film separator thickness should not be less than 2·5 millimetres to obtain satisfactory differentiation of subject intervals. With hypocycloidal movement however subject level differentiation is obtained at 1 mm spacing.

2210

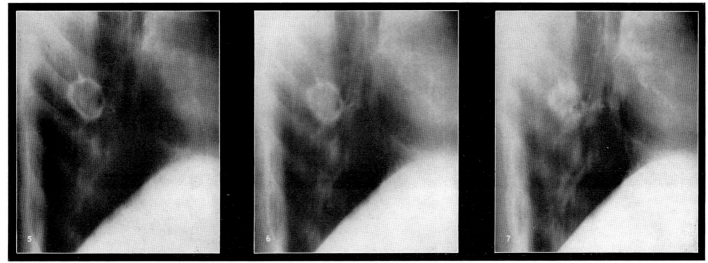

2211

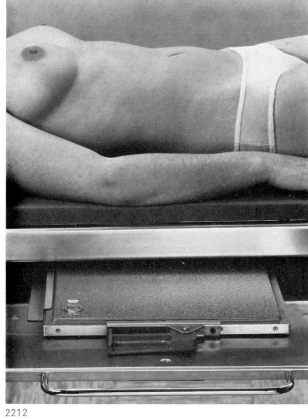

2212

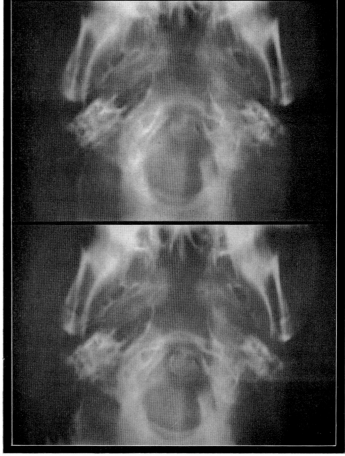

2213

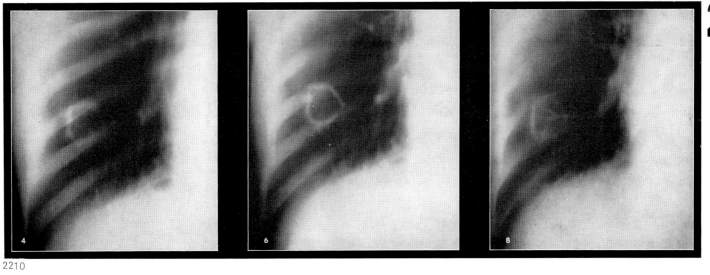

667

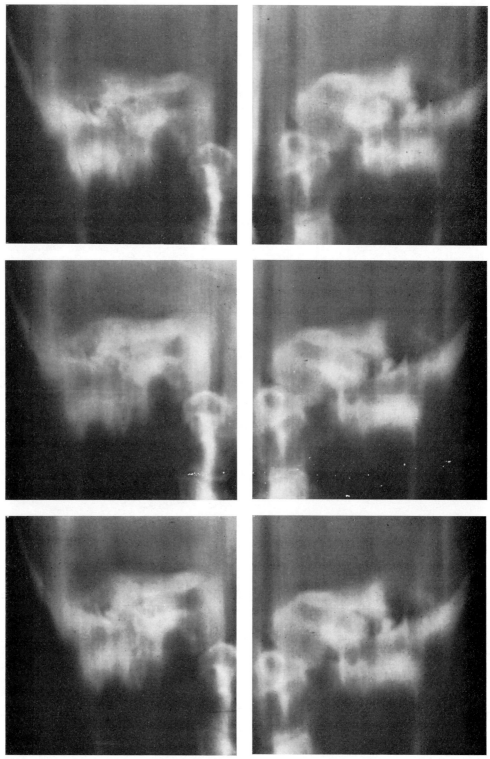

2214

Positioning for suitable orientation of lung structure

Right Lung	Position
R. Main Bronchus	Patient Prone
R. Middle Lobe	55° R. Posterior oblique
Anterior Segmental Bronchus	65° R. Posterior oblique
Apical Segmental Bronchus	Supine
Posterior Segmental Bronchus	20° L. Posterior oblique
R. Lower Lobe Lateral Segmental Bronchus	Supine Position
Posterior Segmental Bronchus	15° L. Posterior oblique
Anterior Basal Segment	15° L. Posterior oblique

Left Lung	Position
Main Bronchus, Upper Lobe Bronchus	35° L. Posterior oblique
Anterior Segmental Bronchus	55° L. Posterior oblique
Posterior Segmental Bronchus	15° R. Posterior oblique
Lower Lobe—Lateral Basal Segmental Bronchus	10° R. Posterior oblique
Anterior Basal Segmental Bronchus	20° L. Posterior oblique
Posterior Basal Segment	Supine raised 10°

Approximate Levels

Orientation of the patient is based on routine positioning, where this necessitates angulation the patient should be adjusted or rotated to this position and maintained in this position.
Initial levels quoted here are based on an average patient and are measured from the table-top.

Skull Approximate Levels

Part	Position	Level
Petrous both sides	A.P. baseline 90°	Measured distance to centre EAM
Internal auditory canal	A.P. baseline 90°	Anterior rim of EAM
Petrous (Single)	A.P. 10–20° rotation away from affected side	1 inch below EAM on affected side
Optic Foramen	A.P. (35° × 35°) Chin raised to bring base-line 35° beyond perpendicular. Rotate head 35° away from affected side	Measured distance on affected side to centre of EAM
Sella Turcica	Lateral	Measured distance to nasion
Antra (facial bones) Frontal Sinuses Upper Orbital Margin	P.A. baseline 70°	6 cm
Lower Orbital Margin fracture	A.P. baseline 20° beyond perpendicular (Raised chin)	Measured distance to lower orbital margin
Ethmoidal Sinuses	P.A. 45° rotation Baseline 30°	5 cm

Respiratory Tract—(Approximate levels)

Part	Position	Level
Larynx	A.P.	1 cm below Thyroid cartilage—14 cm Cephalad tube movement—unsymmetrical exposure
Apical Region	A.P.	4, 6, 8 cm, Routine chest kilovoltages plus 7–10 kVp
Hilar Region	Preferably Prone Supine	P.A. 5, 7, 9 cm A.P. 8, 10, 12 cm
Trachea and Bifurcation	Preferably P.A. A.P.—Partial oblique Lateral	P.A. 7, 9, 11 cm A.P. 9, 11, 13 cm
Lesions at diaphragm level	A.P. Lateral	Caudal tube movement. Unsymmetrical exposure
Peripheral lesions	A.P.—Partial oblique P.A.—Partial oblique	
Lateral Upper Zones	Lateral	Cephalad tube movement. Unsymmetrical exposure
R. Mid-zone	A.P. or P.A. Lateral 35° R. Posterior oblique 55° R. Posterior oblique	 9–14 cm 10–16 cm
L. Mid-zone	A.P. or P.A. Lateral 35° L. Posterior oblique 55° L. Posterior oblique	 9–14 cm 10–16 cm
General for Vascular pattern	R. Posterior oblique 55°	2 cm sections 8–16 cm
1 cm 0·5 cm	Subject intervals Subject intervals	20° operational angle (approximate) 30° operational angle (approximate)

Part	Position	Level
Atlas-Axis	A.P.	10 cm or 1 inch below angle of jaw
Cervical Spine	A.P.	2 cm below Thyroid cartilage
Thoracic Spine	A.P.	3–4 cm
Thoracic Spine	Lateral	Measured distance to spinous process
Lumbar Spine	A.P.	7 cm
Lumbar Spine	Lateral	Measured distance to spinous process
Sacro-Illiac Joints	A.P.	6 cm

Additional Subjects

Part	Position	Level
Sternum	Modified R. Anterior oblique	7 cm
Kidneys	A.P.	7 cm
	20° L. & R. Posterior oblique	9 cm
Gallbladder	P.A.	8 cm
	A.P.	13 cm
	20° L. Anterior oblique	10 cm
	20° R. Posterior oblique	15 cm

General multisection recommendations

3–4 screen unit
Linear movement–operational angles

1 cm spacing	20° angle (approximate)
0.5 cm spacing	30° angle (approximate)
2.5 mm spacing	40°–50° angle (approximate)

Technique

Exposure to suit speed of film and top screen
Kilovoltage—For subject thickness plus 5–7 kVp

Axial Transverse Sections

To obtain a radiograph of a horizontal section of the body, the patient sits on a pedestal which can be rotated on its axis. The film cassette is placed on a turn-table which is linked to the pedestal to enable patient and film to rotate in the same direction. From a distance of 3 metres, the tube is angled downward at approximately 30 degrees. The X-ray beam is directed through the patient at the selected level toward the film on the opposite side. Exposure is made during the complete rotation of patient and film to produce a true cross-sectional image, which can be repeated at any level. Again, stability of equipment together with immobilization of the patient is essential and alignment with focus is most important.

The illustration (2225) gives a diagrammatic representation of the principles involved. Movements of patient and film are geared to rotate through 360 degrees in the same direction. The tube is centred downward at an angle of 30 degrees from a focus–film distance of 3 metres. The level of the section required is adjusted at the objective plane by raising and lowering the patient. The focusing of the tube to obtain a sharp image does not present any difficulty. As will be seen the central ray is directed to pass through the middle of the selected plane in the patient to the centre pivotal point of the film.

On selecting a particular plane for the initial exposure as estimated for an abnormal condition from the preliminary direct radiographs, other planes are exposed at known depths about this level.

A series of horizontal section radiographs (2218 to 2224) shows the thorax at seven different levels from the root of the neck downward at one inch intervals. A lesion is reported in the left lung, confirming the existence of a new growth revealed initially by routine radiography.

Radiographs (2215, 2216) show a new growth in the mandible, following which axial transverse section (2217) was taken for guidance in plotting localized therapy treatment. A fixed position of the jaw restricted other methods of investigation.

The movements required for this technique are similar to those employed for Rotography, except that the patient and film rotate in the same direction.

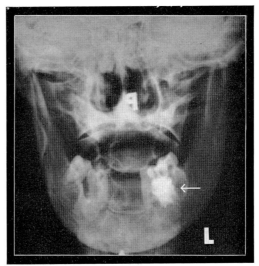

2215

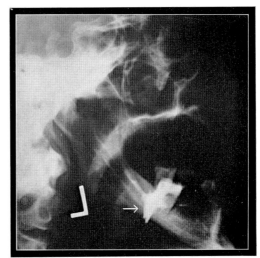

2216

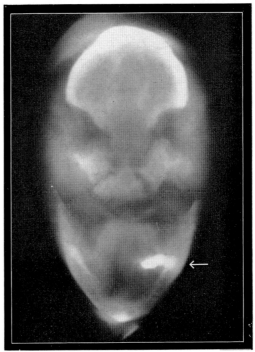

2217

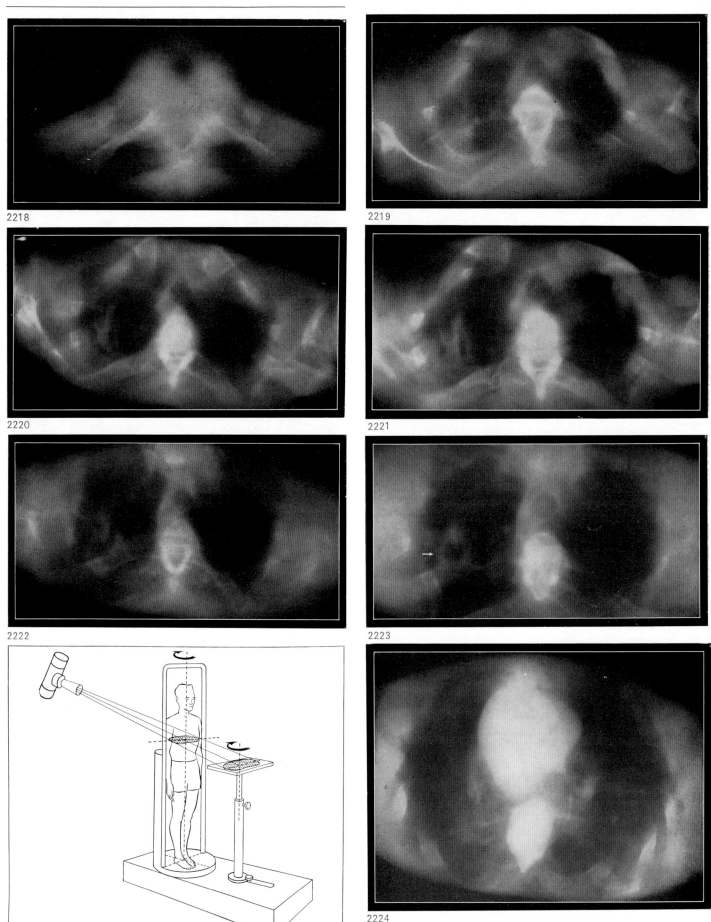

2218

2219

2220

2221

2222

2223

2224

2225

29

STEREOGRAPHY

STEREOGRAPHY

This technique implies the method of taking two radiographs with the tube foci occupying two different view points. The subject and the film position being identical in each of the two exposures. The method is a representation of personal viewing of any subject where the right and left eye are perceiving the subject from their respective positions, and the brain combines the two images to give the impression of depth.

Similarly if the two tube positions are taken as representative of the right and left veiwing of the subject, ultimately if the right eye views the radiograph taken in the right eye position and vice versa with the left eye, the brain resolves the two images as one.

Procedure

The patient having been immobilized the tube is centred and the two films exposed from diametrically opposite points, each $1\frac{1}{2}''$ (3 cms) from the central position (2226).

This tube shift of 6 cms is employed because it is the average inter-pupillary distance of the viewer. To provide satisfactory stereoscopic effect the focus–film distance should be ten times that of the stereoscopic tube shift distance. The 25″ focus–film distance suited to the viewing conditions tends to be impractical due to high radiation dosage. Consequently the focus-film distance may be increased providing the tube shift is also increased, its value being maintained at $\frac{1}{10}$th of the focus–film distance.

For making stereographic exposures, the direction of the tube-shift should be at right angles to that of the predominating lines of the part being examined; when the long bones are the subject, the tube moves at right angles to the long axis; in the case of the chest, where the ribs are the dominant lines, the movement is along the line of the vertebrae, while if the vertebral column is being examined the tube moves across the trunk. In certain exceptions, such as the skull, the direction depends upon the precise area being investigated. Since the purpose of stereography is to secure an impression of perspective, the two exposure points should be chosen with that aim in mind.

In using the tube at ample aperture for coverage it is not necessary to tilt the tube, but when a localizing cone is used the tube should be angled toward the centring point from both positions.

It should be emphasized that each pair of films should be treated as a unit and both films, therefore, taken and processed under identical conditions.

In general radiography, it is possible to immobilize the patient so that movement during the changing of films is reduced to a minimum when tube movement may be controlled by hand. In chest work, however, the two exposures must be made with the least possible interim delay, there being inevitable movement during respiratory or cardiac action. Where stereoscopic films of the chest are taken as a matter of routine, therefore, the uses of apparatus incorporating mechanical tube-shift and film-change is advisable.

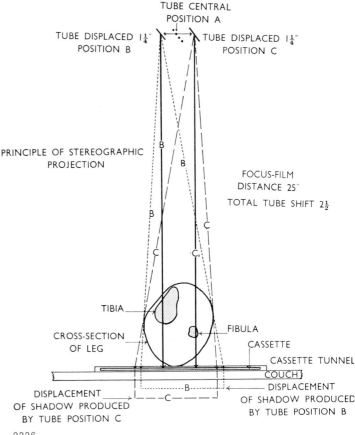

TUBE CENTRAL POSITION A

TUBE DISPLACED $1\frac{1}{4}''$ POSITION B

TUBE DISPLACED $1\frac{1}{4}''$ POSITION C

PRINCIPLE OF STEREOGRAPHIC PROJECTION

FOCUS-FILM DISTANCE 25″
TOTAL TUBE SHIFT $2\frac{1}{2}$

TIBIA

CROSS-SECTION OF LEG

FIBULA

CASSETTE

CASSETTE TUNNEL

COUCH

DISPLACEMENT OF SHADOW PRODUCED BY TUBE POSITION C

DISPLACEMENT OF SHADOW PRODUCED BY TUBE POSITION B

2226

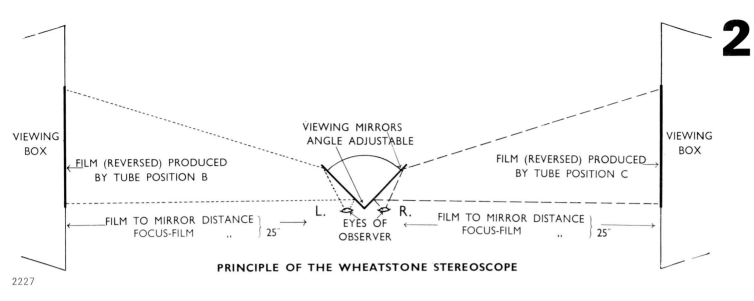

VIEWING BOX

VIEWING MIRRORS ANGLE ADJUSTABLE

FILM (REVERSED) PRODUCED BY TUBE POSITION B

FILM (REVERSED) PRODUCED BY TUBE POSITION C

VIEWING BOX

L. R.

EYES OF OBSERVER

FILM TO MIRROR DISTANCE FOCUS-FILM ,, } 25″

FILM TO MIRROR DISTANCE FOCUS-FILM ,, } 25″

PRINCIPLE OF THE WHEATSTONE STEREOSCOPE

2227

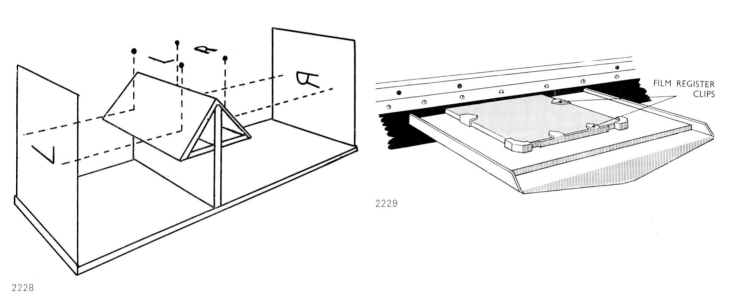

2228

FILM REGISTER CLIPS

2229

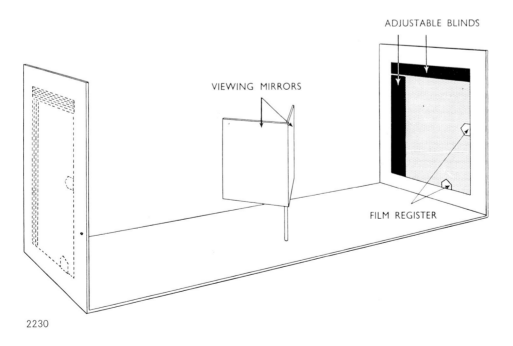

ADJUSTABLE BLINDS

VIEWING MIRRORS

FILM REGISTER

2230

Markers

By marking stereoscopic films with two lead Right and Left letters, the first marker indicates the right or left anatomical aspect of the subject and the second the viewers eye for which the film is intended. It is then possible to ensure that the correct anatomical viewing of the subject is obtained.

Alternatively with one marker only denoting patient aspect, the two films can be superimposed edge to edge, the two images will be slightly out of alignment and the film with the image projected slightly further to the left denotes the film taken with the right tube-shift and vice versa.

If we take stereo-radiographs of the right knee in the antero–posterior position, if the right eye sees the right image and the left eye the left image from the tube aspect the right knee is seen stereoscopically in the A.P. position with the Patella to the front, the aspect as presented in the stereoscope is then said to be orthoscopic. This perspective is correct as seen from the tube position. Due to the nature of the radiographic image, however, if the two films are viewed "face about" the opposite or pseudo-scopic aspect is presented, that is the image would be postero–anterior, with the Patella to the rear.

Transposition of the subject will occur if the films are presented incorrectly due to mounting in the wrong illuminant or incorrect marking of the stereo-pair, i.e. permitting the left eye to view the right shift image, and the right eye the left shift image. This will be viewed as,

(1) the opposite side to that X-rayed.

(2) The image will also be postero–anterior (pseudoscopic) where with correct viewing presentation it is antero–posterior (orthoscopic).

Correcting the latter anatomical viewing fault by reversing the films retains the error of the right side appearing to be the left or vice versa.

The possible danger of such faulty information stresses the care and attention required in this procedure.

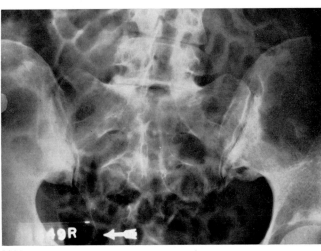

2231

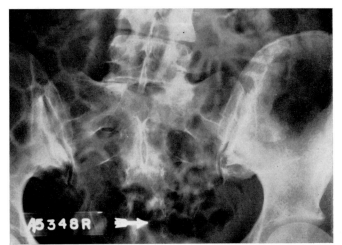

2232

Viewing apparatus

This generally takes the form of one or other of two types.

(1) The Wheatstone Unit as depicted in diagram 2227 enables not only excellent stereoscopic viewing but at the same time accurate measurement if the ratios of FFD to stereo-shift and viewing distance to film coincide. The distance between viewing boxes is adjustable, and the angulation of the mirrors is variable to suit the eyes of the user; the mirrors may be moved across the inter-viewing box line to bring the images into register, and may be raised or lowered as necessitated by the size of the films.

(2) Stereo Binocular Viewing. This takes the form of prismatic binoculars, favoured due to their convenience in use. The films are placed side by side in a rectangular illuminant, the right stereo to the right, the left stereo to the left. With these each eye observes its own particular film by means of a prism in each eye piece, and when the binoculars are adjusted properly the two images become merged into one three–dimensional image.

With both the above units the mirror image is obtained and to off-set this the films should be turned over in their respective viewing boxes, i.e. with the tube aspect of each film facing the illuminant, e.g. the markers were placed to read correctly from the tube they will now read,

_⌐Я Left Viewing Box   ЯЯ Right Viewing Box

A dual stereoscope is shown in (2228) which enables two observers to view a stereoscopic pair of films at the same time. Both see the same aspect, although one sees the image upside down.

Direct-measuring stereoscope

A precision stereoscope enables actual direct readings to be made of internal dimensions, such as for the pelvic diameters. The accuracy of the film positions from taking to viewing must be infallible; the cassettes are clamped into identical positions for each exposure so that metal pointers on the Bucky tray (2229), which appear on the film, coincide with similar pointers on the viewing boxes (2230). An indicator of known dimension, say 4 inches (10·15 centimetres), may consist of two metal arrowheads mounted in a narrow transparent base, with the extreme points exactly four inches apart. The indicator is placed transversely at about the level of the symphysis pubis, to be included on the stereographs. Accurate displacement of the tube between exposures is essential. The stereographs on being viewed in the precision stereoscope, using the known dimension of the 4 inch indicator for guidance to the correct pelvic diameter measurements are projected as a stereoscopic (three-dimensional) image.

The direct-measuring stereoscope enables the pelvis diameters to be read off on the scale attached, as the scale is adjusted to each diameter in turn (2233). The mirrors are semi-transparent so that the scale can be seen as inside the object.

In place of using the precision or direct-measurement stereoscopes, the diameters may be calculated from the stereographs by applying simple mathematical formulae similar to those later discussed for the localization of foreign bodies, Section 32.

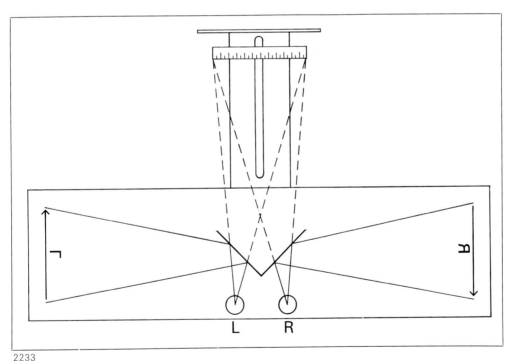

2233

L   R

30

FEMALE REPRODUCTIVE SYSTEM

FEMALE REPRODUCTIVE SYSTEM

The female genital, or reproductive, system consists of the ovaries, the uterine (fallopian) tubes, the uterus and the vagina, shown diagrammatically in (2234) and the external genitals or vulva. The uterus, a thick-walled muscular and expansile organ having a "T"–shaped cavity, is situated in the mid-line of the pelvic cavity, between the bladder and the rectum. It consists of three parts, the fundus, or upper, expanded portion; the cervix or neck, the lower, constricted portion; and the body, this last being the region between fundus and cervix. In the virgin state approximately 3 inches in length and 2 inches in width (2235), the uterus expands during pregnancy into the umbilical region, and then measures 12 inches or more in length and 9 inches to 10 inches in width (2236). The uterus lies between the uterine tubes, which are on either side of and below the level of the fundus, and extends in a backward and downward direction to its junction with the vagina, into which the cervix protrudes. The vagina follows a downward and forward direction (2234, 2235). The ovaries, or reproductive glands, of which there are two, one in each side of the pelvis, vary in position and may lie anywhere from just below the postero-lateral brim of the pelvis —in the ovarian fossa—to close to the side of the uterus. Their position may be indicated on the surface of the body by the mid-point of a line drawn from the upper border of the symphysis pubis to the anterior–superior iliac spines.

Each uterine tube is about 4 inches long and connects the upper and lateral part of the uterus with its respective ovary, the narrow central canal being continuous with the uterine cavity; at the ovarian end, the tube does not quite make contact with the ovary, but expands and opens into the peritoneal cavity, the opening being fringed with processes named fimbriae, one of which makes contact with the ovary (2234).

The vagina encircles the lower part of the cervix and extends downward and forward to the external genitals, or vulva (2234, 2235). The vagina is directed upward and backward, but the uterus is anteverted and anteflexed.

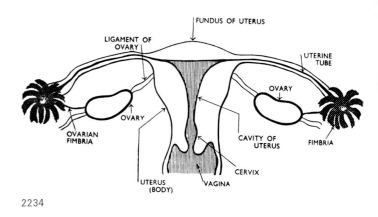

2234

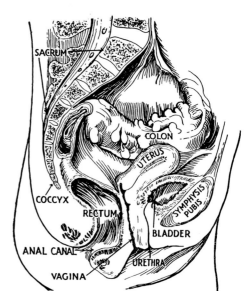

A MEDIAN SAGITTAL SECTION THROUGH THE FEMALE PELVIS
2235

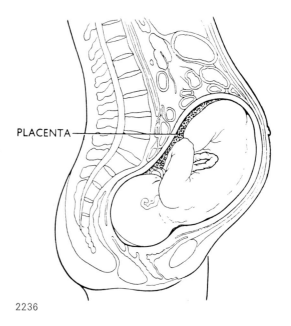

2236

682

Pelvis

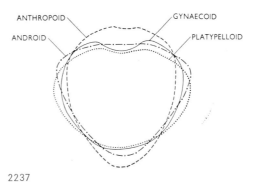

2237

The shape and size of the pelvis is very important in its effect on child-birth. The pelvic brim (2237) may be large and almost circular, this being referred to as the gynaecoid type; elongated and narrow, described as the oval or anthropoid type; broad and shallow with wide subpubic arch, termed the flat or platypelloid type; or almost triangular with narrow subpubic arch, referred to as the android type. Individual consideration is given to the congentially misshapen pelvis.

The shape of the pubic arch must also be considered and three types are shown in (2238). On placing a disc 9·3 centimetres in diameter on the radiograph, within the arch, the distance from the lower border of the symphysis pubis to the uppermost edge of the disc is observed. This is referred to as the "Waste Space of Morris" and normally measures 1 centimetre. The sacral curve varies from subject to subject to affect the capacity of the pelvis, as shown in (2239).

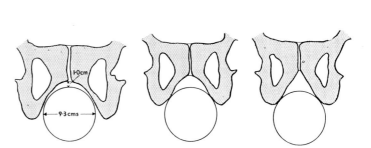

2238

Range of examinations

This section deals chiefly with the examination of the pregnant patient for the presence, number, age, position and condition of the foetus, and for the position of the placenta, when the examination is referred to as placentography. Included also is mensuration of the pelvic apertures, termed pelvimetry, and of the foetal head, termed cephalometry, which in the future may well be related to scanning by ultrasound.

The examination for patency of the uterine tubes is given under hysterosalpingography (uterosalpingography) and of the internal organs generally under gynaecography.

Urography in pregnancy and Radiography of the stillborn foetus are also included.

Although a full range of possible projections for the pregnant subject is given in the following pages, their application is severely limited in view of the radiation hazards involved embracing both mother and infant, the hazard for the infant being greater in the early stages of pregnancy. Thus, X-ray examination of the pregnant patient is confined to subjects when it is essential to the well-being of both mother and child to have this additional aid for guidance to subsequent procedures. The examination is limited to one or maybe two exposures, usually either antero–posterior or postero–anterior and/or the erect lateral projection, but which latter, of necessity, may have to be replaced by horizontal positioning. These four projections are therefore recorded as (BASIC).

From department to department the radiologist may have very different rulings on the X-ray examination of the pregnant subject which must be followed implicitly.

Even so, there is the unusual development in which it can be of greater importance for the well-being of the dual lives concerned to have further X-ray evidence as against a small increase in radiation exposure, the one risk being balanced against the other. Hence, the inclusion of all possible projections for guidance in positioning as required.

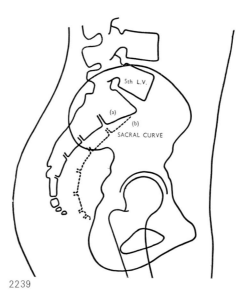

2239

Care of patient

A large three-quarter length gown, with back neck fastening, is comfortable for the patient in moving about the X-ray suite and is readily adjusted to avoid hindrance in the necessarily exacting X-ray positioning. Before the examination, patients should be instructed to evacuate the bladder and, if possible, the bowel.

Every care should be taken to avoid undue discomfort or shock to the patient. Although some of the positions and conditions of examination would appear to be difficult to achieve, the requirements, including possibly compression for certain projections, is readily followed when the patient is given the necessary assistance and encouragement. It should be noted, that when it is acceptable to use compression, the compression band must be broad enough to give even pressure over the whole of the abdomen, necessitating the use of a linen band 16 inches in width. The effect of satisfactory compression is to give all-over even density, with complete immobility, in addition to considerable reduction in exposure.

For demonstration purposes, a plastic band replaces the usual linen band and only moderate compression is shown in the following pages.

All information required by the radiologist should be carefully recorded for each patient, with infallible identification of radiograph with patient concerned.

Exposure conditions

The use of fast intensifying screens and an efficient grid is essential. For certain projections the moving grid in conjunction with sheet tin as a selective filter to give added absorption of scatter improves the result.

Designed for use at a specified distance, a set of rectangular diaphragms should be available to cover each size of film required for these examinations.

The focus–film distance may vary from 36–40 to 48 inches. Combining the advantages of high tube and transformer output with fast film and screens, exposure time is reduced to a minimum to secure a film excluding movement of the foetus; movement being relatively greater when an excess of amniotic fluid (liquor amnii) is present, a condition referred to as hydramnios. Opinion is divided as to whether exposure should be made on arrested inspiration or expiration.

Because opinion is again divided as to the correct penetration for these examinations, two sets of exposure factors for selected positions are included in the table on page 676, at medium and high voltages. Again, it should be mentioned that the conventional use of a 2 millimetre aluminium filter reduces radiation to the patient by approximately 50 per cent.

Radiation protection

Excessive radiation, to be deplored at all times, is particularly to be avoided during the possible reproductive years. Throughout pregnancy, strict precautions are of paramount importance, the use of fast films and fast intensifying screens being clearly indicated. Repeat exposures should be avoided and, in view of genetic hazards, X-ray examination of the pregnant subject should be confined to absolute essentials. Although the limits imposed on such investigations vary somewhat with different authorities, the specific examination for pelvimetry is employed only in exceptional circumstances.

The chief concern for the effects of radiation, although not entirely agreed or proved, is the possibility of mutations which can be hereditary, and malignant disease such as leukaemia. The skin dose received by the mother is also a matter for care. (See supplement 2.)

Note—It is usual for all mothers to have a chest examination to eliminate the possibility of tuberculosis, when a protective apron should cover the abdomen from below the diaphragm.

Hysterosalpingography

The X-ray examination for the patency of the uterine tubes involves the use of an opaque medium by injection through the cervix into the uterus. This examination of the non-pregnant subject, which may also include air insufflation, is used for investigation of sterility, repeated abortion, and for the presence of fibroids or tumours.

Again, radiation exposure must be reduced to a minimum and as a permanent radiographic record is essential, visual screening is considered to be unnecessary except, perhaps, with the image intensifier when it may be important to follow the passage of the opaque medium from the uterus through the tubes to the spill into the peritoneum. One or two exposures in the supine position usually suffice, but occasionally an oblique projection may be required.

The opaque medium may be a water soluble organic iodine compound such as sodium diatrizoate (Urografin 75 per cent or Hypaque 85 per cent) which is rapid in action so that the spill into the peritoneal cavity can be seen almost immediately and it is soon reabsorbed, or alternatively iodized oil which may take up to twenty-four hours to reach the peritoneal cavity and is not readily absorbable. (Refer to supplement 1.)

The patient

It is very necessary to reassure the worried and nervous patient and to create a feeling of friendly understanding. Preparation is important to ensure that the rectum and bladder are evacuated before the injection.

Premedication commences two hours before the X-ray examination so that the patient is well sedated and relaxed at the appointed time. Possibly only 5 per cent of patients may be given a general anaesthetic.

Technique

With the patient in the lithotomy position the special uterine catheter (bulbous backed to prevent leakage) is introduced into the cervix of the uterus. The limbs are then lowered and the patient is moved gently along the couch to be centred in relation to the X-ray tube—2 inches above the symphysis pubis. When all is ready a portable (or hanging) lead protection plaque is placed over the hands of the surgeon (2240). After injection of approximately 12 millilitres of the opaque medium, exposure is made immediately and the film is developed with all speed. When both uterine tubes are patent and show a normal spill into the peritioneal cavity (2241) the catheter is withdrawn. When there is no spill into the peritioneal cavity on one or both sides (2242), up to 20 millilitres of opaque medium may be injected and a further exposure made.

(2243a,b) show the effect (a) of injecting 4 millilitres of Urografin, followed (b) by a further injection to a total of 8 millilitres, shown to be in excess for this subject.

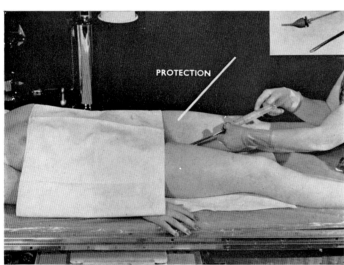

2240

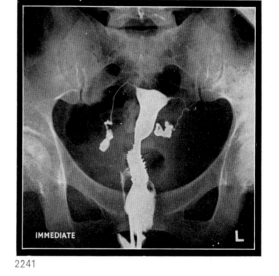

2241

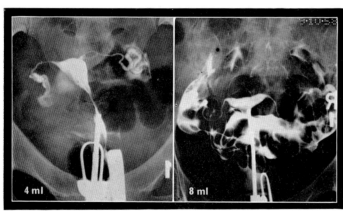

2243a 2243b

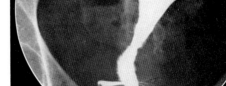

2242

Gynaecography

Air insufflation into the peritoneal cavity with the patient suitably positioned to allow the air to pass into the raised pelvis, enables the uterus, the uterine tubes, the ovaries and sometimes the broad ligament to be demonstrated.

After suitable premedication, with the patient supine, using local anaesthesia the abdominal wall is perforated for the passage of a small rubber catheter into the peritoneal cavity the catheter being attached to an oxygen cylinder. On rotating the patient into the prone position on the tilting table, the head is lowered with the trunk at an angle of approximately 20 degrees. Carbon Dioxide Gas is released into the peritoneal cavity at the rate of 300 millilitres per minute to a total of 2 litres. As there is some discomfort to the patient the unit is in readiness with the tube centred in direction to the coccyx to the level of the anterior–superior iliac spines with cephalid tube angulation of approxi-

mately 10 degrees. Rapid development is essential for the radiograph to be seen in less than two minutes. The gas disperses automatically and fairly rapidly (2244,2245).

For Exposure Factors see page 712.

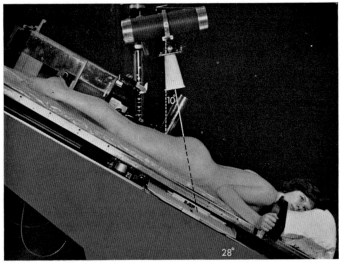

2244

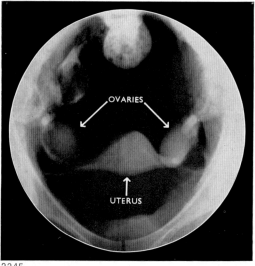

2245

Early Pregnancy

Postero-anterior

The patient is placed in the prone position, in the centre of the couch, with support under the ankles. The broad Bucky band is firmly applied for immobilization.

■ Centre below the coccyx, with the tube angled approximately 15 degrees toward the head to enable the sacral bone to be projected above the level of the foetus. The exposure should be made on arrested respiration

Should the foetus not be detected in the initial film, it may be necessary to increase contrast by reducing the kilovoltage, or an antero–posterior projection may be advisable with a caudal tube angle of 15 degrees.

Radiograph (2247) shows a thirteen to fifteen week foetus lying transversely at the level of the sacro-coccygeal articulation. Radiograph (2248) shows a twenty to twenty-two week foetus.

For Exposure Factors see page 712.

Advanced Pregnancy

During the later stages of pregnancy, and particularly at full term, it is again essential to obtain maximum definition to show the foetus in all its detail, and especially to show the position of the placenta in relation to the foetus and to the maternal pelvis. A high standard of radiography enables decisions to be reached on multiplicity, page 702, presentation, pages 688 to 690, extension of limbs (2293); the presence of excessive fluid obscuring the foetus; on foetal maturity estimated within two weeks aided by epiphyseal development which is important because the foetus is mobile up to thirty-four weeks and can be turned, but later becomes stable. It also facilitates detection of foetal abnormality, including foetal death, page 701, anencephalia (absence of brain), and hydrocephalus (enlarged skull).

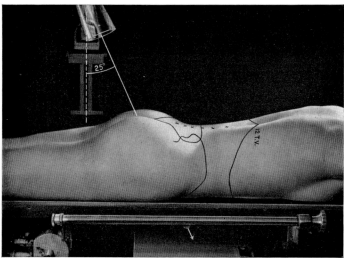

2246

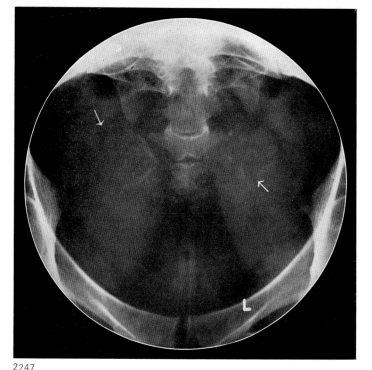

2247

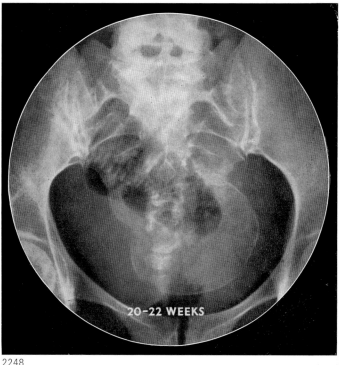

2248

Antero-posterior (Basic)

The patient is placed in the supine position, central to the X-ray couch, with the hands clasped over the upper chest and with a small sandbag under the knees (2249). In applying the 16 inch wide linen band for immobilization on compression being used (2250), the patient is invited to complain on feeling any discomfort and the band is then gradually tightened with a final, firm adjustment just before the exposure is made. The band is released with equal care immediately following the exposure, which is made on arrested respiration.

On using compression, movement of both mother and foetus is limited, and the tissues are reduced to an all-over measured thickness to produce a radiograph showing the maximum definition, detail and contrast.

■ Centre to the apex of the abdominal curve at the approximate level of the fourth to fifth lumbar vertebrae to include the symphysis pubis, using the appropriate rectangular diaphragm for the 14 × 17 inch film. 2249,2250,2251,2252

For Exposure Factors see page 712.

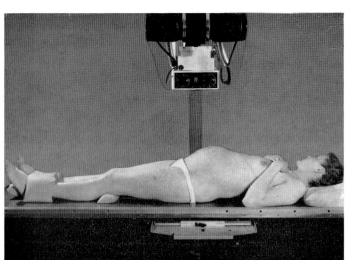

2249

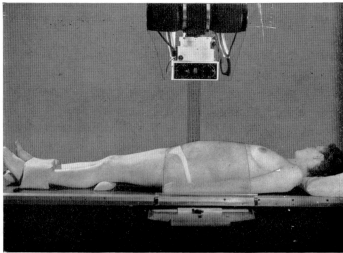

2250

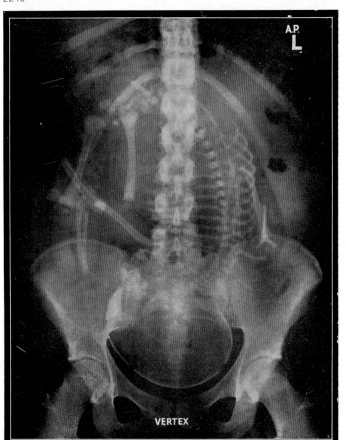

2251

VERTEX

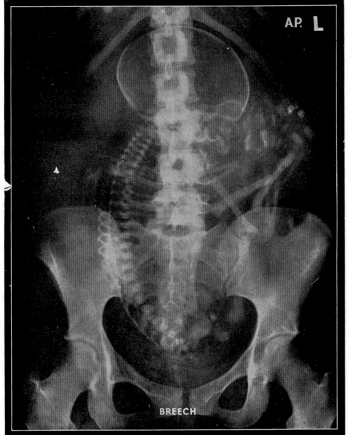

2252

BREECH

Postero-anterior (Basic)

The patient is assisted into the prone position central to the X-ray couch. The head is turned to one side and a sandbag is placed under the ankles. Positioning is continued with the following alternatives: (a) when only gravitational compression is permitted, the position of the arms gives slight support (2253); (b) when full compression is allowed, the arms hang from the sides of the couch and the wide compressor band is used to give general firm pressure (2254); (c) when pressure over the abdomen must be avoided, plastic blocks are placed under the chest and pelvis and the hands are clasped under the chest (2257).

■ Centre to the apex of the abdominal curve, at the approximate level of the fourth to fifth lumbar vertebrae using the appropriate diaphragm for the 14 × 17 inch film. Again, exposure is made on arrested respiration (2253,2254,2255,2256, 2257).

In this position the foetus is very well defined, particularly the foetal head, which is nearer to the film than in 2251. Comparison should be made of the two projections for a vertex presentation (2251,2255) and for a breech presentation (2252,2256).

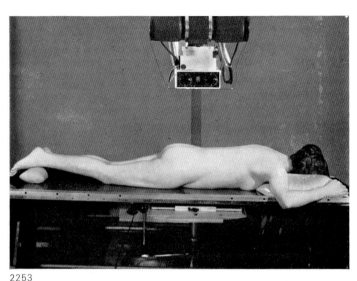

2253

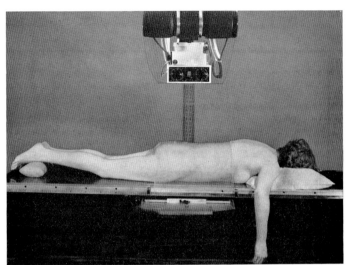

2254

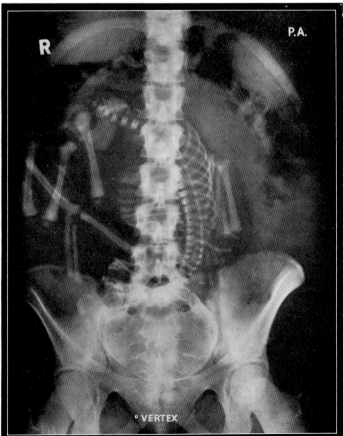

2255

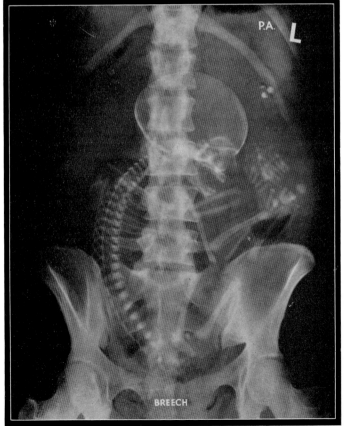

2256

Lateral (Basic)

The patient is turned on to the side toward which the foetal spine is lying as shown in the antero–posterior radiograph (2251), and is supported in this lateral position with the limbs extended. To prevent rotation of the pelvis, the limbs are raised at the ankles to be symmetrical with the pelvis. Sponge pads are placed between the knees and between the ankle joints (2258). The upper arm is raised over the head to clasp the end of the couch for support and, when necessary, the compression band may be used to steady the patient in this position. When the limbs are flexed the symphysis pubis is obscured.

■ Centre at the level of the apex of the abdominal curve, midway between the lumbar vertebrae and the anterior margin of the abdomen. The 14 × 17 inch cassette is placed to include the lower border of the symphysis pubis. Again, exposure is made on arrested respiration

For Exposure Factors see page 712.

It should be noted that when exposure is made on inspiration combined with the raised uppermost arm, the abdomen assumes a very satisfactory lateral position. Two radiographs show a vertex presentation (2259) and a breech presentation (2260) to link appropriately with the subjects shown on pages 688 and 689. In the latter radiograph (2260), the placenta is visible at the anterior wall and fundus of the uterine body and in (2259) anterior to the ventral aspect of the foetus.

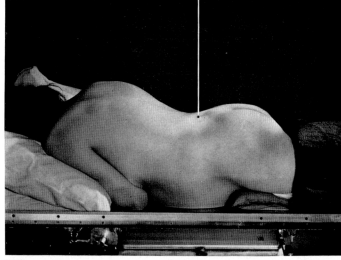

2257

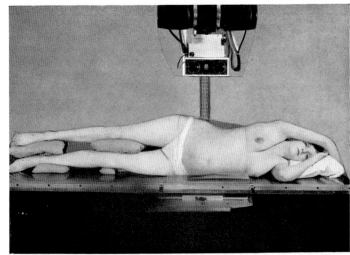

2258

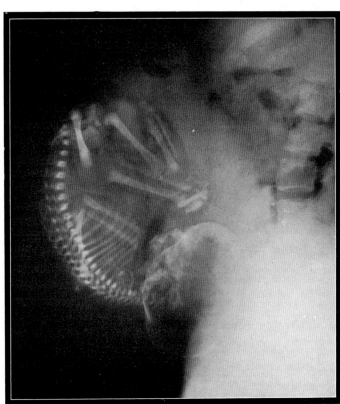

2259

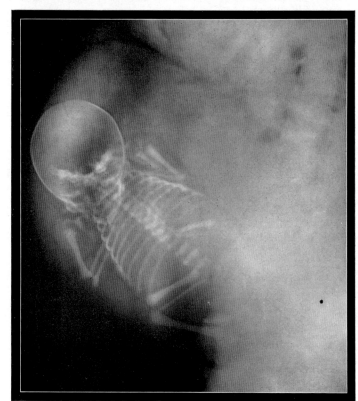

2260

Lateral-supine (1)

For consideration of foetal head measurements, the lateral projection is taken with the patient supine, or prone, to be linked with the antero–posterior and postero-anterior projections respectively.

Having exposed for the antero-posterior position, the tube is lowered for horizontal projection and the pedestal-type Bucky diaphragm is used in the vertical position. The patient is moved across the couch to bring the side of the trunk into contact with the Bucky support.

■ Centre with the X-ray tube lowered for horizontal centring, (a) for a general projection of the subject as indicated on seeing the antero–posterior exposure or (b) for the head of the foetus (2264), usually well down in the pelvis at this stage (2261,2262)

Lateral-supine (2)

An alternative lateral projection may be taken with the couch angled from 20 to 35 degrees toward the feet, when at near term the head may be shown in the "engaged" position.

The patient lies with the feet firmly planted against a foot-rest.

It may be necessary to raise the trunk slightly to ensure that the essential area is included on the film. The cassette and stationary grid are supported in the vertical position against the side of the trunk.

■ Centre laterally to the pelvis to cover the foetal head, using a 10 × 12 inch film (2263,2264)

Note—Radiographs of the foetal head for the two right-angled projections required for cephalometry should be taken without moving the patient between exposures, either in the erect or in the supine position.

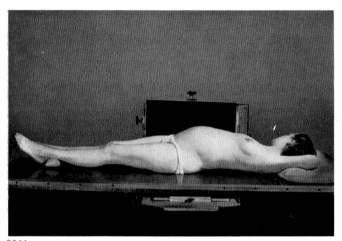

2261

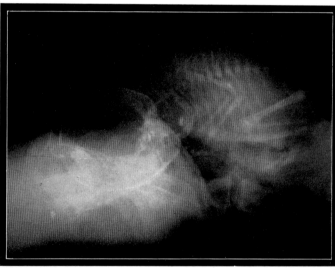

2262

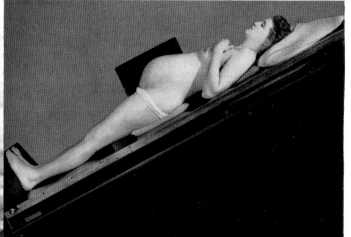

2263

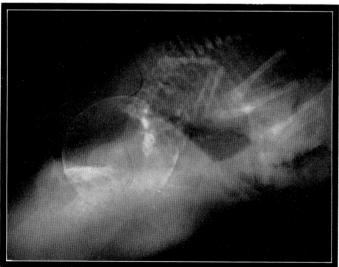

2264

Lateral-erect (Basic)

The effect of gravity at term is, in most subjects, to bring the foetal head well down into the maternal pelvis and the erect lateral position serves this purpose. If this projection is to be used for estimating pelvimetry measurements, it is essential to obtain a true lateral position.

The patient stands sideways with the appropriate near hip against the vertical Bucky stand and with the feet separated to preserve balance. On viewing the patient from side, front and back, careful adjustment is made to avoid any tilting or rotation of the pelvis (2266,a,b,2267).

The prominence of the greater trochanter is placed $2\frac{1}{2}''$ below the centre of the grid, the 10 × 12 inch film and the additional stationary grid being placed transversely (2268). The measured distance between the tube focus and median plane of the pelvis may be recorded to enable the mid-pelvis to fim distance to be established for pelvimetry measurements as required. The immobilizing band is used to steady the patient in position.

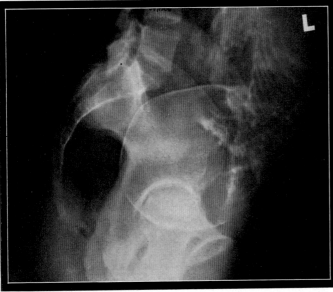

2265

■ Centre two-and-a-half inches above the prominence of the greater trochanter to be central to the grid and film. With careful positioning and centring, the appropriate rectangular diaphragm will include the essential area on the 10 × 12 inch film (2267). In a satisfactory lateral projection, the femoral heads are coincident. The addition of the stationary grid, placed at right angles to the slats of the moving grid, reduces the effect of the considerable scattered radiation occurring in this very dense region (2265)

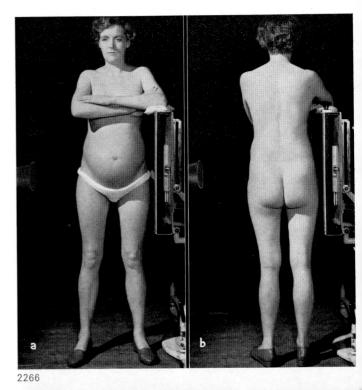

2266

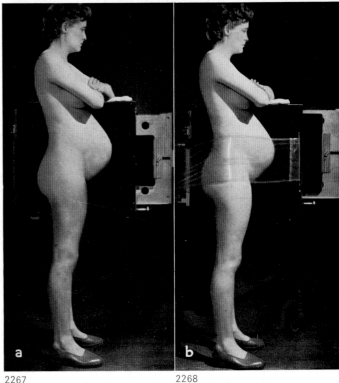

2267   2268

Note—Reference should be made to (2315), page 706 for the essential areas to be defined for pelvimetry measurements which may be the main requirement of this erect lateral projection.

For a general lateral projection, the patient is positioned as shown in (2268), using a 14 × 17 inch film.

Two radiographs (2269,2270) of the same subject, reported as a posterior placenta praevia, show the difference between the erect and horizontal postures.

On studying the antero–posterior (2251) and postero–anterior (2255) radiographs, a following lateral projection would be taken with the foetal spine (left) toward the film (2259); when the foetal spine is obscured in the mid-line, an oblique projection may be necessary (2271).

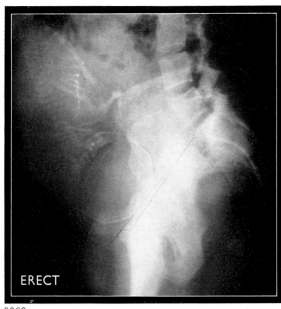

ERECT

2269

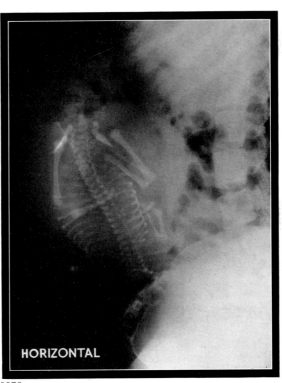

HORIZONTAL

2270

Left posterior oblique

When the shadows of the foetal and maternal vertebrae are not entirely separated in the initial radiograph, a second exposure may be made in the oblique position.

On examining the antero–posterior radiograph, it will be found that the foetus is lying toward the right, or left side (2251), page 675. The patient is then placed laterally with the foetal spine toward the couch, in this instance the left side, and is then rotated backward through approximately 45 degrees with the limbs extended. The foetus tends to fall toward the couch. The patient is supported in position by plastic sponge blocks placed under the hip, shoulder and limb of the raised side, and the use of the compression band assists immobilization (2272). The same position is shown for the right side in the right posterior oblique position (2273).

■ Centre over the side nearest the film, at the level of the estimated mid-point of the foetal spine, to include the whole of the foetus. The 14 × 17 inch film is placed to include the lower border of the symphysis pubis (2272,2273,2271)

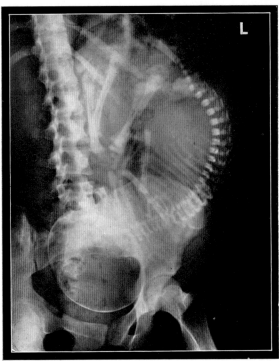

2271

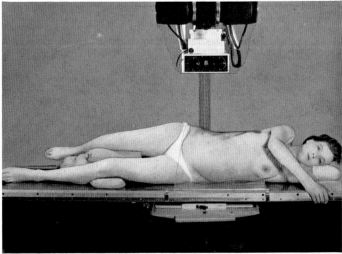

2272

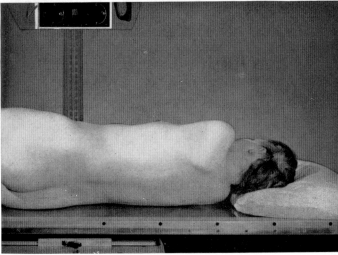

2273

Supero-inferior for pelvic inlet

This projection to show the pelvic inlet can no longer be tolerated as a routine exposure on the pregnant subject. As will be seen, a vertex presentation in this position may well bring the foetal gonads within dangerous range of X-ray source.

This technique is therefore included only as an indication of the possible projection of the foetal head within the pelvic aperture and for guidance on the possibility that the position might be required under very special circumstances to show the shape of the pelvic brim.

The patient sits on the grid with the back supported at an angle of approximately 55 degrees and the feet resting on the floor, or a back rest may be fitted to the X-ray couch to allow the knees to flex over the end of the couch. The back-rest has a cut-away base to allow free access for positioning the pelvis with the brim parallel to the film. This is achieved when the upper surface of the symphysis pubis and the space between the fourth and fifth lumbar spinous processes are equidistant from the film (2274), see also (2318) page 707.

A small localizing cone reduces the effect of the extensive scatter which is inevitable for this projection. A centring plumb-bob is shown in radiograph (2275).

■ Centre between the anterior–superior iliac spines, approximately 2 inches behind the symphysis pubis, using a 10 × 12 inch film. High kilovoltage output will ensure that the whole of the pelvic brim is visible (2274,2275,2276,2277,2278)

For exposure factors see page 712.

30

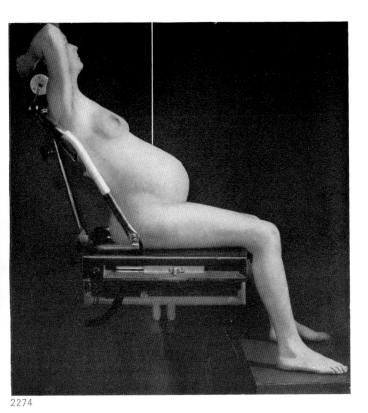

2274

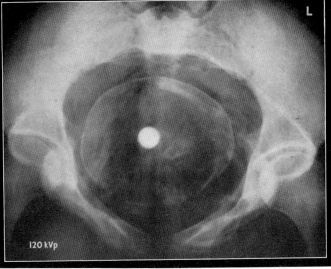

120 kVp

2275

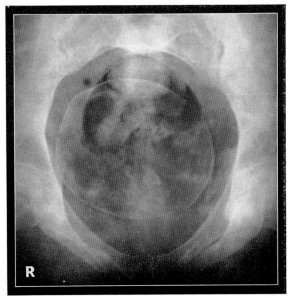

2276

From the antero–posterior radiograph when the obturator foramina appear to be shallow in shape, very little movement is required to a reclining position, but if the rami are widely separated showing the full extent of the obturator foramina, it will be necessary for the patient to sit almost upright to bring the brim of the pelvis into position.

Considerable movement of the upper trunk may take place without changing the established position of the pelvis (2277, 2278), and it may be necessary to lower the back-rest by as much as 10 degrees to avoid the projection of dense breast shadows over the posterior border of the pelvic brim (2274,2275).

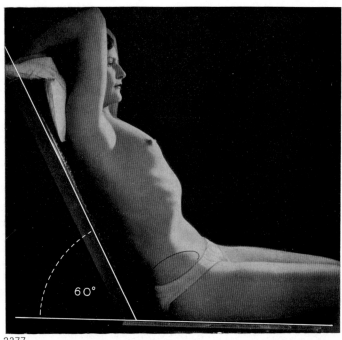

2277

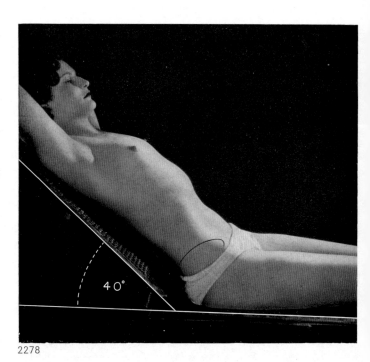

2278

Supero-inferior for pelvic outlet and subpubic arch

Again, this is not a routine projection but of interest in seeing foetal–pelvic relationship in this position and is retained in view of the possibility of such a projection being required under special circumstances.

Seated on the pelvimetry stool, or on the end of the couch with the feet resting on a bench and with the legs widely separated, the patient is asked to flex gently forward from the hip joints, so that the abdomen descends between the legs until it is estimated that the subpubic arch is parallel to the film. The degree of flexion will vary from subject to subject but, with care, a satisfactory projection of the subpubic arch and the intertuberous diameter will be obtained. Unless the arms are unusually short, the hands rest at foot level (2279) rather than on a vertical support (2281).

■ Centre over the apex of the subpubic arch with a compensating tube angulation of 5 to 10 degrees toward the head when the patient is unable to bend forward sufficiently to obtain a satisfactory projection (2279,2281,2280)

As will be noted in (2281), this projection may be made with a stationary grid using an 8 × 10 inch film.

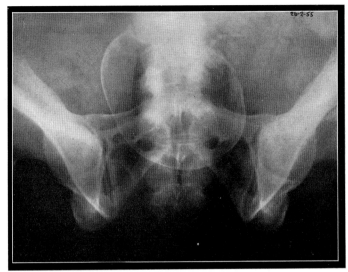

2280

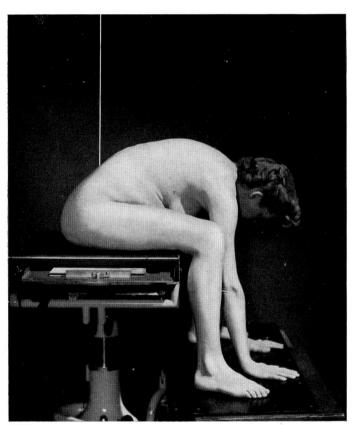

2279

2281

Placentography

At near term, it is essential to know the position of the placenta within the uterus in relation to the foetus and the maternal pelvis (2236), page 670. This fusiform-shaped soft tissue shadow tends to become visible by calcification at from thirty-two to thirty-four weeks. The use of filtration, compression and selective exposure techniques, at short exposure time, enables soft structures to be visualized when the placenta may be shown against the anterior, posterior or lateral uterine wall, at the upper surface or tundus of the uterus, or at the presenting aspect when the position may constitute an anterior, posterior or lateral wall placenta praevia, placenta before foetus. This condition can be demonstrated by cystography, which is not stressed because of the radiation involved except, perhaps, under very special circumstances. However, for guidance to the meaning of placenta praevia two series of cystograms have been retained on page 705, showing a normal presentation (2308 to 2310), and the condition of placenta praevia (2311 to 2313) is reported as a posterior wall placenta praevia with forward displacement of the foetal head and (2283) as an anterior wall placenta praevia with backward displacement of the foetal head.

Technically, the lateral view presents considerable difficulty in view of the steep absorption difference existing between the posterior and anterior soft tissue aspect of the abdomen. Several methods are advocated in order that this difficulty may be overcome.

Exposing normally for the heavy posterior aspect results in excessive exposure to the soft tissue anterior aspect of the abdomen. The total area however can be visualized by providing suitable intensity of illumination to view each aspect. Normal intensity for the correctly exposed area and high intensity viewing (photoflood) to suit the excessive density of the anterior part.

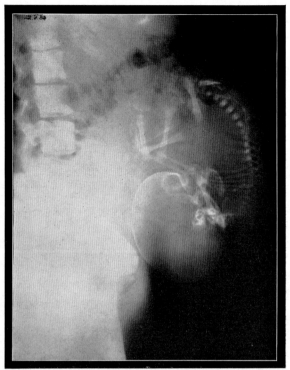

2283

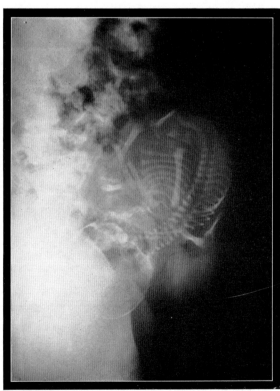

2282

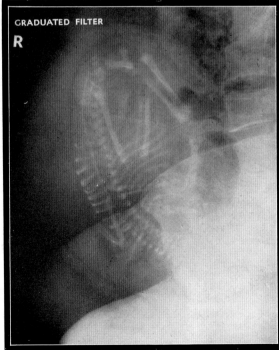

2284

Graduated (Differential) Filter: This method adopts the principle of using a graduated thickness of either aluminium, or a plastic wedge incorporating suitable lead equivalent. This is inserted in the tube outlet with the greatest thickness directed to the anterior soft tissue abdominal aspect. The intensity of the beam will be diminished in accordance with the thickness of the part of the filter through which the beam has traversed. This results in a greater uniformity of density between the respective areas.

(2284) A graduated aluminium filter for the lateral projection shows the placenta against the anterior uterine wall.

(2285,2286,2287) Shows the placenta with confirmation of position against the anterior uterine wall in the right and left lateral views, taken with a plastic lead filter. As the placenta may be shown more clearly in right and left lateral projections both may be included.

(2288,2289,2290) With compression giving all over even density the calcified placenta is shown very clearly.

Compression: This makes the total area more compact but the method may not be generally favoured.

Off-centring: With the patient centred to the table, off-centring of the tube 2 inches from the mid-line towards the spine results in the grid acting as a graduated filter with the effect that there is a greater uniformity of density between the two areas.

The necessity of having to open up the diaphragm to accommodate the greater coverage however may be considered detrimental.

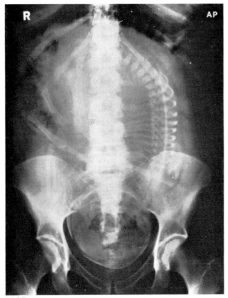

2285

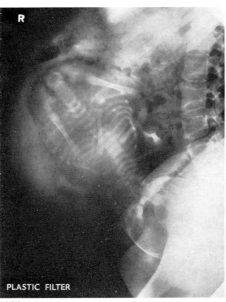

2286

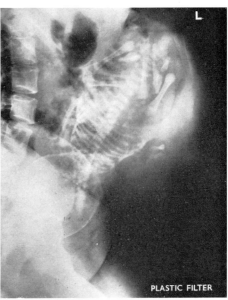

2287

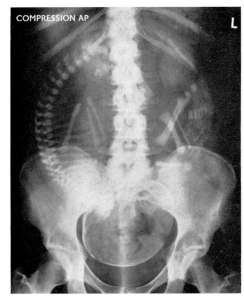

2288

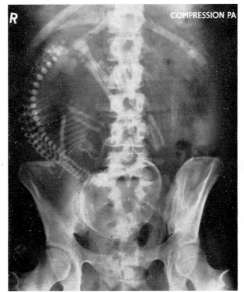

2289

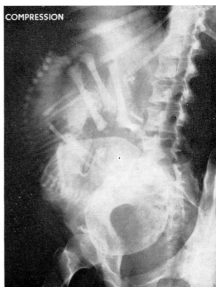

2290

Multiple radiography

A most valuable asset to placentography is the technique for producing two radiographs of differing densities on a single exposure. For this technique two films are placed, one each between two pairs of intensifying screens of different speeds within one cassette. The screens are placed within the cassette in reversed speed order with the fast screen pair towards the top and the slow screens in intimate contact behind. On giving the routine exposure for the heavy posterior aspect the film with the fast screen will record this level of density. The film within the rear screens will automatically record a density level suited to the anterior soft tissue aspect, due to the slower speed of the screens, and the reduced intensity of the beam due to filtration through the first screen pair. Accepted features of this approach are, that patient exposure is reduced in using the fast screen combination to record the heavy density region. The range of information on each film combined is considerably greater than on one film alone.

(2291a,b) Demonstrates the range of densities recorded on each separate film with multiple radiography.

(2292) Shows the placenta after delivery.

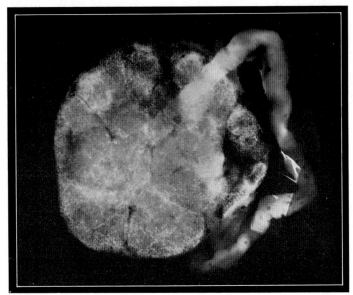

2292

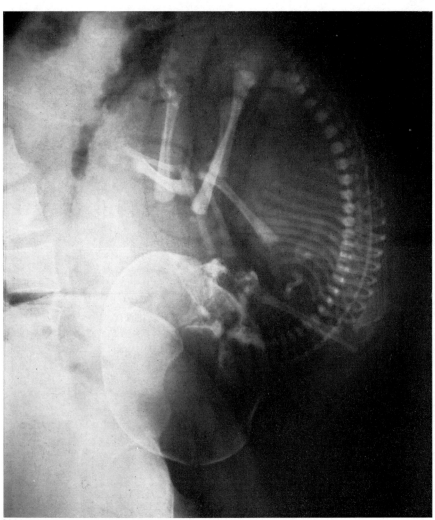

2291a

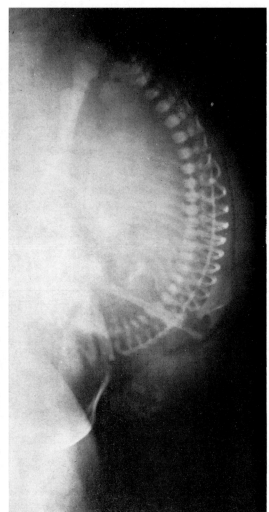

2291b

Female reproductive system
Advanced pregnancy

Foetal maturity

To estimate the age of the foetus by the stage of development of the epiphyses, it is necessary to produce radiographs of the highest quality, with satisfactory definition, suitable density and good contrast. The first essential is complete immobilization. As previously stated the age of the foetus and foetal maturity can be estimated within two weeks. This is important because the foetus is mobile up to thirty-four weeks and can be turned for instance, from the breech position shown in (2293,2252) to a vertex presentation (2251), page 679; after thirty-four weeks the foetus becomes stable.

It is also important to record the position of the limbs, whether extended (2293) or flexed as shown in the majority of the radiographs in this section.

Foetal death

When the death of the foetus is suspected, or it may be unsuspected, it is important to obtain a clear projection of the foetal head for evidence of overlapping of the cranial sutures, a condition which indicates foetal death and is referred to as Spalding's sign, shown in (2294). Gas in the foetal cavities is also an indication of foetal death (2295). Other indications are the unusually small size of the foetus, collapse of the foetus, and hyperextension of the foetal spine.

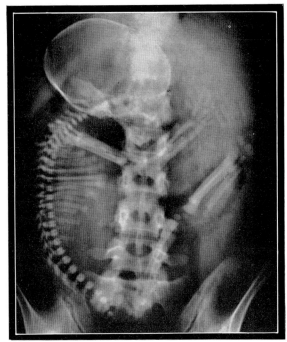

2293

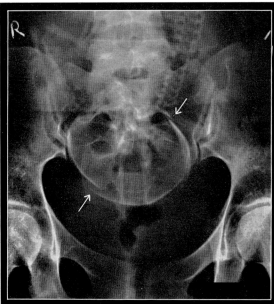

2294

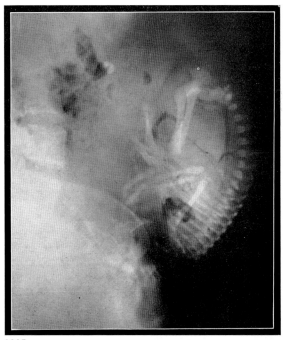

2295

Multiplicity

It is essential to produce radiographs of such quality that both head and vertebrae may be identified in at least two projections. Twins are shown in (2296), quadruplets in (2297,2298) and quintuplets in (2299). As will be seen, except in the case of the twins the antero-posterior projections are inclined to be less informative then the lateral projections. Finally Siamese twins are included, although it will be appreciated that the form of attachment varies (2300).

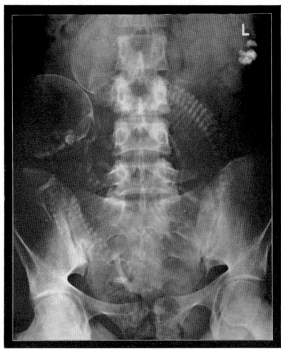

2296

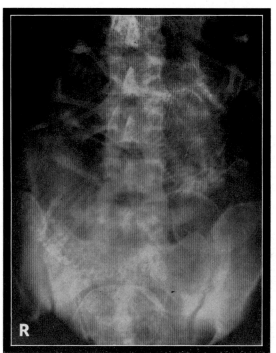

2297

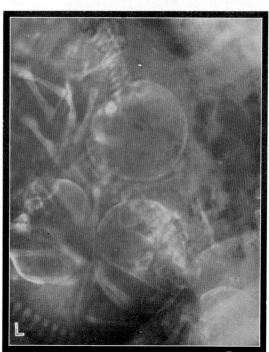

2298

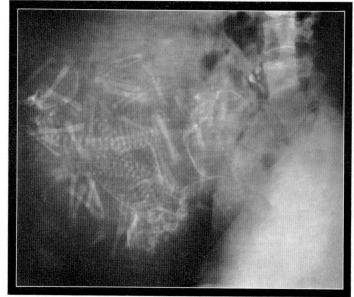

2299

The Foetus (Stillborn)

It may be necessary to examine the stillborn foetus of various ages. The series includes antero–posterior and lateral projections for foetuses of fifteen weeks (2301), of twenty-four to twenty-five weeks (2302) and of thirty-five weeks (2303). In producing these illustrations the relative dimensions have been retained to give the student an appreciation of size and development.

Although experimental exposures can be unlimited except for the cost of materials, a series of exposures is included for guidance to produce the maximum detail and definition.

Age	kVp	mAS	FFD	Film ILFORD	Screens ILFORD	Grid
15 weeks	40	100	30" 75cm	Rapid R (NS)	—	—
24/25 weeks	65	50	36" 90cm	Rapid R	HD	Grid
35 weeks	65	75	36" 90cm	Rapid R	HD	Grid

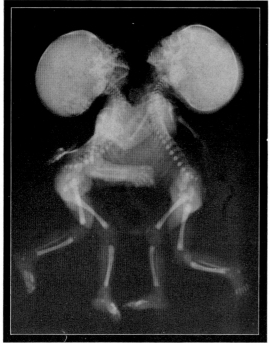

2300

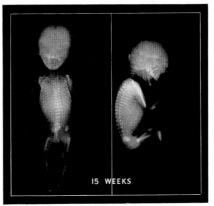

2301

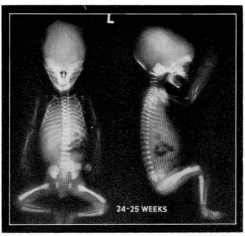

2302

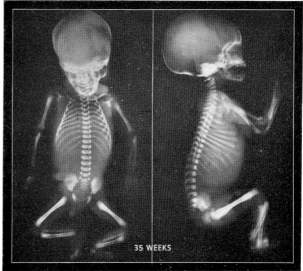

2303

Urography in pregnancy

Although to be avoided for a pregnant subject, nevertheless an examination of the urinary system may become necessary, when great care is taken to keep radiation to a minimum and avoiding undue disturbance to the patient generally. Radiographs are included for guidance as to appearance and radiographic quality and may be anticipated, embracing projections antero–posterior (2304) and postero–anterior (2305) for intravenous pyelography, and antero–posterior (2306) for the retrograde method.

As stated previously, the two series of cystograms on page 705 are included for instruction and guidance only for the condition of placenta praevia. Series (2308 to 2310) shows a normal foetal head to bladder relationship and series (2311 to 2313) was reported as a placenta praevia.

Aminography

Another rare undertaking is the replacement of some of the amniotic fluid surrounding the foetus by a contrast medium, such as diatrizoate (Hypaque 85 per cent or Urografin 75 per cent, see Supplement 1), to show the relative positions of the placenta and the foetus (2307). The amniotic fluid is sometimes present in excess, when the condition is referred to as hydramnios; on account of the added opacity, it may be necessary to increase exposure by from 25 to 50 per cent.

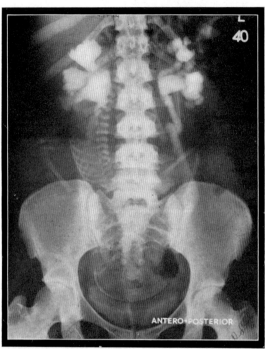

2304

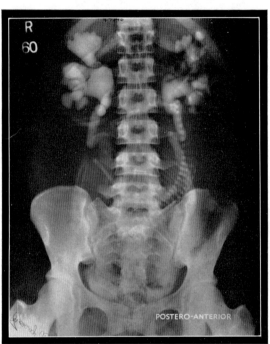

2305

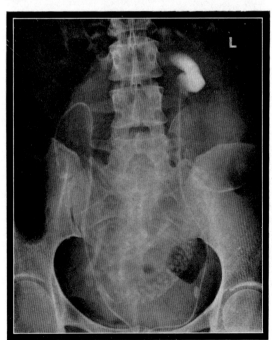

2306

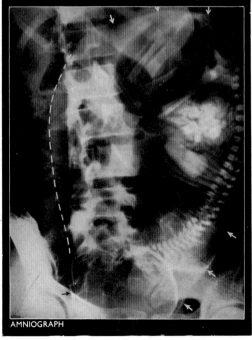

2307

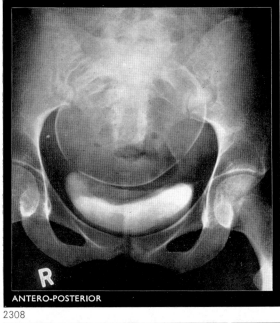

ANTERO-POSTERIOR

2308

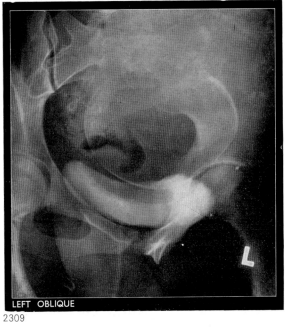

LEFT OBLIQUE

2309

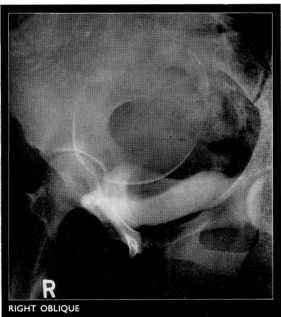

RIGHT OBLIQUE

2310

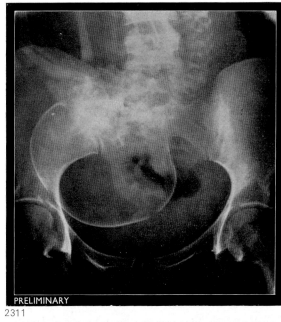

PRELIMINARY

2311

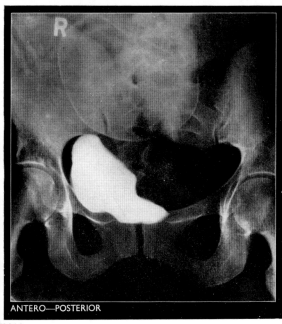

ANTERO—POSTERIOR

2312

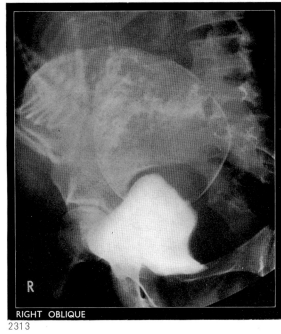

RIGHT OBLIQUE

2313

Pelvimetry

The dimensions of the pelvic inlet and outlet are required for possible disproportion to determine whether the pelvis is large enough for the foetus to pass through and be born in a natural manner; if the pelvis is too small or deformed, or in the presence of a placenta praevia, a Caesarean operation may be necessary, the foetus then being delivered by way of an incision in the abdominal and uterine walls.

As additional exposures for pelvimetry are not permissible, in anticipation of pelvimetry becoming necessary, the essential measurements are recorded for each patient at the initial examination. Before attempting pelvimetry, it is essential to ensure that all measurements indicated on the equipment are reliable.

There are several ways of carrying out this investigation and, according to the method employed, one or two projections are used. These are described in detail in the preceding pages:

(a) antero–posterior with the patient supine (2314),
(b) lateral with the patient erect (2315).

In describing the positions and in giving the exposure factors, a near-term subject is presumed.

Calculations and observations for these radiographs enable the radiologist to give considerable guidance on the conditions for delivery of the foetus.

As the X-ray beam diverges from an almost point source, all radiographs show some enlargement of the subject at the commonly used focus–film distances, and obviously the degree of enlargement depends on the extent of displacement of the subject plane from the film.

Thus, the investigation involves the establishment of the distance away from the film of each essential pelvic plane and thence the estimation of the actual dimensions from the enlarged image shown on the radiograph.

From the antero–posterior radiograph (2314), estimation can be made of:

(1) the transverse diameter of the pelvic inlet;
(2) the bi-ischial spinous diameter.

From the lateral radiograph (2315), estimation can be made of:

(1) the true conjugate, extending from the upper inner border of the symphysis pubis to the sacral promontory;
(2) the mid-plane, antero–posterior, extending from the middle of the inner border of the symphysis pubis to the middle of the third sacral segment;
(3) the outlet, extending from the lower inner border of the symphysis pubis to the tip of the scrum or, in the case of sacro-coccygeal fusion, to the lower inner border of the first coccygeal segment.

The angle of pelvic inclination can be estimated from lateral projections taken on flexion and extension, page 711.

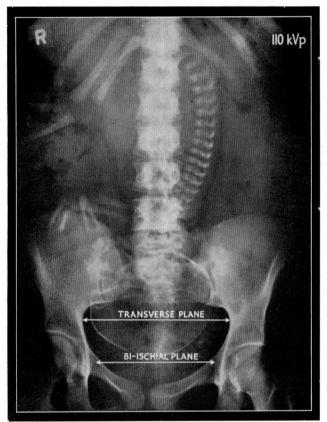

2314

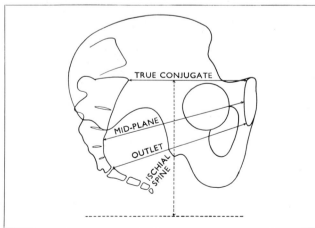

2316

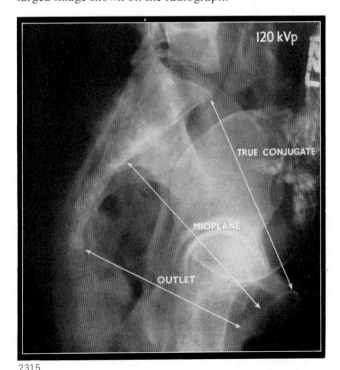

2315

When the foetal head, vertex presentation, is shown to be fully engaged in this lateral projection of the maternal pelvis (2315) and a satisfactory antero–posterior projection of the foetal head is shown in the appropriate projection, estimation may be made of the biparietal diameter of the foetal head. Alternatively, if the foetal head is fully engaged in the occipito–anterior or occipito–posterior position, the occipito–frontal and suboccipito–bregmatic diameters can be estimated.

Although the supero-inferior projection (2317,2318,2319) is no longer employed in view of the excessive radiation involved, it is interesting and informative to see the pelvic dimensions shown:

(1) the transverse diameter, extending from side to side at the widest points of the brim;
(2) the interspinous diameter, extending between the ischial spines (bi-ischial);
(3) the true conjugate, extending from the sacral promontory to the deep surface of the symphysis pubis;
(4) the oblique diameters, if required, extending from the ilio-pubic eminence on the one side to the brim at the sacroiliac articulation on the other side.

Again, although the supero–inferior radiograph to show the pelvic outlet and subpubic arch is rarely included, the following may be of interest; the estimation of the inter-tuberous diameter is considered to be only approximate, because of the difficulty in establishing the plane to film height and the position of the terminating points. On the other hand, it has been found by experiment that, at a focus–film distance of 28 inches, the correction factor for the intertuberous diameter is 0·9, so that on measuring the enlarged diameter on the film (2320) and multiplying by 0·9, the actual dimension is obtained.

Estimation of the normality of the subpubic arch is by experience as to being wide, average, or narrow.

30

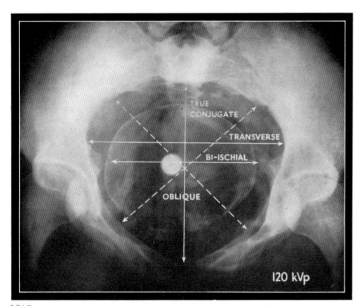

2317

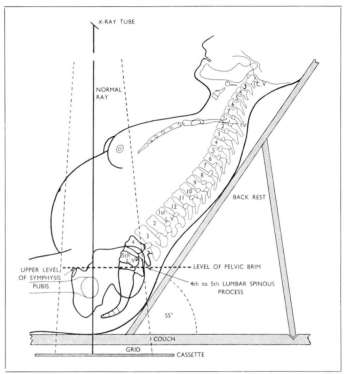

2318

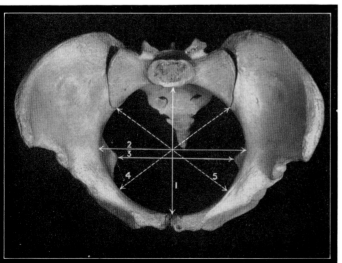

2319

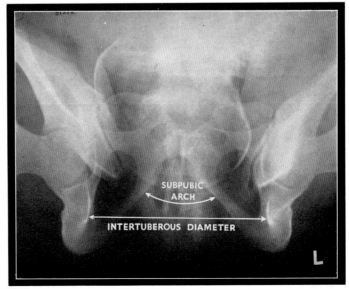

2320

707

Estimation of actual diameters

When all data are available as indicated, the five diameters seen in the antero–posterior and lateral projections may be determined by one of the following methods:

(a) mathematical formula;
(b) the use of a geometrical correction scale;
(c) the use of a perforated ruler.

(a) By mathematical formula:

A pair of dividers and a finely calibrated ruler should be used to take the necessary measurements from the enlarged film image. Then, by applying a corrective formula, the actual pelvic dimensions may be obtained; for example, the transverse diameters:

Actual pelvic measurement

$$= \frac{\text{Film diameter measurement} \times \text{focus–symphysis distance}}{\text{focus–film distance}}$$

For example, when the film diameter measurement is six inches, the focus–symphysis distance thirty-five inches, and the focus–film distance forty inches, then the actual pelvic diameter is:

$$\frac{6 \times 35}{40} = 5\tfrac{1}{4} \text{ inches}$$

It is usual to work to a prepared table embracing the various symphysis-to-film measurements, or to a graph on which these distances have been plotted against the film diameter measurements, thus enabling the actual diameters to be read off at the base of the graph.

For the ischial spines, the distance between the level of the true conjugate and the ischial spines may be ascertained by projection tracing of the lateral view (2315,2322), and this figure is deducted from the symphysis-to-film measurement made on the patient, to give the ischial spines-to-film measurement. The diameter at this level is then calculated as previously.

Pelvimetry calipers: To establish the level of the transverse diameters of the pelvis, it has been found that with the patient supine, the transverse plane of the pelvic inlet is at two-thirds of the distance of the upper border of the symphysis pubis from the table top, and that the bi-ischial diameter is one-third of the pubic-table top distance. The thin, flat base of the metal calipers (2321) slips under the subject from the side while the movable arm, supported on a vertical rod attached to the base, is brought down over the symphysis pubis with compression. The height of the symphysis pubis is read off on the vertical arm, the calibration having taken into account the thickness of the base of the calipers. The calipers are stoutly made so that there is no divergence on applying compression.

As the calipers are used for both couch and vertical stand, the Bucky surface-to-film distance must be identical and, when necessary, an adjustment is made, usually to the stand, by adding a sheet of perspex of appropriate thickness to the Bucky surface.

To establish the levels of the antero–posterior planes from the lateral aspect, the calipers are used to measure the width of the pelvis at the level of the greater trochanters (2322). The calipers are placed over the trochanters and again firmly compressed for accurate measurement. One-half of this distance gives the height of the mid-plane of the pelvis from the table top for the lateral projection and thus, when uniform focus–film distance is employed, no further measurements are required.

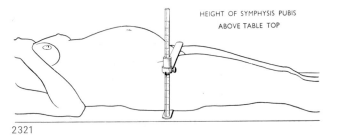

HEIGHT OF SYMPHYSIS PUBIS
ABOVE TABLE TOP

2321

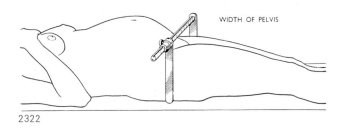

WIDTH OF PELVIS

2322

(b) By geometrical correction scale

This method depends on the use of calipers (2321, 2322) with a geometrical scale and table of distances (2323).

The distance table shows the range of heights of the upper border of the symphysis pubis from the table top at quarter-inch spacing $5\frac{1}{2}$ inches to 9 inches. Against these figures are shown two columns representing the transverse and bi-spinous heights, corresponding respectively to two-thirds and one-third of the pubic height measurement. On establishing the symphysis pubis-table top distance by the use of the calipers, the appropriate levels of the two transverse planes are seen at a glance.

The geometrical correction scale is prepared by radiographing a steel ruler which has been notched at 1 inch, $\frac{1}{2}$ and $\frac{1}{4}$ intervals, (1) at table-top level and (2) at $7\frac{1}{2}$ inches above the table top, using the Potter-Bucky diaphragm and a focus–film distance of 36 inches as employed for taking the routine radiographs.

On placing the two radiographs of the ruler on graph paper, arranging them parallel and $7\frac{1}{2}$ inches apart with the 4 inch points centralized, the chart is completed by ruling lines to connect the corresponding measurement notches at the two levels, and by adding the appropriate figures (2323).

On making an X-ray exposure of the table and chart placed one above the other (2323), the resulting grey background of the film provides a glare-free transparency for use side by side with the patient's radiographs.

To make use of the chart for the transverse planes, having determined the height of each plane in turn by consulting the table of distances, the diameter on the film is recorded with a pair of dividers. If, for instance, the transverse plane height is 4 inches, then on transferring the dividers to the 4 inch level on the correction scale, the actual diameter is indicated at both the upper and lower borders of the scale. This technique is repeated for the bi-spinous diameter.

To make use of the chart for the antero–posterior measurements from the lateral projection, reference is made to the mid-line to table-top distance arrived at by measurement of the width of the pelvis at the level of the trochanters. Take, for example, a bi-trochanteric measurement of 13 inches, giving a mid-line to table-top distance of $6\frac{1}{2}$ inches; then, on recording the length of each film plane in turn with a pair of dividers and placing the dividers at the $6\frac{1}{2}$ inch level on the correction scale, the actual measurements of the true conjugate, the mid-plane and the outlet are indicated on the upper and lower borders of the scale.

HEIGHT OF SYMPHYSIS PUBIS ABOVE TABLE-TOP (IN INCHES)	HEIGHT OF TRANSVERSE DIAMETER ABOVE TABLE-TOP 2/3	HEIGHT OF BI-SPINOUS DIAMETER ABOVE TABLE-TOP 1/3
5·5	3·7	1·85
5·75	3·8	1·9
6·0	4·0	2·0
6·25	4·2	2·1
6·5	4·3	2·15
6·75	4·5	2·25
7·0	4·7	2·35
7·25	4·8	2·4
7·5	5·0	2·5
7·75	5·2	2·6
8·0	5·3	2·65
8·25	5·5	2·75
8·5	5·6	2·8
8·75	5·8	2·9
9·0	6·0	3·0

ENLARGED PELVIC DIAMETERS

2323

(c) By perforated ruler

With the patient in the erect lateral position, a metal ruler which has been holed at 1 centimetre intervals is placed to coincide with the mid-plane of the pelvis, to be recorded radiographically on simultaneous exposure with the subject (2324), as having the same degree of enlargement. This in turn coincides with the enlargement of the three mid-plane dimensions shown in (2315), namely the true conjugate, the mid-plane and the outlet. Thus, measurements of these enlarged planes with the similarly enlarged ruler will give the actual dimensions in centimetres. As for the previous method, separate exposures can be made of the ruler at the varying distances involved to be applied accordingly on measuring the distance of the mid-plane of each subject from the film.

Radigraph (2324) shows the lateral erect projection with the perforated ruler in position and (2325) the enlargement of the ruler being used to measure the essential diameters on the similarly enlarged radiograph.

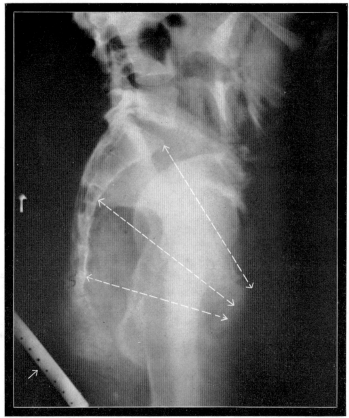

2324

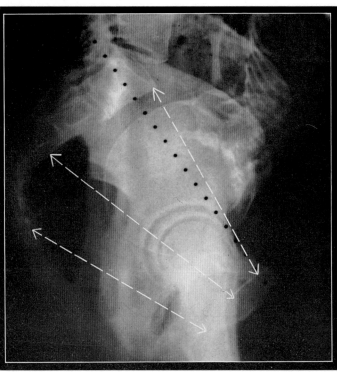

2325

Foetal head mensuration: Approximate foetal head measurement of one or more diameters may be obtained in certain cases by the method applied in determining the pelvic measurements, but complicating factors are involved and the resulting measurements are, therefore, less accurate than for pelvimetry. This process is termed cephalometry.

A pelvicephalometer allows calculations to be made as to pelvic and foetal head dimensions from films taken in the antero–posterior and lateral positions without moving the patient. To reduce the enlargement factor to a minimum, exposures are made at not less than 48 inches.

Angle of pelvic inclination

The angle formed by the plane of the brim of the pelvis and the anterior margin of the fifth lumbar vertebral body is referred to as the angle of pelvic inclination (2326).

The angle varies with posture and from subject to subject as shown in the lateral projection of the pelvis. Postural variations depend on the trunk and limbs being straight (2326) or flexed (2327).

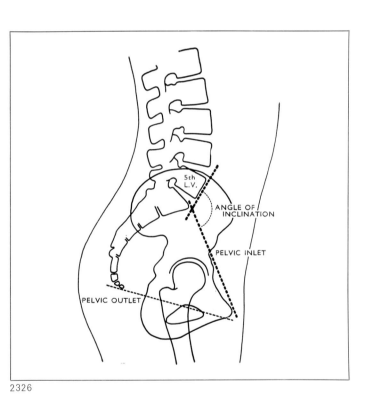

2326

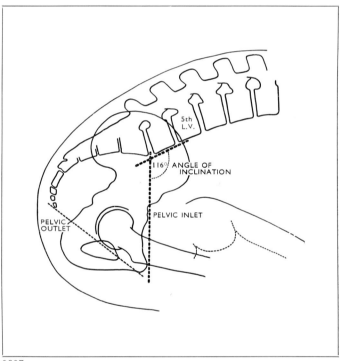

2327

30 Female reproductive system

A summary of exposure conditions for the Female Reproductive System

Region and Position	kVp	mAS	FFD	Film ILFORD	Screens ILFORD	Grid
Hysterosalpingography Antero-posterior	65	40	36"	Rapid R	FT	Grid
Gynaecography Postero-anterior	86	36 (0·12	36"	Rapid R	FT	Grid
Pregnancy-early Postero-anterior/antero-posterior	60	30	36"	Rapid R	FT	Grid
Pregnancy—Full Term	62·5	60	36"	Rapid R	FT	Grid
Antero-posterior-supine	120	15	36"	Rapid R	FT	Grid
Postero-anterior-prone	62·5	50	36"	Rapid R	FT	Grid
Lateral-horizontal	80	40	36"	Rapid R	FT	Grid
Lateral-supine	80	50	36"	Rapid R	FT	Grid
Lateral-tilted	80	40	36"	Rapid R	FT	Grid
Lateral-erect	90	200	36"	Rapid R	FT	Stationary } Moving and Stationary
	120	75	36"	Rapid R	FT	
Oblique-antero-posterior	70	50	36"	Rapid R	FT	Grid
Supero-inferior-inlet	90	125	36"	Rapid R	FT	} Moving and Stationary
	120	40	36"	Rapid R	FT	
	70	60	36"	Rapid R	FT	Grid
Supero-inferior-outlet	120	10	36"	Rapid R	FT	Grid

31

HIGH KILOVOLTAGE
SELECTIVE
FILTRATION

HIGH KILOVOLTAGE AND SELECTIVE FILTRATION

High Kilovoltage

The application of high kilovoltage technique is primarily with a view to obtaining exposure time in the region of milliseconds and the more extensive use of small foci. This effective control of movement unsharpness in subjects influenced by involuntary movement offsets the so often accepted insiduous blurring obtained at longer exposure times.

The differential in contrast within the subject range of opacity is considerably reduced, the visual appearance of bone structure being reduced in opacity to a much greater degree than soft tissue. As a consequence of this an extended range of subject information is obtained at convenient levels of density.

High kilovoltage is suited to subjects of initial steep contrast either present or introduced (opaque media). In such subjects although the scale of subject contrast is reduced, adequate contrast is maintained.

The facility for extensive sequenced exposure as required in Angiography is also possible at short exposure time, in view of the reduced anode temperature loading, compared with milliamperage, control of time and repetition.

Its application to bone radiography is severely limited due to the rapid loss in definition at kilovoltages above 100 kVp.

The efficient collimation of the beam and the effective elimination of the increased scattered radiation are essential. In respect to the latter, the fine-line stationary type of grid at ratios of 10:1 or 12:1 both facilitates the necessary control of scatter and permits the use of the millisecond exposure range.

Exposure time should be adequate to ensure that the subject range of densities is reproduced where the film characteristic produces density proportional to the differences eminating from the subject.

The improvement in definition through the effective control of movement, reduced geometrical unsharpness and the use of high definition screens results in a quality which perhaps is not so aesthetically pleasing due to the lower contrast, but is however superior in diagnostic information.

Applications

Chest radiography—Due to loss of rib opacity and effective penetration of the mediastinum, general survey information is more extensive.

Gastro-intestinal tract—Effective arrest of movement.

Angiography—Short exposure requirements, enables the sequence exposures requirement of the examination to be covered within the tube rating.

Spine—General postural alignment.

Radiation hazards—With the reduction in absorption due to the increased penetration of the beam, it is feasible to accept that both skin surface and depth dosage are reduced, however it must also be realised that increased gonadal dosage is possible in some examinations.

Chest lateral (2328)					
kVp	mAS	FFD	Film	Screens	Grid
140	6	60″(150cm)	Rapid R	HD	Grid
Stomach (2329)					
140	5	36″(90cm)	Rapid R	HD	Grid
Cholangiogram (2330)					
140	4	36″(88cm)	Rapid R	HD	Grid

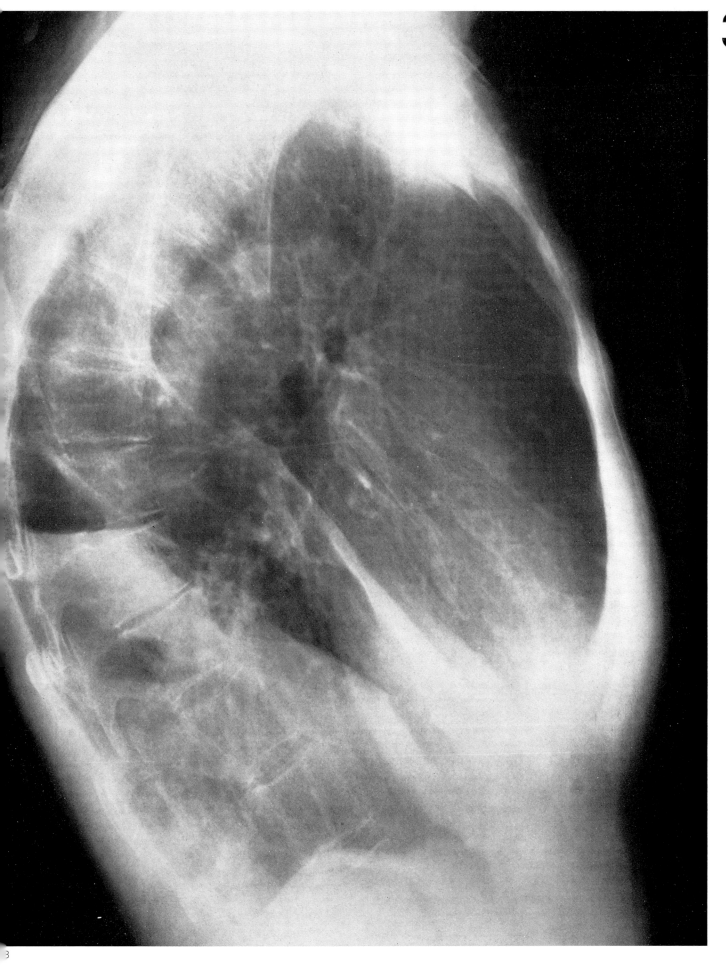

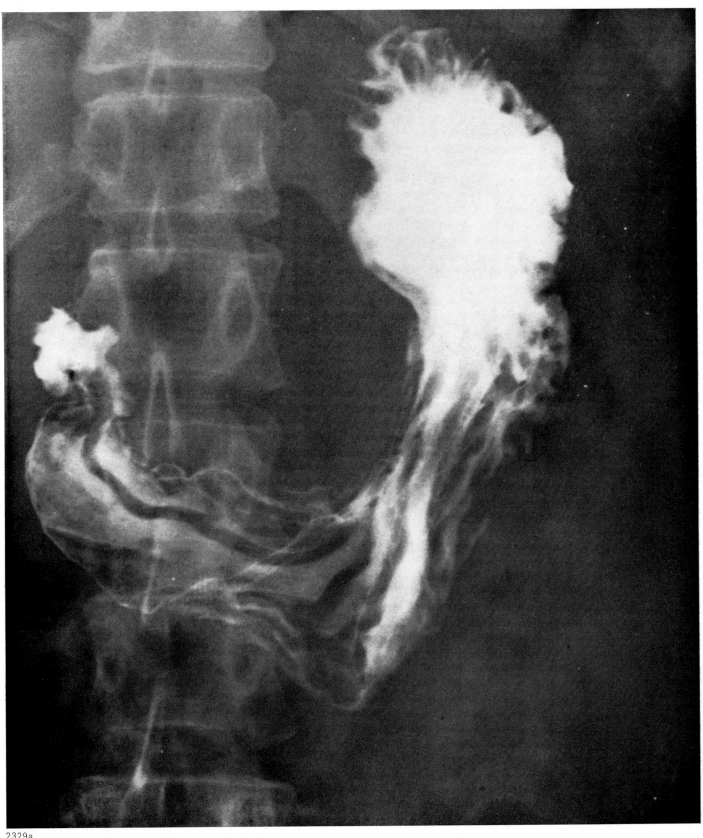

2329a

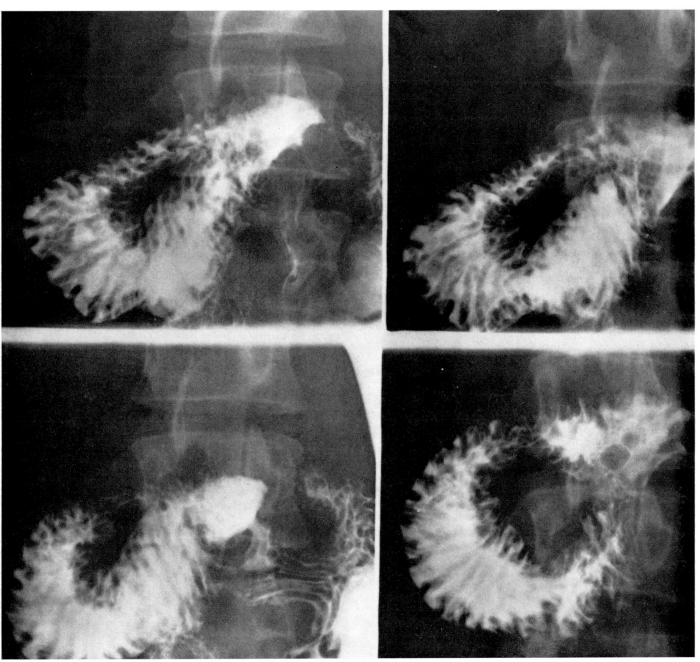

2329b

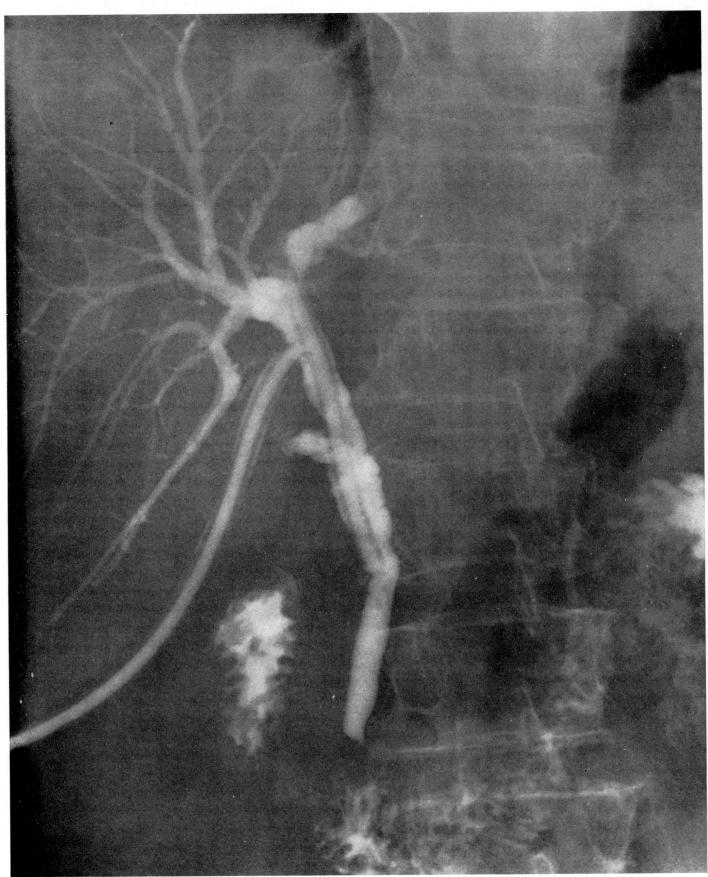

Selective Filtration

A range of radiography has been investigated in which a number of metals singly and collectively could (1) replace the use of grids; (2) be used in conjunction with a grid of 8 : 1 or 10 : 1 ratio, at kilovoltages from 80 and 150 kVp both to eliminate grid scatter and to improve the clean-up of subject scatter; (3) be placed in front of the cassette to increase the possibility of extending the use of the part-film technique.

(1) The use of tin-coated mild steel 29 gauge 1/8000 in. thick or alternatively 0·002 in. thick industrial lead screens alone has been found satisfactory in subjects which border between grid and non-grid techniques, e.g. above average thickness.

(a) Knees and shoulders.

(b) Antero–posterior and oblique views of cervical spines.

(c) Localized sinus and mastoid examinations.

(d) Thick-set subjects for antero–posterior, lateral and oblique views of the chest.

(e) In Smith-Petersen pin operations a lead screen 0·004 in. thick provides adequate contrast at considerably reduced exposure compared with grids.

(2) **Used in conjunction with a grid:** When used in conjunction with tin coated mild steel sheet or lead screens, one or other placed on top of the cassette in the bucky tray the conventional 8 : 1 and 10 : 1 grids produce a decided improvement in "clean-up" in techniques using the higher kilovoltages (80–150 kVp).

The results are virtually comparable to that of ratios in the region of 16 : 1 at reduced exposure and considerably more centring latitude. Tests would tend to indicate that they also eliminate scatter from the grid. At kilovoltages of 80 and above no increase in exposure is necessary when either is used. In conjunction with the grid they are particularly useful in bi-plane angiography and in micturition techniques and all instances where the direction and amount of scatter present a greater problem. In addition to this the filtration effect is useful to producing uniformity through a wide range of subject opacity.

This additional "clean-up" and filtration can also be usefully employed where it is essential to reproduce an extended subject density range simultaneously, e.g. petrous mastoid region, pelvimetry, gastro-intestinal tract, and a number of tomographic examinations, e.g. where it is necessary to demonstrate the bifurcation of the bronchi and lung fields simultaneously.

Recently the advantage of using tin-coated mild steel in conjunction with the space-gap technique has been found useful in radiography of the Petrous. Using the hypocycloidal movement of the Polytome the grid is removed to allow kilovoltage in the region of 70 kVp to be used. This lower kilovoltage maintains maximum subject contrast, and the air gap in conjunction with the selective filter placed on the front of the cassette effectively removes the subject scatter.

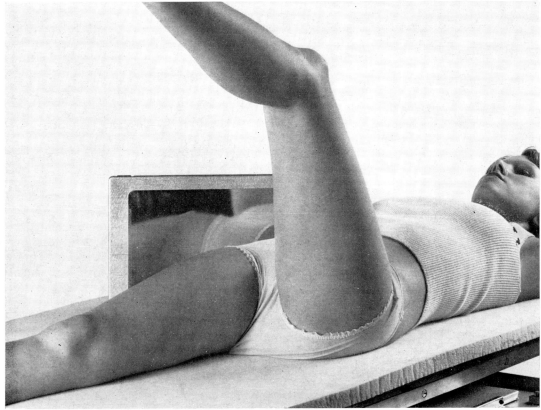

2331

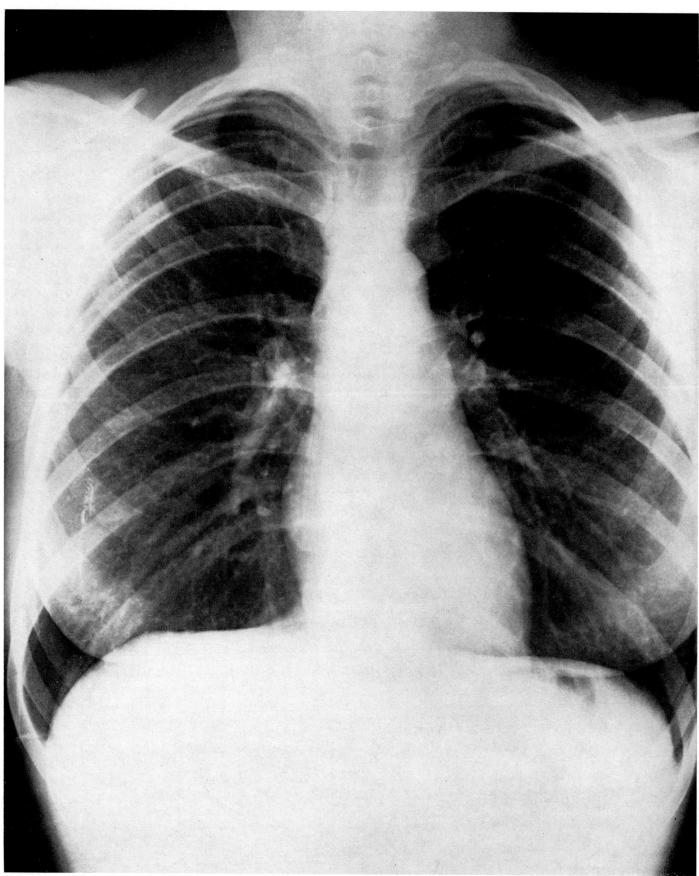

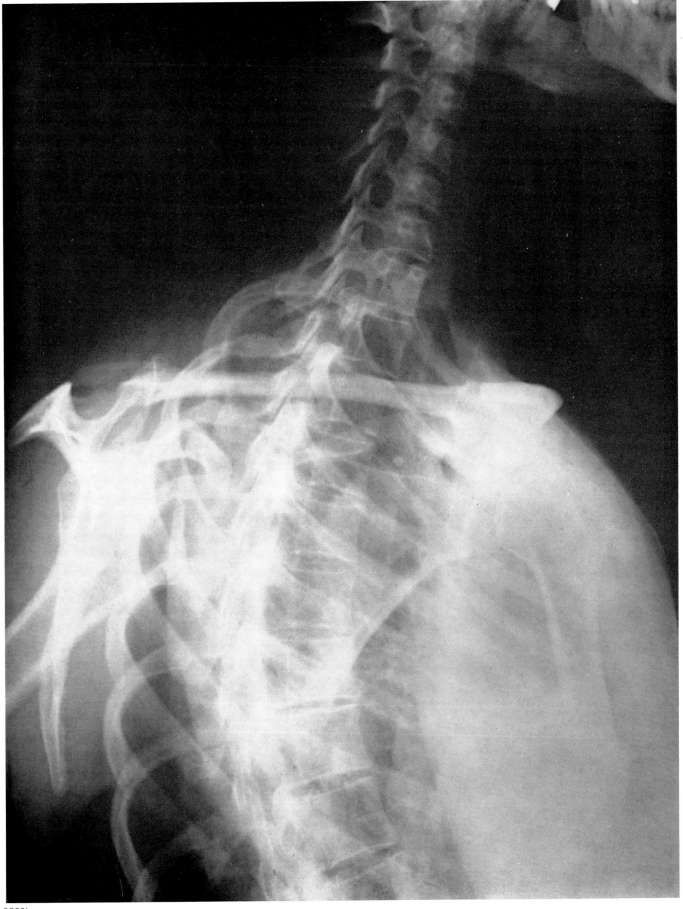

2332b

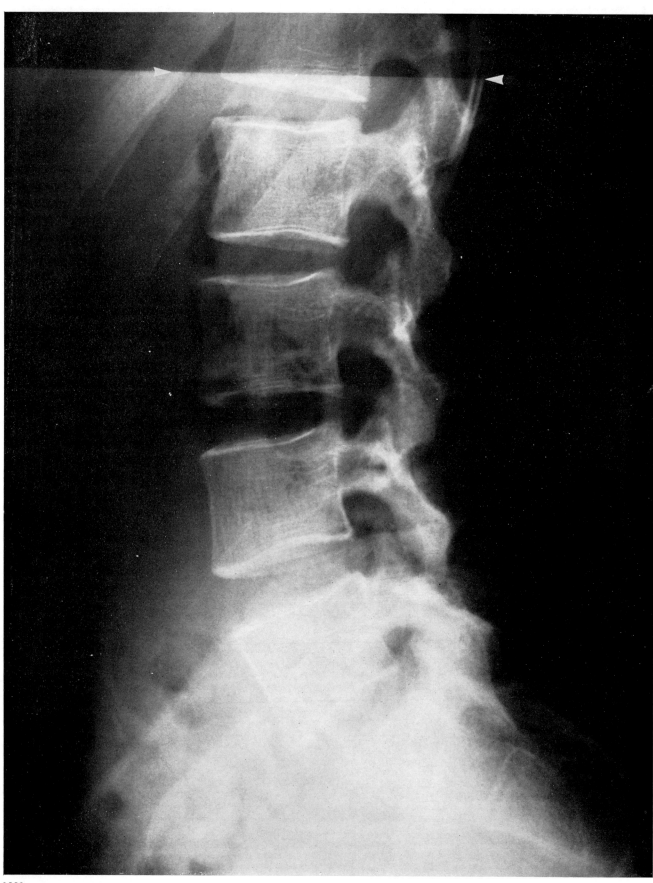

32

FOREIGN BODIES

Head

For descriptive purposes, the head is divided into cranium and face, the latter being again sub-divided into general and localized regions such as the eye, nose, tongue and jaw.

In head work particularly, it is sometimes necessary to demonstrate bone and soft tissues; when suitable, a high kilo-voltage may be applied to show both tissue densities on the one film; or one film may be placed between, and one film in front of, the intensifying screens for each exposure as in (2336), also by wide-range, technique, Multiple Radiography.

In dealing with the face, combined bone and soft tissue radiography is usually necessary (2336), and special note should be made of the soft tissue radiographs of nose and ear in (2337). Projections such as occipito-frontal, occipito-mental, lateral and oblique, with such other projections as may be required, will disclose the position of the foreign body and its relationship to bone and soft tissue structures (2340). Radiography of the facial structures is important also as an aid to plastic surgery.

To identify the presence of a foreign body in the tongue it will be necessary to make exposures with this organ at rest within the mouth (2338) and, if possible, extended outside the mouth, when the relative position of the foreign body will be disclosed.

When examining the cranium, every effort should be made to identify the foreign body as being within the cranium, embedded in the bone wall, or in the scalp or adjacent soft tissues, and additional oblique and sky-line projections should be made to show the foreign body in profile where applicable (2337,2340). In taking stereoscopic pairs, it should be remembered that the head may be rotated in place of the more usual movement of the tube; also, that the direction of the tube shift depends on the region concerned, and movement may be parallel to the median line in the place of the more usual transverse direction. If the apparatus is available, tomography may be invaluable. When the foreign body is proved to be within the bony cranium, a precise depth localization will probably be required immediately.

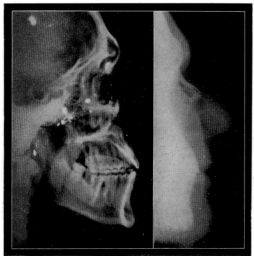

2336

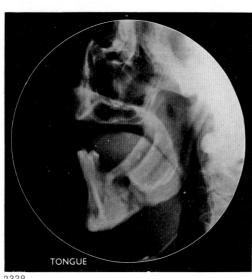

TONGUE

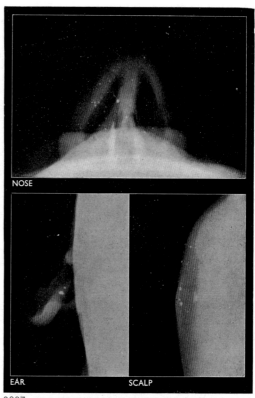

NOSE

EAR   SCALP

2337

Lateral projections should be made of the orbital cavity, one with the eyes raised and the other with the eyes lowered, in order to observe any movement of the foreign body.

Two projections, lateral and 30 degrees occipito-mental, selected from a series of radiographs taken after removal of the eye and replacement by a glass eye, are shown in (2339), the glass eye having been retained to serve as a landmark in identifying the relative position of foreign bodies adjacent to the orbital cavity.

In this instance, the investigation was to identify the precise position of a foreign body in relation to the optic canal, exploratory exposures being followed by localized projections. Note wire ring marking suppurating sinus.

In series (2341), showing a foreign body in the upper cervical region, the additional base projections of the skull was taken to show the plan position of the foreign body in the atlas. These radiographs were selected from a number of projections which left no doubt as to the precise position of the foreign body. Note the additional small foreign body which is not shown in the base projection.

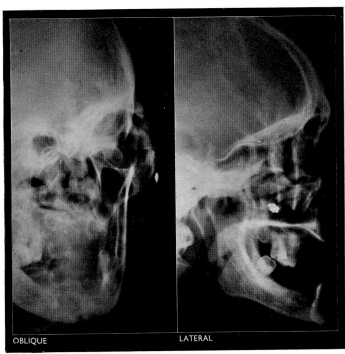

OBLIQUE LATERAL

2340

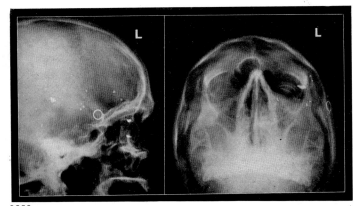

2339

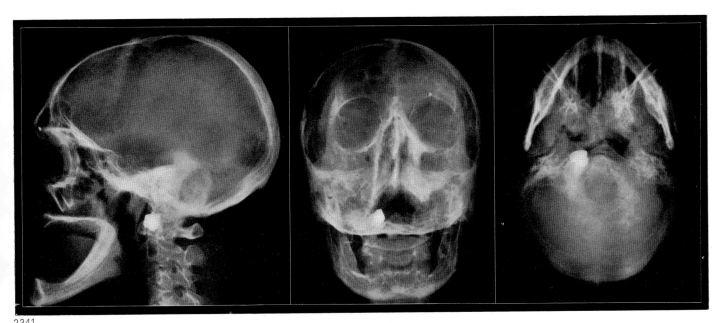

2341

Trunk

Foreign bodies in the *shoulder* region may be difficult to locate, and here again certain skyline projections may be necessary, especially to show foreign bodies in relation to the scapula, as in (2342), where an oblique view has been taken to show that certain opacities appearing in the antero–posterior projection are not in the lung. In (2344), an unusual supero–inferior oblique projection confirms the position of a bullet in the spine of the scapula. Careful screen examination is invaluable in this region to enable the foreign body to be shown in profile.

For the *clavicle*, several additional projections may be made with the patient prone, supine or lateral, and for the prone position with the tube angled at 45 degrees towards the feet thus separating the opaque shadows from other structures, as shown in (2343). These same prone and supine positions are used also to give clear projections of the apices of the lungs.

In dealing with the *vertebral column* (2346) additional oblique projections (2345) and stereoscopic projections are usually necsseary. Initial true antero–posterior and lateral projections (2346) are essential, however, following which very careful screen adjustment is required to disclose a foreign body in a position such as in (2345).

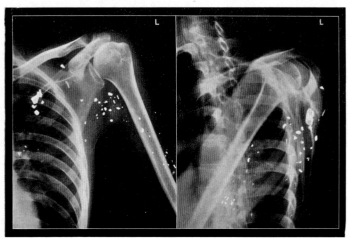

2342

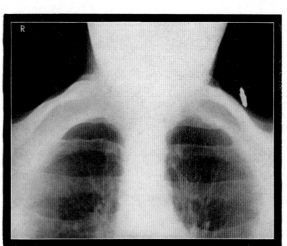

2343

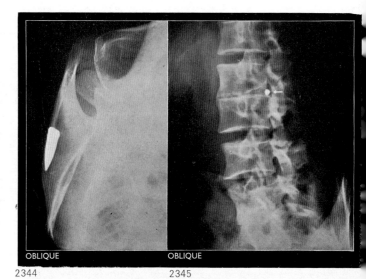

OBLIQUE   OBLIQUE

2344   2345

2346

The *pelvis* lends itself to the taking of various additional oblique projections; axial projections over the anterior brim (2347) and posteriorly over the sacrum (2348) may also be informative, particularly the former, to show the position of foreign bodies in relation to the pubic bones. In (2348), a bullet is shown to be lodged in the sacrum.

For the *hip joint* the general antero–posterior, lateral, lateral neck of femur, general lateral of pelvis oblique and stereoscopic projections may be used.

In one of a stereoscopic pair, metal rings have been placed on the skin surface to show the position of surface wounds, the near-film ring shadow being the smaller (2349).

In the *thorax*, the adjacent scapulae and clavicles have to be considered, as also the position of the foreign body relative to the organs and ribs. In (2350), the foreign bodies marked by arrows are so near to the pleura that only the most critical screen examination disclosed their actual position, enabling them to be recorded radiographically.

Screening for the relationship of foreign body movement and respiratory movement is important.

The *diaphragm*, owing to its ovoid shape and movemenst during respiration, presents its own particular problems. Tangential projections (2354) may be made, also the beam directed parallel to the upper surface, upward, and downward.

In the upper *abdomen*, the position of the foreign body relative to the diaphragm is important and also the relative movements, on respiration, of the foreign body and of the visible organs affected also by respiration.

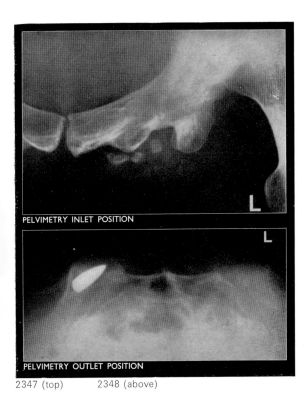

PELVIMETRY INLET POSITION

PELVIMETRY OUTLET POSITION

2347 (top)   2348 (above)

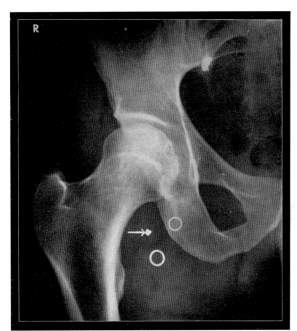

2349

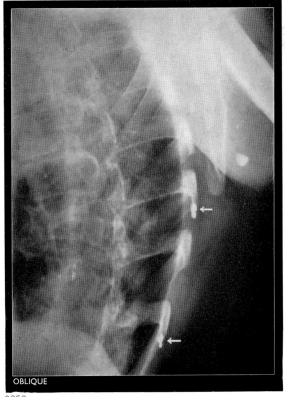

OBLIQUE

2350

Respiratory System

In dealing with the respiratory system the nature of the injury will, in the great majority of cases, indicate the approximate region to be investigated. In the case of gunshot and explosion wounds, the condition of the patient may indicate that there is an injury to the lung or mediastinal viscera, or suggest that the foreign body has been arrested in the superficial tissues. On the other hand, solid matter inhaled into the breathing passages, the larynx, trachea and bronchi, presents another problem; this mishap may occur during operation on the mouth, teeth or throat, but is most frequently sustained by children with the habit of putting things into their mouths, and serious lung injury may follow.

Screening is essential to disclose the movement of the foreign body during respiration; movement coincident with that of the ribs may confirm its presence in the thorax wall.

Tangential projections will serve to locate the position of the foreign body, as shown in (2352,2353) in both cases outside the bony thorax. The principle of tangential projection is shown in cross-sectional diagram (2354).

Initial films should, however, to be taken from two right-angled aspects, postero–anterior or antero–posterior and right or left lateral, according to the near-skin surface of the foreign body.

A bullet or piece of shrapnel piercing the chest wall and entering the pleural cavity may also allow the entry of air and thus cause a pneumothorax, with collapse of the lung, when the foreign body may be free to move about within the pleural cavity with change of posture of the patient.

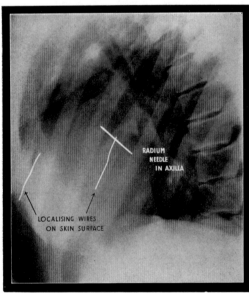

2351

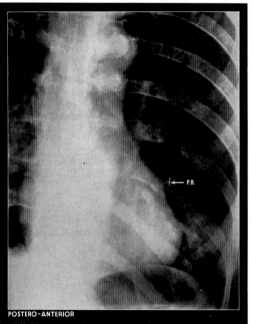

POSTERO-ANTERIOR

2352

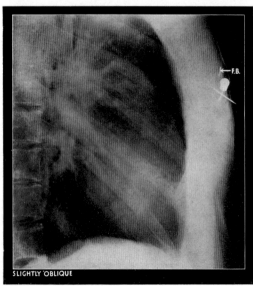

SLIGHTLY OBLIQUE

2353

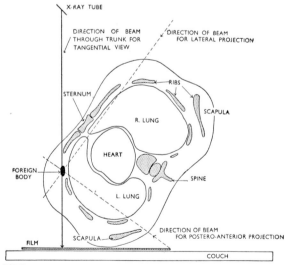

2354

In the case of an opacity overshadowed by the diaphragm, additional projections, tangential to the diaphragm, are made from both aspects to determine its position above or below the diaphragm (2355,2356).

Kymographs may establish the presence of a foreign body in or near to the heart or aorta.

The more opaque bodies will be seen readily and a precise calculation of depth may be necessary, a careful note being made of the phase of respiration. It is recommended that an exposure be made on expiration.

With normal exposure for the lungs, a foreign body may be obscured by the mediastinal viscera in the postero–anterior projection, whereas it will be shown in an oblique or lateral projection. Increased penetration with the use of a grid is therefore essential.

The less opaque foreign bodies—a single tooth is an example—partially obscured as they may be by the dense hilar lung shadows, may not be seen unless the finest possible lung definition is obtained. The examination should, therefore, be most exacting, as the continued presence of a foreign body in the lung (2357), with the probability of its setting up a septic condition, may endanger the life of the patient.

When the patient's symptoms indicate the continued presence in the lungs of a foreign body which has not been identified radiographically, the physician may resort to bronchography to determine the site of the obstruction (2357).

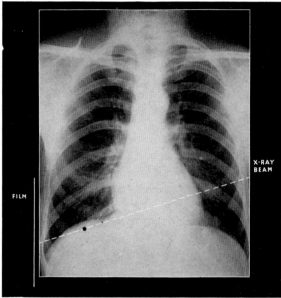

2355

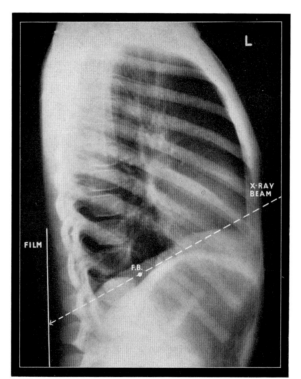

2356

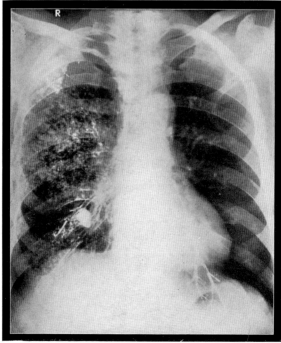

2357

Alimentary tract

It is frequently necessary to examine the alimentary tract for the presence of foreign matter of many kinds which has been swallowed, sometimes intentionally.

For the purpose of this section the alimentary tract is treated in three parts, the pharynx and upper oesophagus, the oesophagus, and the gastro-intestinal tract.

Pharynx and upper oesophagus

The swallowing of small bones is a common occurrence, and these, especially fish bones, may be almost non-opaque and thus require special technique.

These shadows are localized by taking oblique and, particularly, lateral projections of the neck and thoracic inlet to show soft structures only. For this purpose the neck should be extended, the shoulders depressed, and the tube centred high up at the level of the third cervical vertebra in order to show the maximum area of oesophagus above the dense shoulder structures.

A thick barium swallow may be given to show or to confirm the presence of a foreign body, which usually takes a thin, outlining coating. The swallow may be a mixture of barium and cotton wool, termed a bolus, of which the wool may adhere to the foreign body and so indicate its presence. The procedure usually adopted is to take the lateral, soft tissue projection, followed by a second film taken after the passage of the barium swallow has been viewed on the fluorescent screen. Illustration (2358) shows a fish bone in the pharynx, before and after a barium swallow. In (2359), a piece of gristle and in (2360) a coin are seen in the upper oesophagus. (2361) shows a needle in the throat; here the additional postero–anterior projection has replaced the barium swallow.

A patient's complaint of persistent pain in the throat should not be accepted as conclusive evidence of the presence there for a foreign body, as the discomfort may be due to an abrasion caused by its passage to a position lower down in the alimentary tract.

Oesophagus

Apart from X-ray evidence, the patient's symptoms will have indicated to the physician whether the foreign body is in the bronchus or the oseophagus.

The oesophagus is viewed with the patient in the right anterior–oblique position. Unless an opaque foreign body is shown to be present, as in (2362), or if a non-opaque foreign body is anticipated, a thick barium swallow is given to locate the obstruction.

When, however, there is doubt as to the radio-opacity of the foreign body and it is not shown in the screen examination of the oesophagus, a general antero–posterior projection of the abdomen should be taken on the Potter-Bucky couch before administering the barium swallow, as the opaque meal, when it reaches the gastro-intestinal tract, would probably obscure the foreign body should it have passed beyond the oesophagus. It should be noted that when a denture such as shown in (2362) is made of acrylic resin it may not be visible radiographically.

Gastro-intestinal tract

For the remainder of the tract a general radiograph of the abdomen is taken, usually daily, to observe the progress of the foreign body, the chief anxiety being in its possible failure to pass the narrow ileocolic valve at the junction of the small and large intestine. Should operative measures be contemplated, the patient is finally radiographed immediately before the operation to ensure that the foreign body has not been evacuated unnoticed.

The presence of a non-opaque foreign body suspected of causing an obstruction may be confirmed and its position determined by the ingestion of a small barium meal, the flow of which will be wholly or partially arrested by the obstruction. A small meal may also be given to determine the precise position of the opaque foreign body.

In dealing with one or several small opaque bodies, maybe a needle or pin, it is essential to take the general radiograph of the abdomen on the Potter-Bucky couch, using a short-time exposure technique. On taking the fim in the screening stand without a grid, these opacities may be missed, as the secondary radiation is considerable when covering this large area with an open diaphragm which may be sufficient to diffuse the smaller shadows, there being no trace of the foreign bodies either in the film or by screening. The radiograph taken with the grid, however, will show the opacities clearly.

In dealing with young children it is advisable to avoid screening, and to confine the examination to a general projection of the abdomen and thorax (2363). Should further investigation be necessary, an oblique projection of the thorax to show the oesophagus, and a lateral projection of the chest and throat cavity will generally suffice to complete the examination.

In older children, a brief screen examination will serve to locate an opaque foreign body, to be followed by regional confirmatory radiographs. In screening, the whole of the alimentary tract should be covered from the mouth to the anus, as otherwise a nearby foreign body, especially in the throat, may be overlooked.

The progress of a swallowed open safety-pin should be carefully observed from day to day.

In cases of an ingested foreign body, it is usual for instructions to be given for the patient to take thick, stodgy food, and for the faeces to be examined for the presence of the foreign body after each evacuation.

For these investigations of the trunk, the patient's clothing should be replaced by a hospital gown without opaque fastenings.

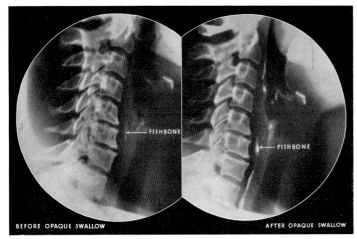

2358

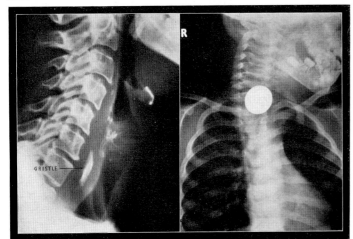

2359 2360

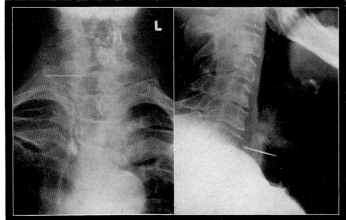

2361

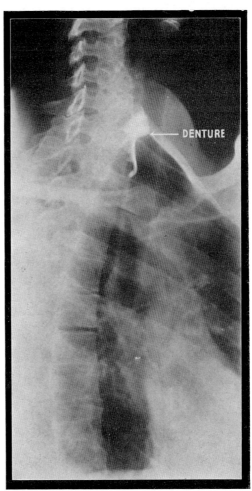

2362

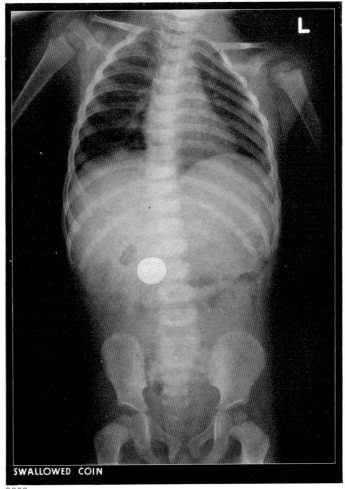

SWALLOWED COIN

2363

32 Foreign bodies
Localization

Preliminaries

Before discussing actual localization methods there are certain preliminaries to be considered such as the patient, operative measures, foreign bodies, equipment, processing, preliminary experiments with a phantom, and geometric principles involved.

Foreign bodies

Any type of material may be included under this heading and, as seen in the various illustrations, there may be present one foreign body or many. In the latter case the surgeon will indicate those to be removed, and these should be carefully noted for identification, (1), (2), (3), etc.

In the case of large foreign bodies, it may be necessary to give numerous depth measurements in order that the general position in the tissues may be known.

Foreign bodies with smooth surfaces, such as a needle or a bullet, may move as the subject moves, passing from one tissue layer to another, hence the importance of immobilizing the patient during the interim between localization and removal. This type of foreign body tends to rotate and alter position when touched by the surgeon's probe, which may thus pass the foreign body. On the other hand, an irregularly shaped mass will probably be fixed in the tissues, moving only with the muscle in which it is embedded.

In dealing with material of which the radiographic density is likely to be doubtful, it is sometimes possible to obtain a piece of similar material for screen examination; this applies particularly when such objects as buttons have been swallowed, or when glass enters the tissues.

Where there is an unavoidable space between film and skin, a marker is attached to the skin and its estimated distance from the film is subtracted from the foreign body to film distance (2364).

For curved surfaces such as the buttock, or over a wound area, the depth measurement should be made from the highest adjacent skin level. The position of a wound and its extent may be indicated by metal markers placed on the film or skin.

The availability of the image intensifier with its very low screening rating at 90–95 kilovolts of 0·3 milliampere and with television viewing greatly reduces the radiation hazard involved.

Marking the Skin Surface: The patient is screened, the diaphragm aperture being reduced to include only a small area, with the tube centred directly through the foreign body.

The skin position may be identified by inserting a metal ring indicator under the screen, over the foreign body, the skin being marked accordingly on the removal of the screen. The metal ring on a convenient handle can be sterilized surgically.

When only the surgical skin surface position of the foreign body is required for immediate operation, the marking of this point may be by a small cross on the skin with a sterile surgical needle.

When the patient is to be moved, after examination, from the X-ray room to the theatre, it may be the practice to mark the skin from three aspects—antero–posterior, medial and lateral—to facilitate the screening position being resumed for the operation. A horizontal tube projection is employed for the medial and lateral markings, and these, being equidistant from the couch, provide the necessary guidance for correct positioning and also indicate the depth of the foreign body A cross in place of a spot may be used to show the near skin surface from both aspects (2364). Care should be taken to ensure that the tube is correctly centred for each of these projections.

On being given a skin marking over the foreign body and the depth of the foreign body below this point, the surgeon is able to determine the correct angle at which to approach the foreign body from any adjacent skin surface position.

Tube centring: Accuracy in depth localization does not depend on the tube focus being centred vertically over the foreign body, as will be seen in several of the examples given, particularly in the orbital cavity. But for skin marking it is most important that the tube focus, the centre of the variable diaphragm, and one edge of the foreign body, are on a line perpendicular to the fluorescent screen. This calls for accurate collimation of the tube focus and diaphragm.

When the tube is tilted longitudinally or rotated about its diameter, the centre of the screen image does not coincide with a vertical ray from the tube but to the axial ray, which is then directed obliquely.

It follows that a skin marking made in such circumstances for the guidance of the surgeon is misleading, any marking being presumed to be, as it should be, vertically over the foreign body (2364).

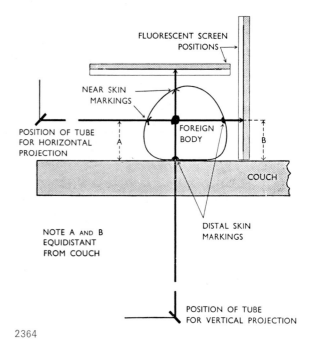

2364

Tube shift: Tube shifts of 6 to 10 centimetres are usually employed. The greater tube shift should be applied in taking a near-film foreign body and also when the focus–film distance is considerable. When these conditions are reversed, however, the lesser tube shift should be employed; it is, indeed, the more commonly used.

It should be understood that the tube movement may be made so that the two exposures are equidistant from the foreign body centring point, as it is necessary when employing the localizer illustrated in (2371,2372) and in spectacle eye localization shown on page 744. Alternatively, the total tube shift may be made to one side of the centring point as shown in (2369). All existing automatic stereoscopic tube shift movements should be checked before being accepted as precise measurements for depth localization.

The tube shift should be made at right angles to the long axis of an elongated foreign body (2365a,2368), and all film shadow-shift measurements should be made between the same two points on the foreign body shadows. It will be understood that only half of the normal exposure is applied for each tube position (2366), when the exposures superimpose on the one film.

Theatre processing: In the absence of a 90 second processor a form of rapid processing should be adopted to enable the surgeon to obtain the required information with the least possible delay. Small theatre processing units are available comprising three compartments suited to the size of film in use and spaced to accommodate developing, rinse and fixing procedure, the film being washed and dried in the department following the termination of the session. The availability, and the rapid developing properties of the concentrated replenishing solutions such as Phenisol replenisher recommends their use. These should be used at a modified dilution of 1 + 2. Developing time can be further reduced by increasing the solution temperature to 75° (25c) but this advantage is generally offset by a constant dropping temperature during the session. In view of this it may be better to base developing time at 68°F (20°) in keeping with room temperature. In conjunction with constant agitation of the film, an added drop of wetting agent to the solution considerably improves uniformity of development. To offset the continued developing activity within the film when removed from the developer an acid rinse is recommended. Rapid fixers (Hypam) with a clearing time of 30 seconds ensure that the film is available in just over a minute for viewing.

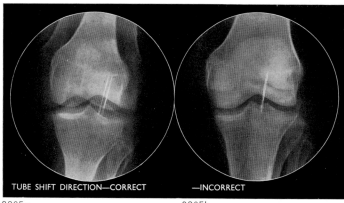

TUBE SHIFT DIRECTION—CORRECT   —INCORRECT

2365a   2365b

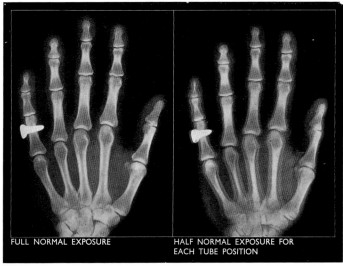

FULL NORMAL EXPOSURE   HALF NORMAL EXPOSURE FOR EACH TUBE POSITION

2366

Focus to table-top distance: To determine the focus to table-top distance, a flat metal object, such as a penny, is placed on the top of the couch. After screening for position, a film is supported horizontally at a known distance above the metal object and an exposure made. The tube is then removed a known distance, 10 centimetres being very convenient, and a second exposure is made (2367).

The displacement between the two shadows of the metal object is measured and the following formula applied:

$$\frac{T \times d}{s} = D$$

where T = tube shift
d = table-top to film distance
s = shadow shift registered on the film; and
D = focus to table-top distance.

In the distance shown in (2367) the distance is found to be:

$$\frac{10 \times 20}{4 \cdot 4} = 45 \cdot 45 \text{ centimetres.}$$

Exposure technique: 50 kilovolts, 30 milliamperes, and 0·5 second exposure for each tube position; Non-screen film.

Preliminary experiments: It is advisable to make initial depth localization on a phantom, the following being suggested for instructional purposes:

(a) Two wooden blocks, six inches high, are placed together with a metal object strapped at various experimental depths to one of the opposing surfaces; exposures being made for the purpose of checking the film or screen to foreign body depth calculations.

Exposure Technique: 50 kilovolts; 30 milliamperes; 60 centimetres focus–film distance; NS film; total exposure, one second, i.e., 0·5 second for each of the two tube positions. As a more realistic subject, a loaf of bread, a marrow, or a turnip may be used, when, on introducing a probe or steel knitting needle to be localized at the tip, subsequent dissection of the object will disclose the degree of accuracy achieved.

(b) To represent the eyeball, a 24 millimetre sphere may be cut from a potato or moulded in paraffin wax, and wedged with cotton wool into an orbital cavity of a dried skull, the "pupil" being outlined on the model eye. Shot or small fragments of metal placed within and behind the model eye provide a satisfactory subject on which to practice the intricacies of eye localization.

Exposure Technique: 50 kilovolts; 40 milliamperes; 50 centimetres focus–film distance; (Standard) Dental Film; total exposure, one-and-a-half seconds, i.e., three-quarters of a second for each of two tube positions.

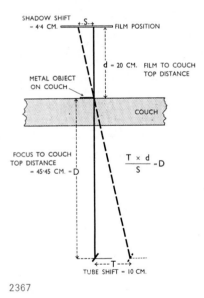

2367

Geometrical projection

Routine radiography is in flat projection, that is, in two dimensions. Localization, however, requires radiographic investigation in three dimensions, as in stereography. Most localization methods utilize the data derived from two or more shadows of the foreign body produced on the screen, film, or films by the displacement of the tube between two exposures. This is the basis of triangulation, on which the majority of localization methods depend. (The Mackenzie Davidson method.)

This localization chart serves as an easy and accurate reference in applying the formula

$$\frac{A \times S}{T + S} = D$$

where A = focus–film distance
  T = tube shift
  S = shadow shift
  D = depth of foreign body.

Margin of error: Radiographic localization, although capable of perfect accuracy in theory, is rarely so in practice, absolute precision being difficult to obtain as the human body cannot be treated as a motionless symmetrical solid. In general work, an error of not more than 5 millimetres is permissible, but in special work, such as the examination of the eye, the variation should not exceed 1 millimetre.

Each method provides for (a) marking or identifying the surface position immediately over the foreign body, and (b) estimating the depth of the foreign body immediately below the skin surface or from a given skin level.

Other methods depend on parallax, i.e., the apparent displacement of an object caused by an actual change of the point of observation.

As seen by screening, when the tube is moved parallel to the screen, any objects between the tube and the screen move in the opposite direction. The extent of movement increases with the increasing distance of the object from the screen. On moving a metal pointer between the screen and couch top, a position can be established at which the two objects—pointer and foreign body—move to the same extent as they are then at the same level. Thus, the position of the pointer can be used to indicate the depth of the foreign body beneath the skin surface.

Localization Chart for a Tube Shift (T) of 60mm, FFD (A) of 500–800 mm, and Shadow Shift (S) of 0·5 – 20 mm Resulting in Depths of Foreign Bodies (D)

SHADOW SHIFT (S) 0·5	1	2	3	4	5	6	7	8	9	10	11	12	13	14	15	16	17	18	19	20
FFD (A) Depths of Foreign Bodies (D)																				
500	4·1	8·2	16·1	23·8	31·2	38·5	45·4	52·2	58·8	65·2	71·4	77·4	83·3	89	94·6	100	105·3	110·4	115·4	120·2	125
510	4·2	8·4	16·5	24·3	32	39·2	46·4	53·3	60	66·5	72·8	79	85	90·8	96·7	102	107·4	112·6	117·7	122·7	127·5
520	4·3	8·5	16·6	24·8	32·5	40	47·3	54·3	61·2	67·8	74·3	80·6	86·6	92·8	98·4	104	109·5	114·8	120	125·1	130
530	4·4	8·7	17	25·2	33·1	40·8	48·2	55·4	62·3	69·1	75·7	82·1	88·3	94·4	100	106	111·6	117	122·3	127·5	132·5
540	4·5	8·9	17·4	25·7	33·8	41·5	49	56·5	63·5	70·4	77·1	83·7	90	96·2	102·2	108	113·7	119·2	124·6	129·9	135
550	4·5	9	17·7	26·1	34·4	42·3	50	57·5	64·7	71·7	78·5	85·2	91·7	98	104	110	115·8	121·4	126·9	132·3	137·5
560	4·6	9·2	18	26·7	35	43·1	50·9	58·5	66	73	80	86·8	93·3	99·8	105·8	112	117·9	123·6	129·2	134·7	140
570	4·7	9·3	18·4	27·1	35·6	43·8	51·8	59·6	67	74·4	81·4	88·3	95	101·5	107·8	114	120	125·8	131·5	137·1	142·5
580	4·8	9·5	18·7	27·6	36·2	44·6	52·7	60·6	68·2	75·7	82·8	89·9	96·6	103·3	109·7	116	122·1	128	133·8	139·5	145
590	4·9	9·7	19	28·1	36·9	45·4	53·6	61·6	69·4	77	84·3	91·4	98·3	105·1	111·6	118	124·2	130·2	136·1	141·9	147·5
600	5	9·8	19·3	28·6	37·5	46·3	54·5	62·7	70·6	78·3	85·7	93	100	106·9	113·5	120	126·3	132·4	138·4	144·3	150
610	5	10	19·7	29·1	38·1	46·9	55·5	63·7	71·7	79·6	87·1	94·5	101·8	108·6	115·4	122	128·4	134·6	140·8	146·7	152·5
620	5·1	10·2	20	29·5	38·7	47·7	56·3	64·8	72·9	80·9	88·5	96·1	103·3	110·4	117·3	124	130·5	136·8	143·2	149·1	155
630	5·2	10·3	20·3	30	39·4	48·5	57	65·8	74·1	82·2	90	97·6	105	112·2	119·2	126	132·6	139	145·4	151·5	157·5
640	5·3	10·5	20·6	30·5	40	49·2	58·2	66·9	75·3	83·5	91·4	98·2	106·6	114	121·1	128	134·7	141·3	147·7	153·9	160
650	5·4	10·7	20·9	31	40·6	50	59	67·9	76·5	84·8	92·8	100·7	108·3	115·7	122·8	130	136·8	143·5	150	156·3	162·5
660	5·5	10·8	21·3	31·4	41·2	50·8	60	69	77·6	86·1	94·3	102·3	110	117·5	124·8	132	139·9	145·7	152·3	158·7	165
670	5·5	11	21·6	31·9	41·9	51·6	61	70	78·8	87·4	95·7	103·8	111·7	119·3	126·7	134	141	147·9	154·6	161·1	167·5
680	5·6	11·1	21·9	32·4	42·5	52·4	61·8	71	80	88·7	97·1	105·4	113·3	121·1	128·7	136	143·1	150·1	157	163·5	170
690	5·7	11·3	22·2	32·9	43·1	53·2	62·7	72·1	81·2	90	98·5	106·9	115	122·9	130·5	138	145·3	152·3	159·2	165·9	172·5
700	5·8	11·5	22·6	33·3	43·7	53·9	63·6	73·1	82·3	91·3	100	108·5	116·6	124·7	132·4	140	147·4	154·5	161·5	168·3	175
710	5·9	11·6	22·9	33·8	44·4	54·7	64·5	74·2	83·5	92·6	101·4	110	118·3	126·4	134·3	142	149·5	156·7	163·8	170·8	177·5
720	6	11·8	23·2	34·3	45	55·4	65·5	75·2	84·7	93·9	102·8	111·6	120	128·2	136·2	144	151·6	158·9	166·2	173·2	180
730	6	11·9	23·5	34·8	45·6	56·2	66·4	76·3	86	95·2	104·3	113·1	121·7	130	138·1	146	153·7	161·2	168·5	175·6	182·5
740	6·1	12·1	23·9	35·2	46·2	57	67·2	77·3	87	96·5	105·7	114·7	123·3	131·8	140	148	155·8	163·4	170·8	178	185
750	6·2	12·3	24·2	35·7	46·8	57·7	68·2	78·2	88·2	97·8	107·1	116·2	125	133·6	141·9	150	157·9	165·6	173·1	180·4	187·5
760	6·3	12·5	24·5	36·2	47·5	58·5	69·1	79·4	89·4	99·1	108·5	117·8	126·6	135·3	143·8	152	160	167·8	175·4	182·8	190
770	6·4	12·6	24·8	36·7	48·1	59·2	70	80·4	90·6	100·4	110	119·3	128·3	137·1	145·8	154	162·1	170	177·7	185·2	192·5
780	6·4	12·8	25	37·1	48·7	60	70·9	81·5	91·8	101·7	111·4	120·9	130	138·9	147·5	156	164·2	172·2	180	187·6	195
790	6·5	13	25·5	37·6	49·4	60·8	71·8	82·5	92·9	103	112·9	122·4	131·7	140·7	149·4	158	166·3	174·4	182·3	190	197·5
800	6·6	13·1	25·8	38·1	50	61·7	72·7	83·6	94·1	104·3	114·3	124	133·3	142·5	151·3	160	168·4	176·6	184·6	192·4	200

Screen and film—triangulation

This is a precise method of depth localization which does not require any special apparatus.

The patient is placed in the position indicated by the surgeon for the removal of the foreign body. On screening, the under couch diaphragm is reduced to a small aperture and the tube is centred directly through the foreign body, the position being marked on the skin surface. The diaphragm is then opened, the film is placed in position, and the first exposure is made, applying half the total normal exposure time. The tube is moved a known distance—for the present purpose 6 centimetres—and the second exposure is made on the same film, again at half the normal time, the total normal exposure time being thus completed to produce the double image (2368,2370). The focus–film distance is noted.

On viewing the processed film, the distance between the foreign body shadows is measured (using the same relative point in each) and from the data now known the depth of the foreign body may be calculated by applying the formula:

$$\frac{A \times S}{T + S} = D$$

where A = focus–film distance
T = tube shift
S = shadow shift; and
D = depth of foreign body.

In the case shown (2368,2369)

$$\frac{600 \times 11}{60 + 11} = 93 \text{ millimetres.}$$

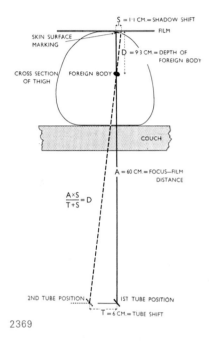

2369

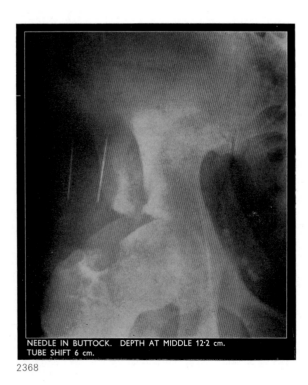

NEEDLE IN BUTTOCK. DEPTH AT MIDDLE 12·2 cm.
TUBE SHIFT 6 cm.

738   2368

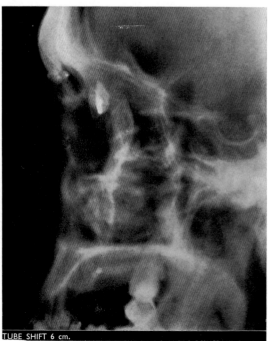

TUBE SHIFT 6 cm.
2370

Screen and film—parallax

Various types of apparatus have been made for the purpose of applying the principle of parallax to the localization of foreign bodies, and the following is chosen for its simplicity of application. This also is a precise method of localization.

The localizer is made of light metal in the form of a right-angled triangle of which the hypotenuse is faced with a brass plate having holes drilled at intervals corresponding to graduated depths in centimetres from the film level. A metal clip allows the film or cassette to be placed horizontally over the localizer holes and the subject (2372).

Application: The patient is placed in the indicated operative position for the removal of the foreign body. Screening is applied and the position of the foreign body is marked on the skin surface. After this, the tube diaphragm is opened sufficiently to cover the whole of the localizer, which is then placed in position with the holes in line with the skin marking and with a cassette in the clip (2372). A convenient focus–film distance is employed, and, although an exact measurement is not necessary, the tube shift should be approximately one-tenth of the focus–film distance—for example, 6 centimetres at 60 centimetres—and the two exposures are made from points equidistant from, and on each side of, the centring point. It is important that the tube movement should be at right angles to the long axis of the localizer; see diagram (2372).

After processing the film, the shadow shift of the foreign body is measured, using dividers, and an equal shadow shift cast by a localizer hole is identified (2504). It is obvious that the foreign body is at the same depth as the hole causing the equal shadow shift; in the elevation view (2372) it is shown to be 6 centimetres. The holes may be numbered from one onwards to indicate the depth scale on the radiograph, and any intermediate hole measurements may be easily calculated. In the localization radiograph (2371), the foreign body was shown to be 7 centimetres deep, which depth the removal operation proved to be correct.

32

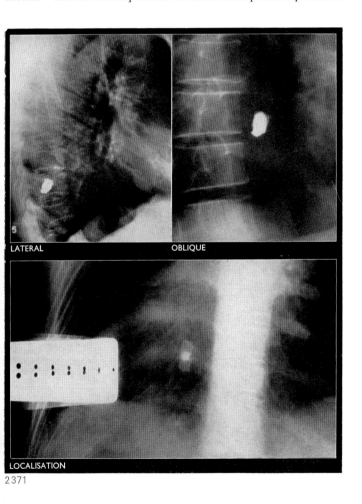

LATERAL   OBLIQUE

LOCALISATION

2371

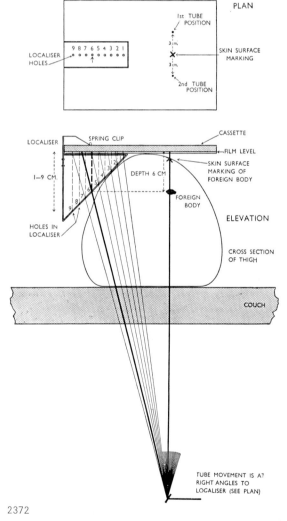

2372

739

General observations

Successful eye localization requires meticulous care and considerable practice by a selected method, and only a limited number of X-ray workers are likely to have the opportunity of becoming proficient in this specialized branch of radiography.

The identification of a foreign body in the orbital cavity—in the eyeball or in close proximity thereto—is only possible when the body is opaque, the examination involving two stages, (a) confirming its presence, and (b) determining its precise position.

Exposures should be made with the head clamped in position—true lateral or occipito-mental, as required.

Soft tissue films showing good detail are essential; intensifying screens when used should be free of any blemishes likely to be confused with foreign body shadows.

The special cassette holder employed has fine cross-wires attached, their point of intersection being adjusted to the centre of the pupil when the sight is directly forward and level, or outside the eyeball, according to the technique applied. The holder may be constructed to accommodate a film large enough for two exposures, the cassette being moved for the purpose, with each half protected in turn (2375).

A focus–film distance of forty inches 100 cm is generally used; while this is usually the maximum possible in ordinary conditions, it is still sufficient to give negligible distortion to near-film shadows.

For the purpose of foreign body localization, the eye is regarded as being an oblate spheroid having a maximum diameter of 24 millimetres.

Confirming the presence of a radio-opaque foreign body

With the patient in the lateral position, two exposures are made on a whole-plate cassette, one exposure with the eyes raised and the other with the eyes lowered.

A typical film thus exposed (2375) reveals an opaque foreign body in two positions in relation to the cross-wires, and indicates also that it is within the orbital cavity, and therefore either in the eyeball or in one of the muscles of the eye. With this information, the precise location of the foreign body may be determined.

To identify a foreign body in the anterior portion of the eyeball, a small dental film may be used, this being firmly held, during exposure, on the nasal aspect of the eye and as nearly as possible parallel to the median plane of the hand (2373,2374). The eye is opened as widely as possible for this exposure.

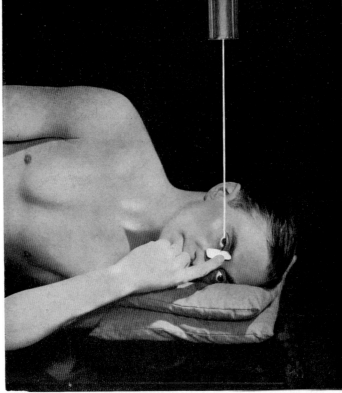

2373

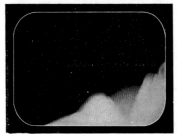

2374

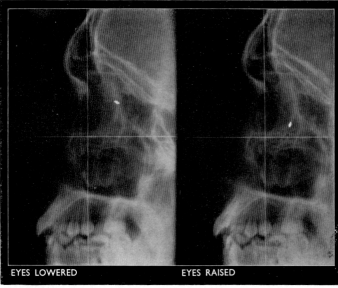

EYES LOWERED   EYES RAISED

2375

kVp	mAS	FFD	Film	Screens ILFORD	Grid
40	42	30″	Fast Dental		

Precise position of foreign body

There are two main methods, (a) determining the position of the foreign body relative to the centre of the eye, for which no special apparatus is required, pages 741–743, (b) determining the depth of the foreign body from the plane tangential to the centre of the cornea, and charting the three dimensions. The several methods employed under (b) necessitate the use of specialized equipment. Two such methods are described namely the localization spectacle method and limbal ring method. These two methods are included with appropriate charting as a summary of three dimensional localization within a sphere and from which the individual worker can appreciate similar procedure and charting of other methods such as the Bromley and Sweet localizing methods.

For these instrumental methods accuracy in localization of orbital foreign bodies depends on precise alignment of the tube focus and given points on the corneal axis and film, also on the corneal axis having a definite known relation to the film; perpendicular in a postero–anterior projection, and parallel in a lateral projection.

There need be no discrepancy in the calculated relation of the foreign body and the corneal axis, but the assumption of 24 millimetres as the diameter of the globe may lead to an error in estimating the relation of a foreign body and the sclera.

Most methods lend themselves to enlargement technique with a fine-focus tube.

Ocular fixation

It should be first ascertained whether the patient is able to keep both eyes fixed on some given mark or object, usually a black disc placed at eye level and directly in front of the eyes, or immediately overhead when the patient is supine: this is termed ocular fixation. Consideration should be given to any impairment of mobility choice of technique being governed by the degree to which mobility is affected.

Position of foreign body
Relative to centre of eye

It will be clear from the diagram (2376), representing the eye from the lateral aspect, that if a foreign body is anterior to the centre of the eye, it will move upward when the eye is raised and, if posterior, it will move downward; there will be no apparent change of position of a circular body at the centre, while the re-orientation of an irregular outline will be obvious.

Similarly in (2377), the foreign body in an anterior hemisphere will turn in direction with the eye when the eye is adducted, that in the posterior hemisphere moving in the opposite direction, while the body at the centre will remain apparently stationary.

Five films are therefore exposed to show the displacement of the shadow about the centre of the eye.

The patient should look steadily at some predetermined mark or small object which, as previously mentioned, usually takes the form of a prominent black disc placed at the level of the eyes, and on wall or ceiling according to whether vertical or horizontal technique is employed.

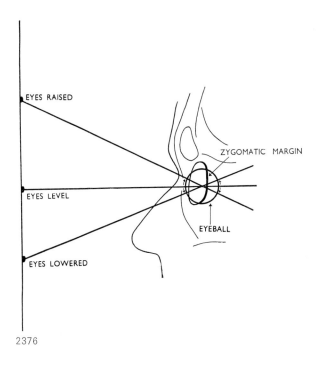

2376

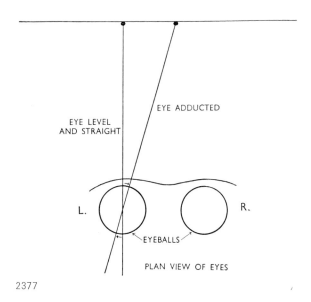

2377

For postero–anterior exposures, the frame supporting the fine cross-wires is placed with the point of intersection of the wires in line with the centre of the pupil, while for lateral exposures the horizontal wire is adjusted to the level of the centre of the pupil.

The head is carefully immobilized before the following two postero–anterior and three lateral exposures are made:

(a) Modified Ocpt-mental (25°) with eyes level and straight toward disc (2378).

(b) Modified Ocpt-mental (25°) with affected eye adducted (turned toward the nose) (2379).

(c) Lateral, with patient looking at disc (2381).

(d) Lateral, with eyes raised (2382).

(e) Lateral, with eyes lowered (2383).

These five films enable the body to be localized, whether it be in the eyeball or in the adjacent muscles (2380).

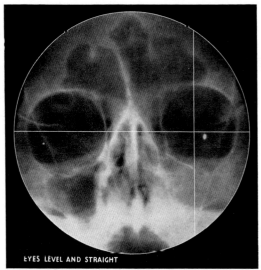

EYES LEVEL AND STRAIGHT

2378

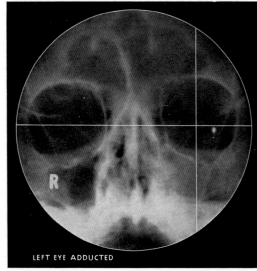

LEFT EYE ADDUCTED

2379

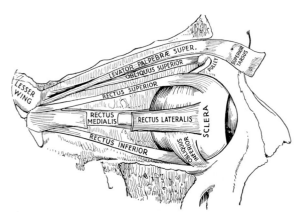

THE MUSCLES OF THE RIGHT ORBIT.
LATERAL ASPECT

2380

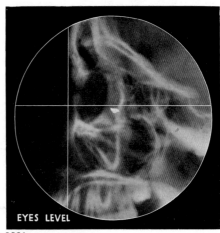

EYES LEVEL

2381

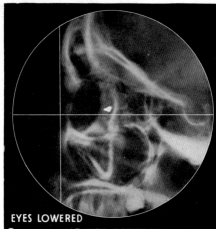

EYES RAISED

2382

EYES LOWERED

2383

From the three lateral projections, a tracing is made showing the three shadows of the foreign body; straight lines are drawn to join them, and these being chords of the arc described by the body during eye movement, lines bisecting them at right angles, midway between the shadows, will, at their point of intersection, indicate the centre of the eyeball if the point of intersection falls slightly anterior to the zygomatic border of the orbit (2384), in which case the foreign body is indicated as being in the eyeball. If, however, the point of intersection should be remote from the zygomatic border, it will be an indication that the foreign body is not the eyeball but in the surrounding tissue or muscles (2387).

A second tracing, prepared from the two postero–anterior films, enable the lateral movement of the foreign body to be plotted, and will disclose its antero–posterior position relative to the centre of the pupil, indicated by the intersection of the cross-wires (2385).

The five films, therefore, will be found to disclose the latitude and longitude, as it were, of the foreign body.

When the foreign body is shown by the tracing to be outside the eyeball, the particular muscle in which it is situated may be identified by reference to the anatomical diagram showing the muscle attachments of the eye (2380).

Two diagrams show (2386) a foreign body (in this case a pellet from an airgun) in the rectus superior muscle, and (2387) its movement, from the lateral aspect, in the three eye positions and also its centre of movement in relation to the centre of the eye.

Although this method has certain drawbacks, a knowledge of its possibilities will allow it to be applied, in part, when other methods have been found to be inconclusive because of the possible variation in the size or shape of the eye.

32

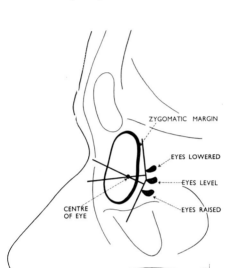

ZYGOMATIC MARGIN

EYES LOWERED

EYES LEVEL

EYES RAISED

CENTRE OF EYE

2384

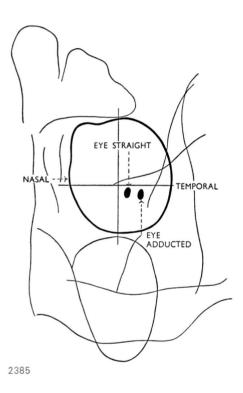

EYE STRAIGHT

NASAL

TEMPORAL

EYE ADDUCTED

2385

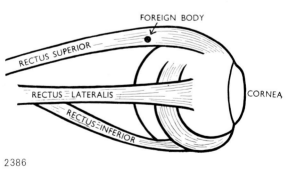

FOREIGN BODY

RECTUS SUPERIOR

RECTUS LATERALIS

RECTUS INFERIOR

CORNEA

2386

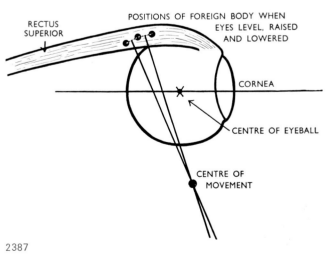

POSITIONS OF FOREIGN BODY WHEN EYES LEVEL, RAISED AND LOWERED

RECTUS SUPERIOR

CORNEA

CENTRE OF EYEBALL

CENTRE OF MOVEMENT

2387

Spectacles method

After determining that an opaque foreign body is present in the orbital cavity and confirming that ocular fixation, described earlier, is possible, the spectacles technique follows a course which, for convenience, is discussed in the following stages:

(a) Taking the shadow-shift film.

(b) Estimating the surface position of the foreign body.

(c) Calculating the depth measurement.

(d) Charting the actual position of the foreign body.

(a) **Taking the shadow-shift film.** A specially designed form of spectacles frame is used, having an adjustable nose-piece and cross-wired eyepieces. By means of a side with screw control each eyepiece can be lowered to the level of the eye where it serves as a rest for the film during the exposure. When correctly in position, the eyepiece is parallel to the couch and to the direction of the tube movement, with the raised indicator vertically over the intersection of the cross-wires (2388,2389).

The patient's head is immobilized with the neck resting on a sandbag and the eyes fixed on the overhead mark. The eyepiece over the eye being examined is adjusted so that the point of intersection of the cross-wires is immediately over the pupil; the eyes are then closed, the eyepiece is lowered until it touches the eyelid, gentle compression is applied, and by means of screening the tube is centred to the point of intersection of the cross-wires with the raised indicator immediately above; the diaphragm is then opened, the film—dental size—is rested upon the eyepiece, the sound eye again looks at the overhead mark, and the two tube-shift exposures are made on the one film, the tube positions being 3 centimetres on each side of the centring point and in line with one of the cross-wires. A small weight, a penny is suitable, placed on the film serves to maintain good contact (2389). The position of the film is recorded by a small metal projection on the eyepiece, which indicates a particular quadrant of the eye—lower temporal, right or left: careful record should be made of the focus–film distance and tube-shift employed, and these examinations will be facilitated if conditions are standardized as far as possible. After processing the film, the presence of a foreign body in a particular quadrant is noted.

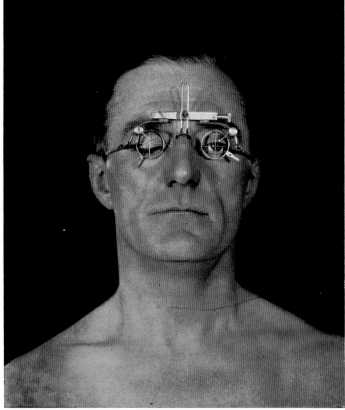

2388

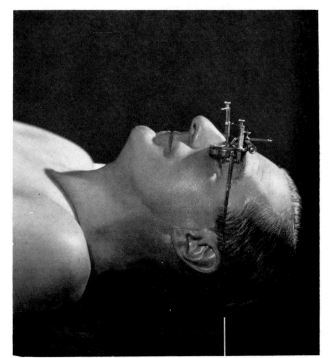

2389

(b) Estimating the surface position of the foreign body. The film distance of the foreign body shadows from the cross-wires is measured in millimetres and, with a sharp pencil, the position of the foreign body is marked on the Chart C (2390), which is lined in units to represent millimetres.

The four points, tube-centre positions T_1 and T_2 to foreign body shadows S_1 and S_2, are joined, the lines intersecting to give the actual position of the foreign body as seen from the anterior viewing aspect (elevation) of the eye (2391). The points S_1 and S_2 are similar to those referred to earlier as F_1 and F_2.

(c) Calculation of Depth. The film–shadow shift of the foreign body is measured, and by applying the formula

$$\frac{A \times S}{T + S} = D,$$

or by referring to the table of depths, the depth of the foreign body in the case shown (2391) is

$$\frac{550 \times 2 \cdot 5}{60 + 2 \cdot 5} = 22 \text{ millimetres}$$

this being its distance from the film plane tangential to the cornea.

(d) Charting the actual position of the foreign body. It will be seen that the Chart D (2391) embraces two diagrams, representing elevation and plan views of the eyeball respectively, with the exposure position of the film indicated by the line XY in the latter view. The position, of the foreign body F, is transferred from the Chart C (2390) to the elevation diagram (2391) as P, and through P a horizontal line a–c is drawn of which the part within the circumference of the circle represents the diameter of the section of the eye in which the foreign body lies. From the points at which a–c cuts the circumference, perpendiculars are dropped to d–e, the major axis of the lower diagram, and between the feet of the perpendiculars the plan view of the section is completed (shaded).

From the point P (elevation), a perpendicular is dropped to the plan film line, XY, which it meets at P and from this point the ascertained depth of the foreign body from the film P to P_1, is set off along the perpendicular, P_1 being the actual position of the foreign body. When P_1 is within the shaded section the foreign body is actually within the eyeball, and a position such as that shown in (2391), therefore, is outside the eyeball although within the orbital cavity.

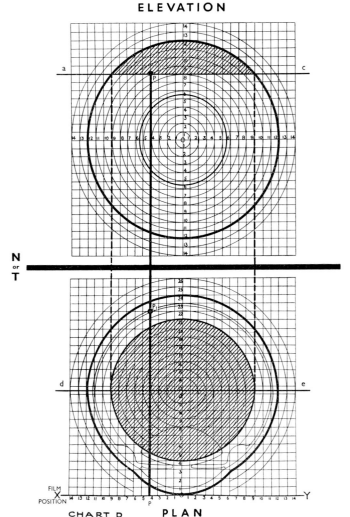

ELEVATION

N or T

FILM X POSITION

CHART D   PLAN

2391

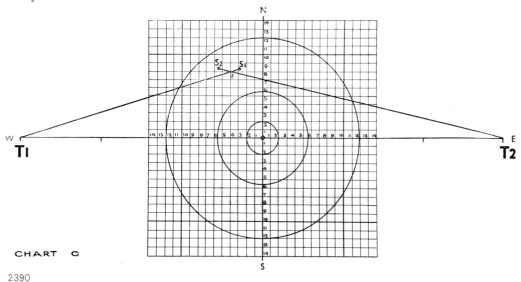

CHART C

2390

The position of the foreign body would be reported as follows:

A foreign body, radiologically opaque, is present in the right eye.

The foreign body is:
  8 mm above the central corneal axis;
  4 mm to the temporal side of the central corneal axis;
  22 mm deep to the plane tangential to the centre of the anterior surface of the cornea.
The charts show the foreign body to be external to the outer surface of the eyeball.

A clear understanding of the procedure may be gained by practising the full technique on a dry skull with phantom eye inserted in a small brass curtain ring fitted with fine cross-wires and an improvised "quadrant indicator" serves as a substitute for the spectacles eyepiece (2388).

Illustration (2392a) shows the type of chart supplied for the spectacles localization method. The actual form, however, is a littler larger than the reproduction and includes also the patient's particulars.

This same form is equally suitable for charting eye localization by other methods.

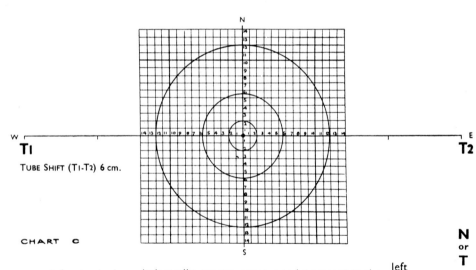

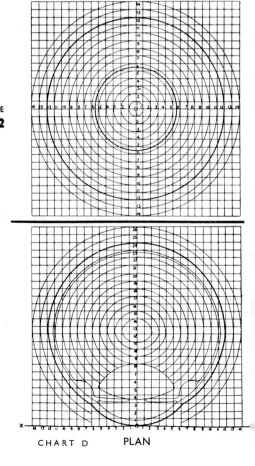

ELEVATION

TUBE SHIFT (T1-T2) 6 cm.

CHART C

A foreign body, radiologically opaque, appears to be present in the $\frac{left}{right}$ eye.

The foreign body is:

  mm. $\frac{above}{below}$ the central corneal axis.

  mm. to the $\frac{nasal}{temporal}$ side of the central corneal axis.

  mm. deep to the plane tangential to the centre of the anterior surface of the cornea.

The charts show the foreign body to be $\frac{internal}{external}$ **to the outer surface of the eyeball.**

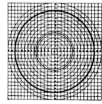

Note. Actual diameter of eyeball 24 mm.

CHART D   PLAN

    2392a

The Limbal Ring method

The position of a foreign body, whether within or outside the eyeball, may be established by the Limbal Ring method which consists of a metal wire ring, 12 millimetres in diameter, which is first sutured to the junction of the cornea and conjunctiva. Alternatively, using a contact lens, the metal ring is embedded in the lens, or maybe four small metal balls, or short lengths of wire, are embedded at N, S, E and W positions. The fixing involves local anaesthesia and/or surgery. This method is independent of focus to film distance.

Lateral and antero–posterior projections are made with the tube centred to the centre of the ring of wire, or circle of markers (2393a,b).

Diagram (2392b) enables a template to be cut in actual size and proportions for the preparation of a chart on squared paper about ×2 the actual size of the eyeball (2392a), each square representing 1 mm.

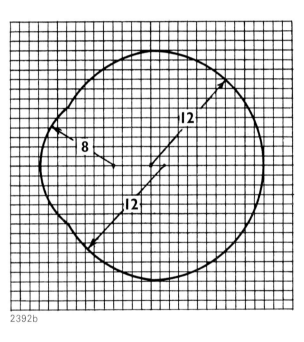

2392b

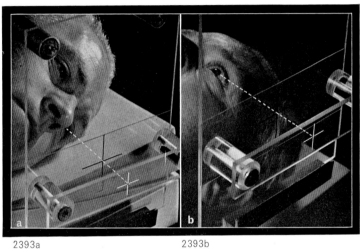

2393a   2393b

When processed and dry the radiographs are scribed as shown in (2394) and (2396a). The position of the foreign body in relation to the centring points is then transferred to squared paper using a scale of ×2 or more; any squared paper divided in tens is suitable. In (2395,2396b) side, frontal and plan projections are shown. The oblate side and plan views were drawn with a template made to the radii shown in (2392b), page 747.

Points S_1 and S_2 are then joined to their respective centring points, T_1 and T_2. The actual position of the foreign body is somewhere along these lines, and is found from

$$\frac{\text{diameter ring} \times T_1 S_1}{\text{diameter of ring image}} = T_1 B_1$$

This distance is then marked along the line from T_1. A line parallel to the corneal axis through this point intersects the line $T_2 S_2$ and so fixes the position of the foreign body in the frontal aspect.

The localization is then completed by projecting on to the chart plan similar to that used for the spectacles method (2392a).

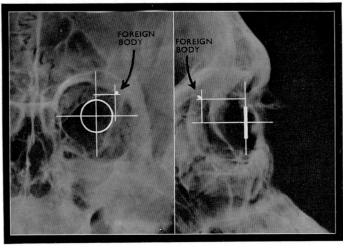

2394

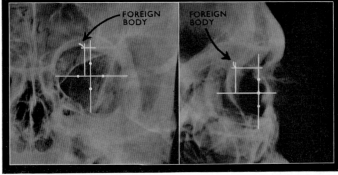

2396a

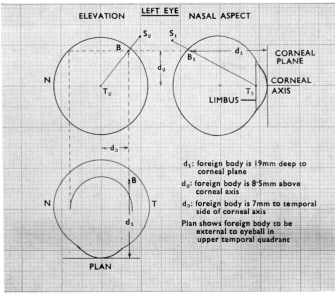

ELEVATION LEFT EYE NASAL ASPECT

d_1: foreign body is 19mm deep to corneal plane

d_2: foreign body is 8·5mm above corneal axis

d_3: foreign body is 7mm to temporal side of corneal axis

Plan shows foreign body to be external to eyeball in upper temporal quadrant

PLAN

2395

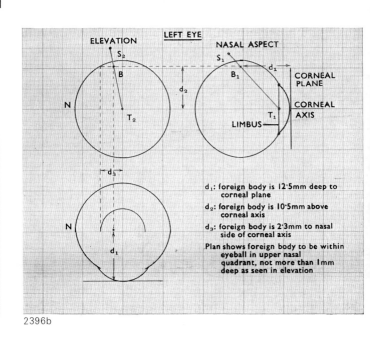

ELEVATION LEFT EYE NASAL ASPECT

d_1: foreign body is 12·5mm deep to corneal plane

d_2: foreign body is 10·5mm above corneal axis

d_3: foreign body is 2·3mm to nasal side of corneal axis

Plan shows foreign body to be within eyeball in upper nasal quadrant, not more than 1mm deep as seen in elevation

2396b

33

MINIATURE RADIOGRAPHY

MINIATURE RADIOGRAPHY

Photographic recording of the X-ray fluorescent screen image is employed in two ways:

(a) **Miniature radiography.** The recording of a single exposure of each subject.

(b) **Cineradiography.** A method of making a rapid series of exposures of one subject which, on projection, forms a "moving" picture; see Section 34.

Miniature radiography

Miniature radiography—fluorography or radio-photography— is similar to the indirect method of cineradiography, except that it is concerned only with the taking of "stills" of the fluorescent screen image. While the question of definition is perhaps of even greater importance than in cineradiography, the procedure in miniature radiography is simpler because only one exposure of each subject is required. This method of examination is applied chiefly to the lungs, although there is a tendency to use miniature radiography in the larger sizes for the abdominal viscera and for angiography.

Before undertaking this work, however, it is essential to appreciate the necessity for a very high standard of quality and uniformity of result, and to realize also its limitations. At present nothing can replace in precision and completeness the radiological investigation of the lungs by a combination of fluoroscopy and direct radiography, but miniature radiography does, nevertheless, render possible an intermediate form of examination which has the great advantage over screening alone of providing, in a comparatively short time, permanent records of many subjects. This method is referred to as Mass Radiography.

Mass miniature radiography is at present applied to the examination of the chests of large numbers of people who otherwise would not be examined, and it permits of the rapid survey of the inhabitants of a district, of large groups of workers, or of members of the armed forces. It has been found in such surveys that approximately 0·04 per cent of those examined are in need of immediate treatment and possibly 2 per cent may be given medical advice.

Miniature Units for the larger film sizes 70 and 100 millimetres are established in centres such as hospitals where all patients have a precautionary routine X-ray lung exposure, and in chest clinics for routine and follow-up contact examination, also to be available to local medical practitioners for direct reference of patients as required.

General procedure

Briefly, the image shown on the fluorescent screen is photographed on a small film, which may be in the form of *roll* film, 35 or 70 millimetres wide, and also of *cut* film, 100 millimetres square.

Certain cameras for roll films provide for the maximum size of image by eliminating the need for film edge perforations (2404,2406a,b).

The subjects are examined in the erect position, the whole apparatus being designed to facilitate positioning and the quick passage of each person, while at the same time providing full protection for the operator against excessive X radiation. Although the examinees no longer remove all clothing to the waist, the photographs on pages 751 and 754 showing the earlier routine with clothing removed, are retained to demonstrate positioning.

A plan diagram shows the relative arrangement for taking the miniature (indirect) radiographs and the re-examination large (direct) radiographs (2397).

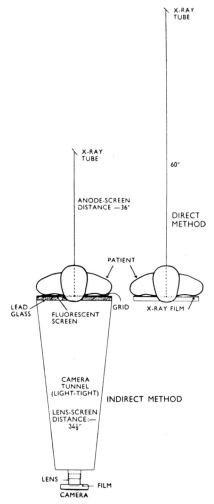

2397

X-ray equipment

Apparatus for miniature radiography may be considered briefly in three parts—the X-ray Power Unit, the Camera Unit, and the Control Table.

The power unit may consist of a four-valve transformer built for transportability and having an output of at least 200 milliamperes at 90 kilovolts-peak, using a standard rotating anode tube; an adjustable diaphragm enables the tube aperture to be varied to suit the several X-ray focus–screen and focus–film distances required for miniature and large films (2400).

On using the faster optical systems and the larger size films, and on eliminating the taking of full-size X-ray films as a part of the survey, a low-power self-rectified unit may be used, 85 kilovolts-peak at 30 to 50 milliamperes. Miniature units for mass radiography are constructed for mobility and two types are shown in (2400) and (2401,2402). These units provide for the protection of the operator against excessive radiation exposure, particularly in view of the large number of exposures made in a single day.

The camera unit consists of a light-proof pyramid-shaped tunnel fitted at the smaller end with the camera and at the larger end with the fluorescent screen, protective lead glass and radiographic grid. The tunnel also carries the identification device (2399,2403). For the 35 millimetre method, the camera accommodates 25 metres of miniature film (2398), movement of the film in the camera, following each exposure, being controlled automatically from the switch table: a cutting device enables the exposed length of film to be divided into suitable lengths for removal in the take-up cassette for subsequent development. For the conventional lens system the camera is fitted with a fluoride-coated two-inch $f/1\cdot5$ lens. The coating of the surfaces of the lens eliminates internal reflection and thus ensures maximum definition, contrast and speed. Focusing of the lens is a precision adjustment.

The introduction of the mirror optical system with its improved definition and increased speed has largely replaced the lens system. For certain units, the fast mirror optical system is being used to provide mobile equipment of low output for use on limited electrical mains supply. This type of equipment, built for compactness, makes use of a right-angled reflecting system which enables the camera tunnel to be placed vertically (2402) instead of projecting horizontally as in (2401).

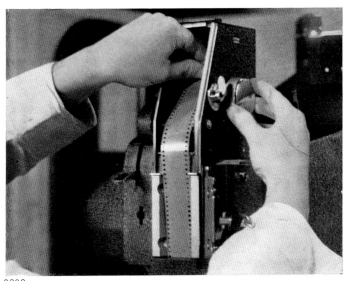

2398

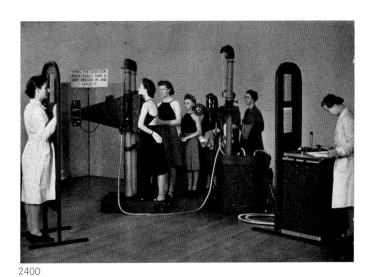

2400

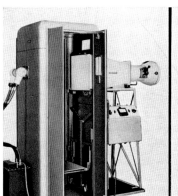

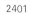

2399

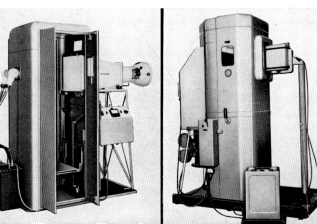

2401   2402

The development of the Schmidt mirror system from the original astronomical version to its present application to miniature radiography in the form of the Schmidt-Helm, or more generally the Odelca camera, is will known. Diagram (2403) shows the mirror system within the camera tunnel. The cylindrical curve of the screen is not shown.

The 70 millimetre Odelca unit accommodates a 50-exposure roll film magazine and also the Rapidex motorized cassette for rapid consecutive exposures as required for angiography.

The Odelca mirror camera for 100 millimetre square cut film provides for the packing of 100 films into a Separator cassette (2403). A blue-sensitive film is used with the appropriate blue-fluorescing screen. Or alternatively with a yellow-green emitting screen, orthochromatic or panchromatic film is used.

The *fluorescent screen*, of the yellow-green or blue fluorescent type, is sixteen inches square so that it may include the whole of the largest chest, there being some enlargement of the screen image owing to the short X-ray focus–screen distance employed,

which is usually thirty six inches, but is reduced to twenty-seven inches for the 70 millimetre small-output mobile unit. To reduce scattered radiation, thereby improving definition and contrast, and also as a protective measure, the tube diaphragm is adjusted to limit the X-ray beam to the area of the screen.

The *protective lead glass*, which is on the camera side of the screen, absorbs approximately 10 per cent of the fluorescent screen illumination, but this is not considered to be a sufficient loss to warrant its disuse for the 35-millimetre unit. Indeed, this relatively small loss in speed is of little consequence and is far outweighed by the protective value of the lead glass.

Identification of a chest radiograph with the subject is achieved by photographing on to the lower border of the radiograph the serial number on the individual's record card (2403) which is placed in a slot provided on the apparatus, the exposure being made automatically. It should be noted that the apparatus cannot function unless the record card is placed in the correct position.

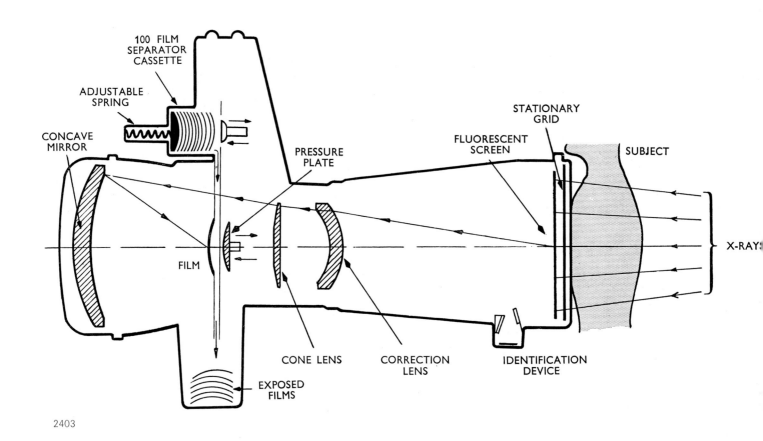

2403

A *stationary grid* of suitable characteristics is used to reduce scattered radiation which, if allowed to reach the film, would cause diffusion of detail and a lowering of contrast. The resultant loss of definition and general veiling would be particularly objectionable on projection. The grid is placed in contact with the front of the fluorescent screen and is therefore between the patient and the screen. The grid lines are not visible on the 35 millimetre lens-unit film, even when projected; on the other hand, they are clearly visible when radiographs taken by the later mirror-type optical system, with its superior resolving power, are viewed at any considerable degree of enlargement.

Miniature film perforations

Films (2404,2406a,b) show advantage in size when the perforations are eliminated. 70 millimetre film cameras having been made to take perforated film (2405) and others unperforated film (2404,2406a,b).

(2407) 100 mm cut film.

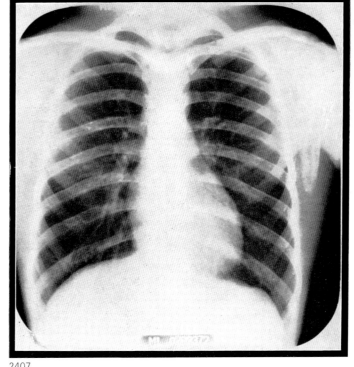

2407

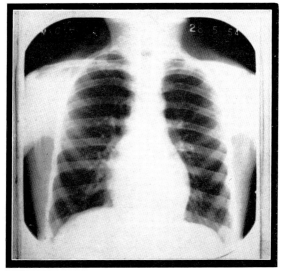

2404

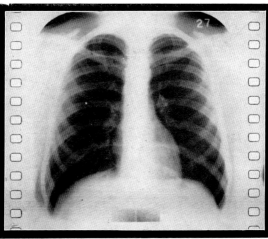

2405

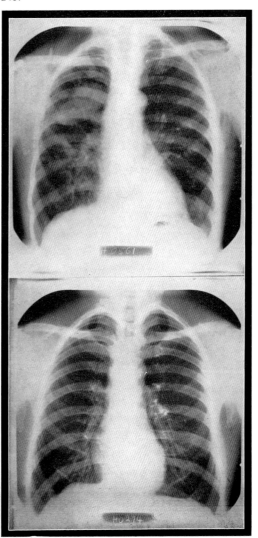

2406a/2406b

Positioning

In miniature radiography, the short focus–screen distance renders positioning critical. In a well-designed unit, the positioner is able to move freely behind the subject, positioning for symmetry being thus simplified. The subject is "moulded" to the screen by pressing the shoulders downward and forward, the arms being adjusted in the most satisfactory position to enable the clavicles to be depressed and the shadows of the scapulae to be projected outside the lung field. It should be remembered that, when working at a distance of thirty-six inches, the smallest fault in positioning is magnified in the radiograph, and the utmost care should therefore be taken to follow closely the positioning described and shown on this page. See also (2408) showing the hands at waist level as is necessary with subjects having *short* arms; (2409) with the arms extended, brought forward and rotated, as may be necessary for elderly subjects who are inclined to be stiff, in order to bring the shoulders near to the screen; and (2410) with the hands low down over the buttocks as required for subjects with *long* arms.

It should be remembered that the shoulder position is of first importance and that the position of the arms and hands is adapted accordingly.

Correct alignment between X-ray tube and screen is important and may be checked by means of an optical centring device or other method incorporated in the unit. Simultaneous adjustment of the level of the two units—X-ray tube and camera tunnel—to suit the varying heights of the examinees, is obtained in one type of unit (2400) by the use of a flexible cable system and in another type (2401), by a lift for moving the patient in relation to tube and screen.

The control table is so designed that when set for the appropriate exposure, the single control switch automatically brings into operation, in correct sequence, the rotor of the X-ray tube, the exposure of the number on the record card, the X-ray exposure and, finally, the winding-on of the film in the camera. Meters and light indicators enable the operator to detect failure in any part of the apparatus, and limiting devices prevent overloading of the X-ray tube.

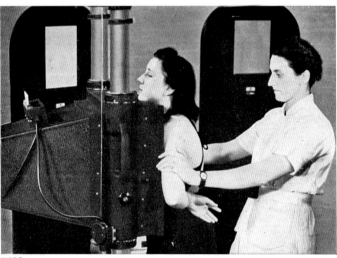

2408

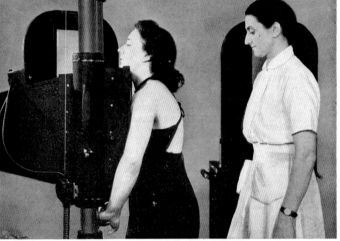

2409

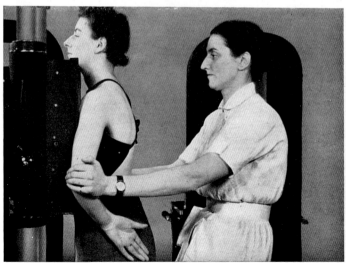

2410

Comparison of Large Film and Miniature Techniques

Direct Large Film	Indirect Miniature
Double coated film	Single coated film
Double intensifying screens	Single screen
No-grid technique	Grid technique
Grid technique	
Film and Screens in Contact	Reduction in light intensity due to optical system. Reduction in light intensity due to inverse square law, loss between screen and film.

Light intensity losses are greater in the miniature system. The 35 mm system requiring an increase of ×9 times the normal X-ray large film exposure.

To maintain an exposure time suitable, to offset subject movement, the focus–film distance of 5 or 6 feet as used for direct radiographs is reduced to a focus–screen distance of 3 feet (2397) for the miniature technique. Where the large film technique is a non-grid technique an increase of 20 kilovolts is required to compensate for the use of the grid in the miniature technique.

With the faster mirror optics the disparity in exposure required between the miniature and large film approach is reduced to a factor of ×3.

Essentials in the miniature system

(a) A large aperture lens, and short focal length lens system is required.
(b) The speed of the single screen should be such as to provide maximum emission with acceptable sharpness.
(c) Processing should be with a view to obtaining maximum speed, low grain and fog.

Processing

Development of the miniature film is standardized by employing a spiral daylight tank or frame for roll film lengths of from 3 to 25 metres and slotted carriers or frames for cut film. Development is for 6 minutes at 68°F (20°C) in a conventional X-ray manual developer, which not only serves to reduce exposure time but gives clean results with good contrast, essential both for satisfactory projection and for direct viewing with or without magnification. Recent trend however in 70 millimetre roll-film size has been to adopt films suited to 90 second automatic processing.

The colour sensitivity of the film chosen, generally either monochromatic or orthochromatic is dependent on the spectral emission colour of the unit screen.

Films should not be handled unnecessarily as all surface blemishes are magnified on enlargement for viewing.

Viewing

A suitable projector and viewing screen enable the 35 millimetre miniature radiographs to be seen at a size of 5 × 5 inches or larger, as may be chosen.

It is essential that the projector should have a well-corrected lens, simple mechanism for the easy and scratch-free manipulation of the miniature film, and satisfactory illumination, usually with a 100-watt lamp.

The *projection screen* has a white matt surface which is masked to the size of the projected image. When many miniature radiographs are to be examined at one viewing, it is found that eye-strain may be reduced by confining projection to the smaller size of 5 × 5 inches. A further factor is the better definition of lung detail shown in the smaller and more concentrated image, thus enabling the radiologist to sit very near to the screen.

Both 45 millimetre and 70 millimetre films are viewed by direct magnification to one-and-a-half times the original size, although the latter may be viewed without enlargement. The 100 millimetre and 4 × 5 inch size films are not enlarged, but should be inspected in a masked viewing box.

When numbered at the ends and filed in shallow drawers with cardboard partitions, the roll-film records are readily accessible for reference, many thousands of chest radiographs occupying only a very small space.

As its name implies, *mass* miniature radiography is undertaken with a large number of subjects and, therefore, the need for satisfactory organization and technical uniformity becomes imperative. It is essential that the staff should work as a team and, within limits, be able to interchange readily.

With examinations being made at the rate of 500 and more per day, and working to standard development of the film strips standardized exposure to produce uniformity of results assumes great importance, and is achieved by the use of a photo-timer which automatically adjusts the exposure to the density of the subject, using three alternative kilovoltage settings for average, large and small subjects. The alternative is to base the exposure technique on the chest thickness measurement.

33 Miniature radiography

Confirmation on large films

35 millimetre miniature ML 8951 (2411) this subject having been recalled for a full-sized film to be taken as shown in (2412) postero–anterior, a lesion in the upper lobe of the right lung being confirmed. Similarly a lesion suspected in miniature (2413) is confirmed both in the large film (2414) and follow-up tomograms (2415).

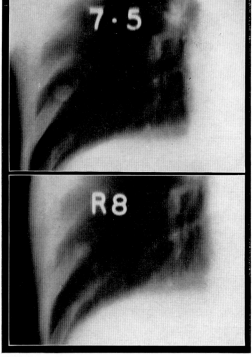

2415

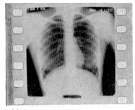

2411

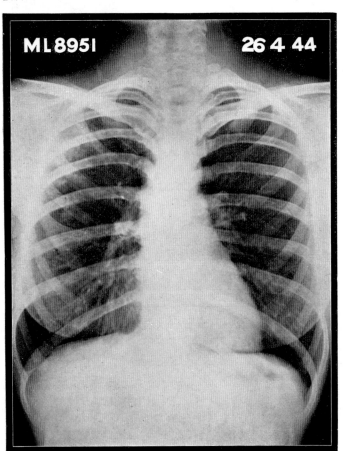

2412

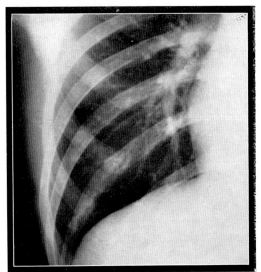

2414

2413

34

CINERADIOGRAPHY

CINERADIOGRAPHY

Cine-fluorography is the process of recording by cine-photography the X-ray fluorescent screen image on film or tape, of organs in continuous movement, producing a changing pattern in accordance with the normality and motility of the organ.

Its main application is to regions such as the heart—circulatory and (abdominal) G.I.T. system to demonstrate functional disorder. Where the pattern change is slow and motion need not be recorded the allied technique of spot filming provides a succession of still pictures of the fluoroscopic image in such rapid succession that the necessary continuous evidence is provided.

Cine radiography employing the conventional fluorescent type of screen would necessitate a prohibitive dosage rate to the patient, it is necessary therefore to have a system which gives a much brighter screen image to achieve the desired result. There are two main types of equipment available for achieving this. The first being in the form of an image intensifier, and the second is based on the intensity of the screen image being amplified through a T.V. camera system.

This small image is photographed through the cine camera lens system on to 16 or 35 millimetre film.

Intensification of the screen image is by a combination of acceleration and linear reduction of the electrons in their passage between the two screens. These two effects, multiplied together, result in an overall intensification factor of the order of up to × 5000.

The image intensifier

The image intensifier is shown diagrammatically in (2416). The components are in a sealed, bottle-necked, glass container, the X-ray activated surface being at the broad end and the cine photographic elements at the neck.

Referring to diagram (2416), it will be seen that the input screen on a thin curved aluminium support, is mounted at the broad end of the container, with the convex surface facing the subject and X-ray tube. The concave surface, facing the neck, carries a fluorescent screen coating which is in turn covered by a photoelectron emitting layer. This layer is connected to the cathode side of a 25 kilovolt direct-current supply.

A small fine grain fluorescent screen, the output screen is placed at the neck of the container with the fluorescent surface facing the lens system of the 16 or 35 millimetre cine camera.

To enable free electrons to be directed from the larger to the smaller screen, an electron-focusing device is placed just ahead of the small fluorescent screen.

In action, the X-rays project the patient's image on to the larger fluorescent screen. Photo-electrons, following this same image pattern, are freed from the negatively charged photo-electron layer, their passage being accelerated by the direct-current charge. The electrons converge toward the electron-focusing device to impinge on the small viewing screen, there to produce an image of the original subject.

Units differ in input screen diameter between 5″ and 9″ and 12″. The 5″ input screen while suited to children tends to be too restricted in adult subject coverage, the tendency therefore has been toward the larger screen units or a combination of small and larger size input screen coverage.

This equipment can provide for the attachment of a cine camera, a spot-film camera, a T.V. camera and associated monitor or an optical viewer for fluoroscopy. Up to any three of these instruments can be attached at one time. An optical beam-splitting device or image-distributor enables the image to be switched rapidly from one to another or shared between two to allow simultaneous observation and recording. Recording can be by cine-film, spot-film, or video-tape; observation can be carried out by means of the optical viewer or the attached T.V. monitor system.

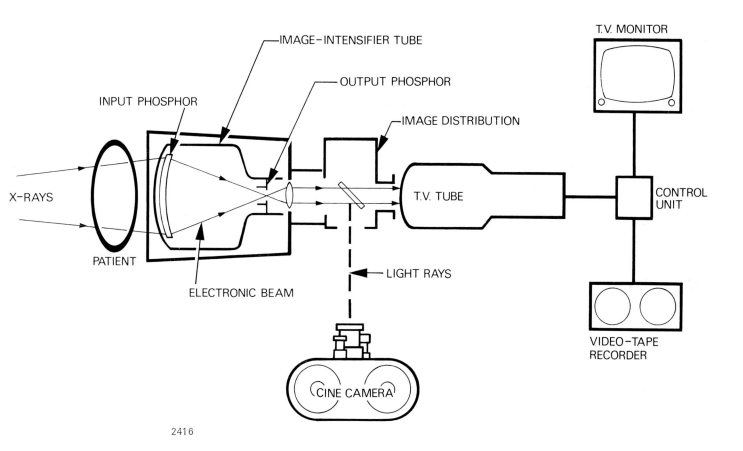

IMAGE—INTENSIFIER TUBE

OUTPUT PHOSPHOR

INPUT PHOSPHOR

IMAGE DISTRIBUTION

T.V. MONITOR

X-RAYS

PATIENT

T.V. TUBE

CONTROL UNIT

ELECTRONIC BEAM

LIGHT RAYS

CINE CAMERA

VIDEO—TAPE RECORDER

2416

20 20pp.

34 Cineradiography

The T.V. camera system shown in figure 2417 is based on the Orthicon T.V. camera tube. The image formed on a 12 inch diameter fluorescent screen is focused by a high speed concentric mirror optical system on the T.V. camera tube which transforms the image into an electronic signal. This is amplified and produces a T.V. monitor screen image of sufficient brightness to be recorded by a cine, video-tape or spot-film camera. A separate monitor screen is provided for viewing purposes.

Television monitoring: Incorporating television in the procedure has had far reaching effects. The brilliant television screen image may be viewed in subdued room lighting. Television monitors in the X-ray room, and placed remotely in other parts of the building, enable the radiological procedure to be followed and discussed on a two-way talking system, as appropriate, being useful also for educational purposes for medical students, for interested observers, and furthermore for the remote selective recording of the examination by cine film or by continuous recording on magnetic tape, all phases being under the manipulative control of the operating radiologist.

In addition to conventional viewing by television, provision is made for various alternatives to give a choice for better viewing or recording—reversal of the image from positive to negative; enlargement of a selected area; reversal from right to left, also from above downward, enabling the region to be seen in the conventional anatomical position. Image storage methods which enable the image to be retained up to thirty minutes for study or for copying, is another important development.

The fine-focus tube: The increased luminosity of the screen enables visual fluoroscopy and television viewing to be made at currents from 0·2 to 2mA. Dosage-rates to patients over a wide range of examinations are quoted for the 12″ unit as being from 7·5 to 140 millirads. With image intensifying fluoroscopy as compared with conventional the X-ray dose is reduced to approximately 10–20 per cent for the thorax and 20 to 30 per cent for the abdomen.

The low milliamperage required allows the use of fine foci 0·3 × 0·3 or 0·6 × 0·6 millimetre to provide a high standard of definition for screening, cine and spot filming.

16 mm and 35 mm cameras: Although a 16 mm camera unit is fully capable of resolving the detail of a 5″ screen image, definition is progressively superior with the 35 mm unit, as the image size increases, further to this for the same projected image the 35 mm format requires smaller enlargement and is sharper as a consequence.

Irrespective of this however other factors not the least being the greater economy of the 16 mm system can influence the eventual choice, e.g. faster lens systems tend to be more readily available in 16 mm size than in 35 mm, and for a given output screen size the 35 mm system can be up to four times slower.

The greater speed of the 16 mm system due to the availability of lenses of wider aperture also provides a greater latitude in the use of shorter exposure times, extended coverage or dosage rates can be reduced. Alternatively it permits a greater choice of slower type film to improve definition and uniformity of the image.

The ever increasing efficiency of the image intensifier system has however tended to nullify many of the previous advantages afforded to the 16 mm format.

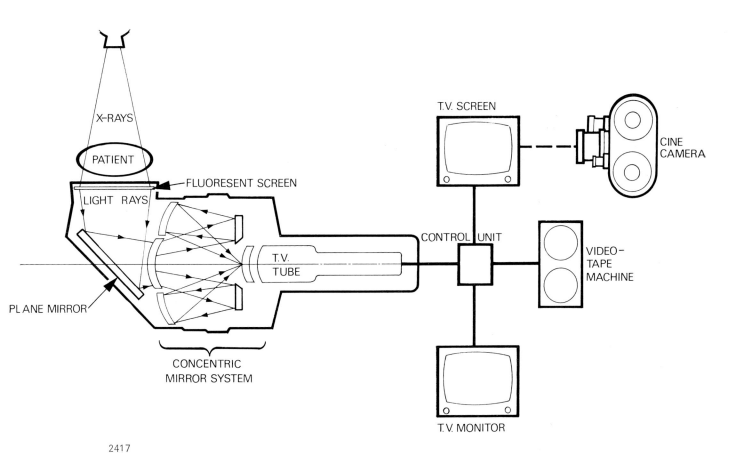

X-RAYS

PATIENT

FLUORESENT SCREEN

LIGHT RAYS

PLANE MIRROR

CONCENTRIC
MIRROR SYSTEM

T.V.
TUBE

T.V. SCREEN

CINE
CAMERA

CONTROL UNIT

VIDEO-
TAPE
MACHINE

T.V. MONITOR

2417

34 Cineradiography

Cine frame speeds: Most cine cameras provide a choice of framing speeds of 8, 48, and 64 frames per second. 16 mm cameras are now available with speeds up to 200 per second, and recently introduced 35 mm cameras have the capability of framing speeds of 80 and 150 frames per second.

The footage of film required for the duration of the cine run can be appreciated from the fact that 16 mm film size takes 40 frames per foot of film and 35 mm takes 16 frames per foot of film. In the above film sizes therefore 16 mm at a framing rate of 200 frames per second would require 5 feet of film per second and 35 mm at a framing rate of 64 frames per second would require 4 feet of film per second. Multiplied by the duration of the cine run will then give the total length of film required.

A high rate of frames per second and projected at a conventional rate can be used to advantage in the evaluation of rapid subject movement whereas a slower rate of framing at conventional projection rate is suited to subjects of slower motility.

In high speed subjects such as Angiography the greater the number of frames per second will determine how complete the continuity of the information is, between each successive frame. Slower framing speed increases the intervening time interval between each frame during which no information is recorded, and although on projection the movement appears continuous, phases of subject movement and information will be absent.

Frame speeds greater than 50 can only be achieved with a constant high voltage and a camera independent of the television viewing screen.

Where the camera records direct from a monitor the frame speed must synchronize with the television system. The system in (2147) has a triple scan of a thousand lines. With a pulsating high tension, a frame speed of 50 requires careful synchronizing of the camera, and lower frame speeds must be submultiples of 50 where the frequency is 50 cycles per second.

Likewise, although slower speeds 8–16 frames are suitable for recording the slower moving parts such as the Alimentary and Urinary Tract, 25–50 frames per second is common practice to coincide with convenient simultaneous television viewing.

Exposure Control: Exposure to the film is determined by the frame speed or alternatively by pulsed exposure to each single frame. Three systems are in use:

(a) Continuous—where the X-ray tube is energized during the complete cine run.
(b) Synchronized—where the tube is energized to coincide with the shutter-open, film stationary period.
(c) Grid Tube Pulse Control—Provision of pulsed millisecond exposure within the shutter open, film stationary phase.

It will be appreciated that dosage to the patient is progressively decreased from a–c.

The arrest of subject movement in each frame by millisecond exposure enables each frame to be studied individually, and provides for sharper definition of the projected image, due to the absence of kinetic blurring.

In systems a & b with a frame speed of 64 per second the duration of the exposure to the film would be 1/128th second.

In system c Pulsed X-ray exposure is generally from 2–5 milliseconds.

Selection of Film: Features essential in the choice of film are that it should have the ability to record the light intensity differences and detail of the screen image. Its speed should be in keeping with the exposure requirements of the subject and have the required contrast.

The increasing efficiency of the image intensifier has tended to make the medium speed, e.g. FP4 film the film of choice whereby obtaining a pleasing compromise in all factors. Where this procedure is not adopted or in special circumstances where the preference may be toward slower material to provide the maximum in fine detail, e.g. Pan F, or alternatively where speed is the criteria (e.g. Mark V) a choice of one or the other will ensure the optimum conditions of the remaining factors when one is chosen specifically.

Processing: Cine film in lengths up to 10 feet can be wound in vertical loops around an X-ray hanger, the film should be wound on the hanger so that the base of the film and not the emulsion side is touching the hanger. These can then be processed by hand in conventional X-ray processing tanks, spiral film-processing outfits or automatic processing outfits are available for greater lengths. Processing procedure is determined by the eventual usage of this, the original.

If required for immediate diagnostic purposes, processing to high contrast is generally recommended, if however intended as a "Master" from which subsequent contact or reduced copies are required, a lower gamma presents a more controllable printing quality.

70 mm Technique: The above type of camera can be adapted to the image intensifier as a means of taking single frame or continuing frames at a rapidity of 3 or 6 second. Its major application has been in connection with the Gastro intestinal tract although considerable investigation as to its practicability in examination for coronary arteriography has been undertaken. In Gastro intestinal work due to the speed of the intensifier system, exposure times are in the region of $\frac{1}{10}$th that required for large film. This advantage tends to be somewhat nullified in that with the small field coverage afforded by the intensifier, multiple films are required to cover the same area as the single large films. This in turn however may be advantageous in that the examination tends to be more detailed over specific locations.

Magnification techniques can be adapted to ensure that small areas, e.g. the duodenal cap fills the full 70mm frame. It is necessary to ensure however that repetitive exposure below 0·04 seconds is available in order that exposure occurs while the film is stationary in the gate.

The absence of heavy cassette manipulation is an asset each magazine roll of film taking a film length of 150 feet or more depending on the film base thickness.

100 mm spot film technique: The above is available at present at a framing speed of 3 per second.

Applications

For angiocardiography by selective catheterization, the 20 millimetre injection of an opaque medium may be arranged in three or four intermittent stages, possibly 25 per cent of the injection in each of four locations within the heart, each followed by a brief cine recording to provide a detailed and localized functional survey, again with a minimum of radiation to the patient.

For gastric examinations the follow-up by cinefluorography is most important as quite often only motility will disclose the pathology.

The majority of cine recordings involve techniques requiring the use of an opaque medium which in itself provides ample contrast at high kilovoltage, but the technique needs to be modified when the contrast medium either disperses so rapidly that its passage cannot be recorded, or so slowly that it fails to achieve sufficient density or contrast to enable a satisfactory cine recording to be made at the high kilovoltage.

Cineradiographs

For all but two strips of cine recordings appearing in this section, the first two or three frames show the full width of the film, including the perforations; the remaining frames are enlarged and, to permit this, the perforations have been omitted.

(2420) is of cerebral angiography following injection of 10 millilitres of 35 per cent diodone. Exposures were at the rate of sixteen frames per second.

(2421) showing the passage of barium through the lower oesophagus, was taken at the rate of eight frames per second.

(2422) showing movements of the antrum, and with an ulcer at the lesser curvature of the pylorus, again taken at the rate of eight frames per second.

(2423) shows the calyces of the kidneys exposed at the rate of eight frames per second; a positive reproduction.

For the alimentary and renal tracts, the conditions of exposure, using a grid, are from 90 to 120 kVp, 6mA, at from eight to twelve frames per second.

(2424) embraces three extracts from a cine recording of an adult subject exposed during micturition, following retrograde filling of the bladder with diodone 50 per cent diluted by 50 per cent distilled water, 500 millilitres of the dilute solution being prepared to each examination.

(2418) showing cardiac angiography of an infant, reported as a patient ductus arteriosus.

Equipment is available for enlarging single selected cine frames—four on an 8 × 10 inch film (2419)—for record purposes, possibly for convenience of inclusion in the patient's notes.

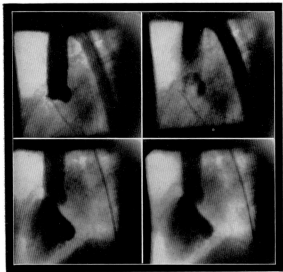

2419

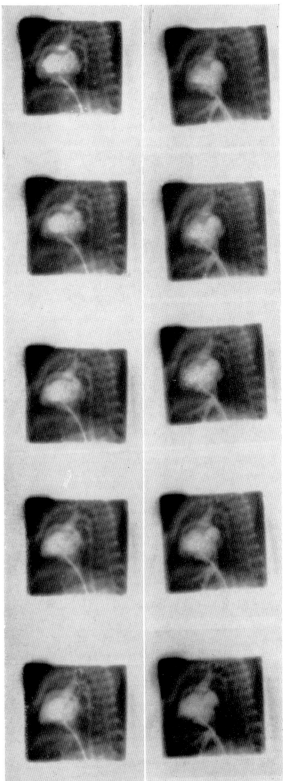

2418

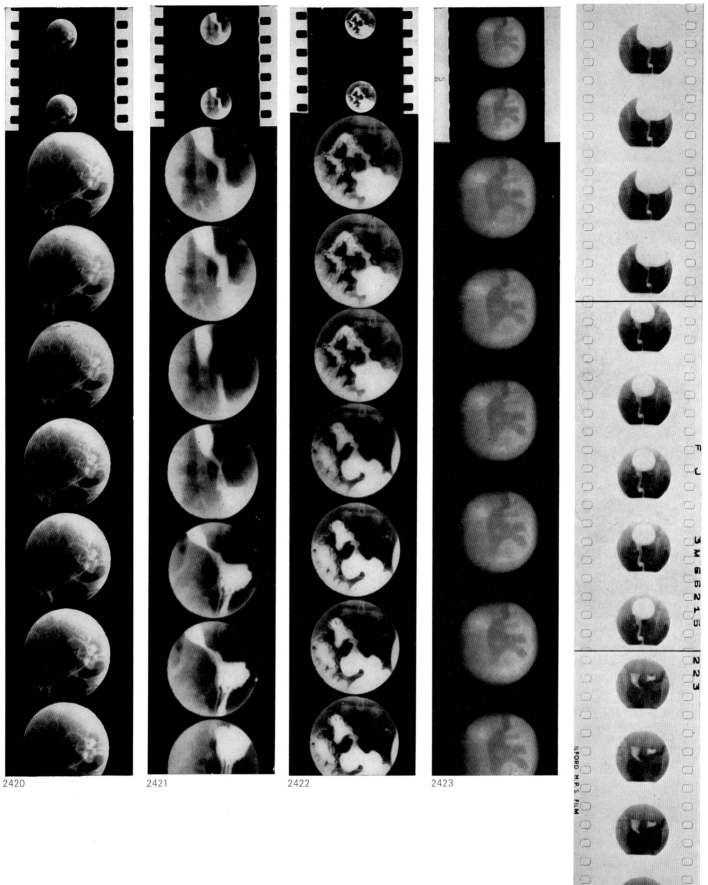

34

2420

2421

2422

2423

2424

765

CONTRAST
AND OPAQUE MEDIA

CONTRAST AND OPAQUE MEDIA

Tissue differentiation

The visualization of adjacent structures within the body is determined by the differences in their absorption of the X-ray beam as it passes through the body. This is dependent on both the nature and thickness of the absorbing tissues—the characteristic of bone, muscle and soft tissue and the air cavities of the body are such that their X-ray absorption differences are sufficient to be recognized as changes in exposure to the film. The film responds to these differences in exposure, producing changes in film blackening (density) and this constitutes what is termed the radiographic contrast between the structures. Altered opacity, however, resulting from disease or atrophy of the tissues affect these differences in absorption. A fluid-filled lung greatly increases the absorption of the X-ray beam, whereas a partially atrophied bone is much less opaque than the normal. Similarly the muscular tone of the patient will have a noticeable affect on the radiographic contrast between muscle and soft tissue.

In many regions of the body, however, the difference in opacity between adjacent structures is not sufficient for them to be distinguishable on the radiograph. The oesophagus, stomach, colon, kidney, urinary bladder, gall bladder and blood vessels are examples of organs which generally require an introduction of substances having a greater or reduced opacity than the tissues surrounding these areas.

Thus this enhanced distinction may be acquired in one or other of two approaches namely the introduction of contrast media or the introduction of opaque media. Contrast media is a term used to describe substances of low molecular weight such as oxygen or air which show radiographically in contrast with the surrounding body tissues as a dark shadow. Opaque media are substances which contain elements of high atomic weight which show radiographically as light shadows against the body tissues, for example, barium and iodine.

The approximate atomic weights of the elements concerned are included for references:

Element	Atomic Weight
Hydrogen	1
Carbon	12
Nitrogen	14
Oxygen	16
Calcium	40
Bromine	80
Iodine	127
Barium	137

Barium preparations

Barium sulphate ($BaSO_4$)

Barium sulphate is supplied both as a powder and as a 50 per cent. w/v (weight/volume) or 100 per cent. w/v suspension, either plain for enemata or suitably flavoured for ingestion. These preparations, in some of which the barium sulphate is kept in suspension by the use of water-soluble gums, are available from the hospital dispensary, and are usually the 50 per cent. w/v preparations.

Colloidal barium sulphate is available in powder form and as a 100 per cent. w/v suspension. These preparations do not contain a suspending agent.

Proprietary names under which barium preparations are supplied include:

Micropaque, Micropaque Powder, Raybar.

Applications

Barium swallow

Special preparations are available, or barium sulphate powder and water are mixed together to obtain the desired consistency.

Barium meal

Using the 50 per cent. w/v preparations, eight fluid ounces of barium sulphate are diluted with water to make a total volume of one pint. For obese patients, the barium sulphate is increased to twelve fluid ounces, again diluted to make up a total volume of one pint.

When using the 100 per cent. w/v preparation or powdered colloidal barium sulphate, only four ounces are required in making up a total volume of one pint.

Barium enema (plain)

Barium sulphate	1 pound
Water up to	1 pint

Preparation: mix the barium with a small quantity of hot water and make up to three pints with tepid water.

Iodine preparations

The iodine preparations can be divided into three groups, the *organic* iodine compounds, the *inorganic* iodine compounds and the *iodized oils*.

The *organic iodine compounds* have two main components, the iodine and the carrier. While iodine provides the necessary radiographic opacity, the carrier holds the iodine in chemical combination and furthermore, by its constitution, determines the chemical and physical properties of the preparation.

In use, these organic iodine compounds can be classified in three groups:

(1)	(2)	(3)
For Urography and Angiography (water soluble)	For Cholecystography	For the mechanical filling of tracts and cavities

Sensitivity to the water-soluble organic iodine compounds

The cause of reactions to these compounds when injected intravenously is not fully known. Preliminary testing with small quantities is unreliable as an indication of how a patient will react when the full injection is given for the X-ray examination. However, a careful study of the medical history to find patients known to suffer from cardiovascular disease or to have an allergy, or suffer from hay fever or asthma, will eliminate most of those likely to be sensitive. For all patients, as a precaution against reactions the first 1–2 ml. of the compound are injected very slowly and the patient carefully watched for any sign of reaction such as flushing, nausea and urticaria. There should always be at hand in the X-ray department an emergency tray containing sterilized syringes, needles and dressings, together with an anti-histamine drug and heart stimulant. A cylinder of oxygen should also be available. Patients known to be allergic may be desensitized with an antihistamine drug prior to an examination requiring the use of an organic iodine compound.

Patients with a previous history of adverse reaction to an intravenous injection of one of the water-soluble organic iodine compounds will need to be questioned carefully to ascertain the nature of the previous reaction, then, unless absolutely necessary, the examination should not be repeated.

Sensitivity tests for the inorganic iodine preparations, and iodized oils

A few patients are sensitive to iodine: for these it is advisable not to use the inorganic preparations, or iodized oil, until the patient has been tested for iodine sensitivity. This may be done by either a skin test or an oral test.

(*a*) *Skin Test.* An area on the forearm is painted with a 2 per cent. solution of iodine. If there is no reaction after one hour, the examination with the opaque medium may follow.

(*b*) *Oral Test.* One ounce of 10 per cent. potassium iodide is ingested. If there is no reaction after half-an-hour, the opaque medium may be used for the examination.

Excretion of organic iodine compounds

It is the solubility of the compound that determines the route of excretion. The water soluble organic iodine compounds containing acetic and/or benzoic acid in the molecular structure are excreted from the body via the kidneys, the maximum concentration being reached 3 to 5 minutes after injection.

The ingested organic iodine compounds are less soluble, containing either propionic or butyric acid in the molecular structure; these are excreted from the body chiefly via the biliary system, but helped at the same time by the urinary system. The maximum concentration in the gall bladder is approximately 12 hours after ingestion.

The time taken for an organic iodine compound to be eliminated from the body varies with the compound. The water soluble compounds take approximately 12 to 16 weeks and the ingested group of compounds approximately 16 to 20 weeks.

Organic iodine compounds

1. Water-soluble group for urography and angiography

Iodoxyl. A water-soluble diiodo organic iodine compound.

Iodoxyl is the di-sodium salt of N-methyl-3:5-diiodo-4-pyridone-2:6-dicarboxylic acid. Its structural formula is:

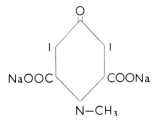

Iodoxyl contains 51·5 per cent. iodine. It is available in 20 per cent. and 75 per cent. solutions:

20 per cent. solution contains 10·3 per cent. w/v iodine.

75 per cent. solution contains 38·7 per cent. w/v iodine.

This preparation is supplied under the proprietary name of Uropac.

Iodine preparations

Diodine. A water-soluble diiodo organic iodine substance.

This is a preparation of di-ethanolamine and 3:5-diiodo-4-pyridone-N-acetic acid.

The structural formula is:

$$CH_2COOH—NH(C_2H_4OH)_2$$

Diodone contains about 50 per cent. of iodine. It is available as a 35, 45, 50 and 75 per cent. solution:

35 per cent. solution contains 17·5 per cent. w/v iodine.
45 per cent. solution contains 21·2 per cent. w/v iodine.
50 per cent. solution contains 25 per cent. w/v iodine.
70 per cent. solution contains 35 per cent. w/v iodine.

This preparation is supplied under the proprietary name: Vasiodone.

Diodone (viscous preparation). A 35 per cent. solution of Diodone, rendered viscous with carboxy methyl cellulose, and containing approximately 17·5 per cent. of iodine, is available under the proprietary name of Umbradil Viscous "U". It also contains an anaesthetic, xylocaine.

Sodium Acetrizoate. A water-soluble triiodo organic iodine compound.

This is the sodium salt of 3-acetylamino-2:4:6-triiodo-benzoic acid, and has the following structural formula:

COONa

N—COCH$_3$
H

This preparation has an iodine content of approximately 65·8 per cent. It is available in 25, 30, 50 and 70 per cent. solutions:

30 per cent. solution contains 20 per cent w/v iodine.
50 per cent. solution contains 33 per cent. w/v iodine.
70 per cent. solution contains 46 per cent. w/v iodine.

Sodium acetrizoate is supplied under the proprietary name of Diaginol.

It is also available as a viscous preparation, supplied under the proprietary name of Diaginal Viscous. This contains 40 per cent. of sodium acetrizoate, which is equivalent to 26·3 per cent. w/v iodine, rendered viscous by dextran solution.

Sodium Diatrizoate. A water-soluble triiodo organic iodine compound.

This is the sodium salt of 3:5-diacetamido-2:4:6-triiodo-benzoate and has the following structural formula:

COONa

CH$_3$.CO.NH   NH.CO.CH$_3$

This preparation has an iodine content of approximately 60 per cent. It is available as a 25, 45, 65 and 85 per cent. solution:

25 per cent. solution contains 15 per cent. iodine.
45 per cent. solution contains 27 per cent. iodine.
65 per cent. solution contains 39 per cent. iodine.
85 per cent. solution contains 44 per cent. iodine.

Sodium diatrizoate is supplied under the proprietary name of Hypaque.

Urografin. A water-soluble triiodo organic iodine preparation.

Supplies as a solution of the sodium and methylglucamine salts of N,N′diacetyl-3:5-diamino-2:4:6-triiodo-benzoic acid in the ratio of 10:66.

The structural formula of the free acid is:

CH$_3$.CO.NH   NH.CO.CH$_3$

COOH

Urografin has an iodine content of 62·1 per cent. It is available in 30, 45, 60 and 76 per cent. solutions:

30 per cent. solution contains 18·6 per cent. w/v iodine.
45 per cent. solution contains 28 per cent. w/v iodine.
60 per cent. solution contains 37 per cent. w/v iodine.
76 per cent. solution contains 47 per cent. w/v iodine.

Urografin is a proprietary name. The viscous form Gastrografin is for the gastrointestinal tract.

Sodium Metrizoate. A triiodo water-soluble organic iodine compound.

Sodium metrizoate is sodium 3-acetamido-2:4:6-triiodo-5-N-methyl-acetamidobenzoate.

The structural formula is:

COONa

CH$_3$OCHN   N(CH$_3$)COCH$_3$

This has an iodine content of approximately 58·5 per cent. It is available in 25, 45, 60 and 70 per cent. solutions:

25 per cent. solution contains 14·6 per cent. w/v iodine.
45 per cent. solution contains 26 per cent. w/v iodine.
60 per cent. solution contains 35 per cent. w/v iodine.
75 per cent. solution contains 44 per cent. w/v iodine.

The proprietary name is Triosil.

2. Cholecystography group

Biligrafin. A triiodo organic iodine compound (for intravenous injection).

Biligrafin is the methylglucamine salt of N,N′-adipic-di(3-amino-2:4:6-triiodebenzoic acid).

It has the following structural formula:

The iodine content of this preparation is 48·1 per cent., and it is available as 30 and 50 per cent. solutions:

30 per cent. solution contains 14·4 per cent. w/v iodine.
50 per cent. solution contains 24 per cent. w/v iodine.

The proprietary names are Biligrafin (30 per cent. solution) and Biligrafin Forte (50 per cent. solution).

Endografin. This is chemically identical with Biligrafin, available as a 70 per cent. solution.

Telepaque. A triiodo organic iodine compound.

This is described as 3-(3-amino-2:4:6-triiodophenyl)-2-ethyl propanoic acid, and has the following structural formula:

The iodine content is 66 per cent. The proprietary name is Telepaque.

Biloptin. A triiodo organic iodine compound.

Biloptin is the sodium salt of β-(3-dimethylamino-methyl-enamino-2,4,6-triiodophenyl)-propionic acid.

The structural formula is:

The iodine content of the salt is 61·4 per cent.
The proprietary name is Biloptin, supplied in capsule form.

Solu-Biloptin. A triiodo organic iodine compound.

Solu-Biloptin is the calcium salt of β-(3-dimethylamino-methylenamino-2:4:6-triiodophenyl)-propionic acid.

The iodine content of the salt is 61·7 per cent.
The proprietary name is Solu-Biloptin, supplied in powder form.

Phenobutiodyl. This is a triiodo organic iodine compound and is described as 1-(2:4:6-triiodo-phenoxy)-butyric acid and has the following structural formula:

Phenobutiodyl contains 68·2 per cent. iodine. The proprietary name is Biliodyl.

3. Group used for the mechanical filling of tracts and cavities

Propyliodone. This compound is similar to Diodone and is available as either an aqueous or an oily suspension, combined with a suspending and bacteriostatic agent. It is the n-propyl ester of 3:5-diiodo-4-pyridone-N-acetic acid.

The structural formula is:

Propyliodone contains approximately 50 per cent. iodine. The aqueous preparation is a 50 per cent. suspension containing 771

Iodine preparations

about 25 per cent. iodine; the oily preparation is a 60 per cent. suspension containing approximately 30 per cent. iodine.

These preparations are available under the proprietary names of Dionosil and Dionosil Oily.

Ethyliodophenylundecylate. A non-soluble organic iodine compound.

The structural formula is:

I—⟨hexagon⟩—$CH_2-(CH_2)_9COOH_2H_5$

This compound contains approximately 30 per cent. of iodine. It is available under the proprietary name of Myodil.

NOTE—In the foregoing descriptions of the organic iodine compounds used as opaque media, the structural formulae and chemical descriptions are those published by the respective manufacturers.

Inorganic iodine compounds

Sodium iodide

Contains approximately 85 per cent. of iodine and may be used as a 10, 12·5 or 15 per cent. solution.

10 per cent. solution contains about 7·6 per cent. iodine.
12·5 per cent. solution contains about 9·5 per cent. iodine.
15 per cent. solution contains about 11·4 per cent. iodine.

NOTE—These solutions need to be made up freshly, as they slowly liberate iodine and will not keep.

Iodized oils (viscous)

For the viscous form of iodized oil, iodine is combined with oil of poppy seed; it is available in three strengths with iodine contents of 10 per cent., 20 per cent. and 40 per cent.—Lipiodol Viscous.

Iodized oil (fluid)

This alternative fluid form of iodized oil is prepared from the iodized ethyl esters of the fatty acids of poppy seed oil and iodine; it has an iodine content of 40 per cent.

The proprietary name is Lipiodol Ultra-fluid.

Iodized oil and myodil are very slowly absorbed, over a period of several years.

Bromide compounds

Potassium bromide

This is usually made up as a 10 per cent. solution and can be used in place of potassium or sodium iodide when the patient is allergic to iodine.

Brominized oil

Brominized oil is a preparation of poppy seed oil and bromine, containing about 35 per cent. of bromine in organic combination. It has a viscosity similar to that of iodized oil, but is not so radio-opaque. Brominized oil may be used to replace iodized oil when the patient is allergic to iodine.

The preparation is available under the proprietary name of Brominized Oil.

Examination	Opaque Media	Working Strength of Solution	Approximate Iodine Content
Angiocardiography Aortography	Angiografin Cardio-Conray		305·8 mg. per ml. 400 mg. per ml.
(Renal Arteriography)	Conray 280 Conray 420	70%	280 mg. per ml. 420 mg. per ml.
(Coronary Arteriography)	Hypaque Triosil Urografin Vasiodone	65%; 85% 75% 76% 70%	280 & 440 mg. per ml. 439 mg. per ml. 370 mg. per ml. 350 mg. per ml.
Arthrography	Hypaque Urografin	25%; 45% 30%	150 & 270 mg. per ml. 146 mg. per ml.
Barium Examinations	Micropaque Microtrast Raybar 75	95% 66·5% 71·25%	
(Abdomen acute)	Gastrografin	76%	370 mg. per ml.
Brachial Arteriography	Conray 280 Hypaque	45%	280 mg. per ml. 270 mg. per ml.
(Femoral Arteriography)	Urografin Urovision	45%; 60% 58%	220 & 292 mg. per ml. 325 mg. per ml.
Bronchography	Dionosil aqueous Dionosil oily Hytrast Iodatol Lipiodol viscous Steripaque—Br	50% 60% 46%/iopydone 30·5% 50%	284 mg. per ml. 340 mg. per ml.
Cerebral angiography	Angiografin Conray 280 Hypaque Urografin	 45% 45%; 60%	305·8 mg. per ml. 280 mg. per ml. 270 mg. per ml. 220 & 292 mg. per ml.
Cholecystography (oral)	Biliodyl Biloptin Osbil Solu-biloptin Telepaque	 0·5 g. 3 g. 0·5 g.	
Cholecystangiography (I.V.)	Biligrafin Biligrafin (forte)	30% 50%	150 mg. per ml. 250 mg. per ml.
Cholangiography (direct)	Biligrafin Biligrafin (forte) Diaginol viscous Hypaque Steripaque V Urografin	30% 50% 40% 45% 30% 60%	150 mg. per ml. 250 mg. per ml. 263 mg. per ml. 270 mg. per ml. 292 mg. per ml.
Cysto-urethrography (urethography)	Diaginol viscous Lipiodol ultra fluid Umbradil viscous U Urografin Uropac	40% 35% 60%; 76% 75%	263 mg. per ml. 220 mg. per ml. 292 & 370 mg. per ml. 380 mg. per ml.

Examination	Opaque Media	Working Strength of Solution	Approximate Iodine Content
Discography	Hypaque	45%	270 mg. per ml.
	Urografin	60%	292 mg. per ml.
Hystero-salpingography	Diaginol viscous	40%	263 mg. per ml.
	Hypaque	45%	270 mg. per ml.
	Lipiodol ultra fluid		
	Salpix	53%	345 mg. per ml.
	Urografin	76%	370 mg. per ml.
Intravenous Pyelography	Conray 280		280 mg. per ml.
	Conray 325	54%	325 mg. per ml.
	Conray 420	70%	420 mg. per ml.
	Hypaque	45%	270 mg. per ml.
	Triosil	75%	439 mg. per ml.
	Urografin	60%; 76%	292 & 370 mg. per ml.
	Urovision	58%	325 mg. per ml.
Lymphography	Lipiodol ultra fluid		
Myelography (Ventriculography)	Myodil		300 mg. per ml.
	Conray 280		280 mg. per ml.
Portal Venography	Conray 280		280 mg. per ml.
	Hypaque	85%	440 mg. per ml.
	Triosil	75%	439 mg. per ml.
	Urografin	76%	470 mg. per ml.
Retrograde pyelography	Hypaque	25%	150 mg. per ml.
	Retro-conray	35%	163 mg. per ml.
	Urografin	30%	146 mg. per ml.
	Uropac (retrograde dilution)	20%	102 mg. per ml.
Sialography	Endografin	70%	350 mg. per ml.
	Hypaque	45%	270 mg. per ml.
	Lipiodol ultra fluid		
	Triosil	75%	439 mg. per ml.
	Urografin	60%	292 mg. per ml.
Sinography	Diaginol viscous	40%	263 mg. per ml.
	Dionosil aqueous	50%	284 mg. per ml.
	Endografin	70%	350 mg. per ml.
	Hypaque	45%	270 mg. per ml.
	Lipiodol ultra fluid		
	Lipiodol viscous		
	Steripaque V	30%	
	Urografin	76%	370 mg. per ml.
Venography	Hypaque	45%	270 mg. per ml.
	Urografin	45%; 60%	220 & 292 mg. per ml.

EFFECTS OF RADIATION AND PROTECTION METHODS IN DIAGNOSTIC RADIOLOGY

THE EFFECTS OF RADIATION, AND PROTECTION METHODS IN DIAGNOSTIC RADIOLOGY

Introduction

In recent years a great deal has been said about the hazards of radiation, especially in connection with the "fall-out" from nuclear weapon tests. Much of this is exaggerated and has led to a general fear of radiation by the public at large, and refusal, in some cases, of patients to undergo diagnostic radiography, the benefits of which far outweigh the adverse effects. It is right, therefore, that all of those engaged in exposing members of the public to radiation should understand the extent of these hazards and how to reduce them to a minimum in the course of their work.

Doses of radiation will be referred to in rems, rads and roentgens (r). The rem, or "Rad-Equivalent-Man", takes into account the different biological effects produced by different types of radiation, following the same dose measured in rads. When considering the effects of X-rays on soft tissue, however, there is little difference between rems, rads and roentgens. For definitions of these units see page 781.

The effects of exposure to radiation can be divided into two classes: somatic effects (those experienced by the exposed individual) and genetic effects (those passed on to later generations). Each of these will be considered in some detail.

Somatic effects of radiation

Only relatively large doses of radiation can produce serious effects and such large doses should never be encountered in diagnostic radiography.

High doses of radiation to the whole body, such as those received by the victims of the atomic bombs in Japan in 1945, produce an acute illness within a few hours of exposure, with subsequent death in many instances. A dose of 500r produces this illness in all cases and about 50 per cent. die. Small parts of the body can tolerate much higher doses of radiation. 500r to an area of skin received during radiotherapy only produces a reddening and loss of hair. 4000r or more may be given in radiotherapy, when the skin becomes very sensitive and prone to infection, and at this stage is covered with dilated blood vessels.

Apart from the above effects, which appear soon after exposure, doses of radiation can cause leukaemia and many forms of cancer at a later date. Leukaemia, which may appear as much as 10 years after exposure is a very rare disease, and even after exposure to large doses of radiation the likelihood of suffering from it is still small. Cancer has been known to occur 54 years after exposure, so that individuals exposed in later life will probably die from some other cause before any radiation-induced cancer has had time to appear.

Some parts of the body are more sensitive to radiation than others, particularly the blood forming organs, the lens of the eye and the reproductive organs. A whole-body dose as low as 25r can produce a temporary change in the blood count. 200r to the eye will occasionally cause cataract formation and with 750r this will occur in most cases. Doses to the gonads of 200r will produce temporary sterility and 300r to 600r may cause permanent sterility.

It seems relevant here to quote from the 1956 report of the Medical Research Council, "The Hazards to Man of Nuclear and Allied Radiations" (paragraph 99, page 23): "Under modern conditions of occupational exposure, for example, among radiologists and radiographers, there is no evidence of any impairment of fertility. Furthermore there is no suggestion that female radiographers suffer from radiation-induced menstrual disturbances which might be accompanied by diminished fertility."

Doses of radiation to pregnant women as high as those received during radiotherapy or by the Japanese in 1945 can cause miscarriage or stillbirth. There is some evidence to show that, occasionally, irradiation of the foetus at a particular stage of early pregnancy may cause developmental abnormalities in the child. Thus, irradiation of the foetus in pregnant women should only be carried out when really necessary.

Genetic effects of radiation

All cells in the body have in the nucleus a number of chromosomes, each of which contains a very large number of genes. These genes determine the hereditary nature of the individual. The selection of genes in all cells of an individual's body is identical, half being inherited from each parent. The exception to this is the sperm or egg cell which contains only half the number of chromosomes and genes. For this reason, on average, a particular gene is passed on to half of one's children, to a quarter of one's grandchildren, to an eighth of one's great grandchildren, etc., and after a large number of generations it will be spread widely in the population.

Genes can occasionally undergo a sudden change into a different form. This is known as mutation. If this happens in a sperm or egg cell, the gene will be passed on to later generations in its changed form. Mutation occurs normally at a certain low rate caused, among other things, by natural background radiation coming from cosmic rays and small amounts of radioactive substances in our bodies and in the surroundings. Most mutations result in genes which have harmful effects on the population. The worst of these effects are severe mental defects, mental illness, blindness and neonatal deaths, stillbirths and congenital malformations. The existing levels of these conditions are due to the natural mutation rate to which mankind has always been subjected. However, any additional radiation to the reproductive organs from the time of one's own conception until the conception of one's child, increases the mutation rate and therefore the occurrence of these harmful genetic effects in later generations.

The additional dose of radiation to double the natural mutation rate has been estimated to be between 30r and 80r to the reproductive organs up to the age of 30 years, this age being taken as the average age of reproduction. As background radiation in this country contributes only about 3r in 30 years it must account for less than 10 per cent. of natural mutations. The genetic effect has been shown to be negligible if a relatively small group of prospective parents receives this "doubling" dose or even somewhat more; but if the average dose throughout the population were as high as this, then all genetic effects would eventually be doubled. One can see that, should a large scale nuclear war ever occur, the average dose throughout the population of the world could be greater than the doubling dose, even for those who survive the somatic effects, and the increase of harmful genetic effects on subsequent generations would be very great indeed.

Permissible doses of radiation

In view of the harmful genetic effects produced by relatively small doses of radiation to the whole population, it is obviously necessary that rules should be made to ensure that such effects are kept within acceptable limits. Today, when radiation is widely used in diagnosis and treatment of disease and in industry, a balance must be found between the advantage of using radiation in certain circumstances and the possible risks. A report of the International Commission on Radiological Protection published in 1960 gives a number of recommendations on maximum permissible levels of radiation, in addition to background radiation, to different groups of people, based on the most up-to-date information. Table 1, page 782, summarizes these recommendations. It was decided that a dose of 5 rems to the gonads up to the age of 30, averaged throughout the population, would produce a genetic effect small enough to be acceptable, and that a small group of radiation workers could be allowed to receive 60 rems to the gonads between the ages of 18 and 30 years. The average dose of 5 rems is somewhat less than twice the normal background radiation and 60 rems is roughly equal to the doubling dose. In order to limit the average gonad dose in the population to 5 rems it is obvious that members of the general public must have a maximum permissible dose in 30 years of less than 5 rems. It is emphasized in the recommendations that these are all *maximum* doses and that every effort should be made to keep all doses to the minimum possible. It will be seen in Table 1 that radiation workers are permitted to receive somewhat larger doses of radiation to some parts of the body other than the gonads. This is because no genetic effect is produced except when the gonads are irradiated, and any somatic effects to the other parts of the body will not in general be produced by such low doses.

The maximum permissible doses laid down in these recommendations do not include radiation doses received from medical exposure. The International Commission recommends that, ". . . the genetic dose to the whole population from all sources additional to natural background radiation should not exceed 5 rems (per 30 years) plus the lowest practicable contribution from medical exposure".

Responsibility for dose reduction in diagnostic radiology

The last sentence, together with all that has gone before, should make all those having any connection with diagnostic radiography very much aware of their grave responsibility for any additional genetic effects produced in the population, and the need for the greatest care to protect all persons from radiation, especially to the gonads, by all possible means. Dose reduction

is so important that it is essential for radiographers to know in some detail all methods of minimizing radiation exposure to themselves, to other radiation workers and to patients.

Protection for the radiologist and the radiographer

All diagnostic X-ray departments should conform with requirements laid down in the Ministry of Health's "Code of Practice for the Protection of Persons Exposed to Ionizing Radiations". This involves the protective thickening of walls, floors, ceilings and doors where necessary to shield persons in adjacent rooms, and using modern equipment with adequate protection around the X-ray tube (except in the main beam) and with protection for the radiologist during fluoroscopy. Protective body aprons and gloves should also be available for use during fluoroscopy.

In addition to these protective measures, there are a number of ways in which radiographers can actively help to keep radiation to themselves and to fellow workers to a minimum. These are:

(1) Always to remember the "inverse square law" and keep as far as possible away from all sources of radiation, whether primary or scattered. *Never* to stand in the primary beam. If a child or unsteady patient needs to be supported this should be done by an accompanying parent or person not concerned with the X-ray department who should be provided with protective clothing and positioned so as to avoid the primary beam.

(2) Always to use the smallest possible X-ray beam. As well as minimizing radiation to the patient this reduces scattered radiation to the radiographer. The main source of scattered radiation is the area of the patient directly irradiated by the X-ray beam, the amount of scatter produced being approximately proportional to this area. Therefore, in a very small room it is essential to provide a protective screen with a lead glass window to reduce the scatter to the radiographer.

(3) Never to remain in the X-ray room unnecessarily during exposures.

(4) During erect fluoroscopy to stand, whenever possible, behind the radiologist where protection is provided by the lead glass of the screen and by the apron suspended from it. During horizontal screening, when the radiographer stands on the opposite side of the couch to the radiologist, there may be no protection provided for the radiographer and therefore a protective body apron should be worn.

(5) To make regular inspections (say, every six months) of all protective gloves and aprons to detect any splitting or holes. Aprons can be inspected simply by screening, but the easiest way to inspect gloves is to lay them on a double-wrapped film and expose to X-rays sufficient to penetrate them slightly, using the highest kilovoltage available. Examples of such radiographs of gloves are reproduced by Osborn in "X-ray Focus", Vol. 4, No. 1, 1963, p. 11.

Every radiation worker is required by the "Code of Practice" to wear either a film badge or a pocket ionization chamber which is normally worn outside any protective clothing, usually on the lapel or in the breast pocket, thus giving an indication of the dose received by unprotected parts of the body. The radiographer should co-operate in wearing these badges or ionization chambers and in returning them at the required time for dose assessment. A continuous personal record can then be kept of every worker's doses. Investigation into any doses higher than normal may point to improvements needed in general technique or may be an early indication of faulty equipment.

Protection of the patient

The use of up-to-date equipment and accessories helps to reduce radiation to the patient. Recommendations in this connection have been made in "The Code of Practice", in the report "Radiological Hazards to Patients" and by the International Commission on Radiological Protection. These recommendations include the use of light beam localizers, accurate timing devices and aluminium filters. A permanent total filter of 2 mm aluminium should be fitted to all radiographic and fluoroscopic equipment. An unfiltered X-ray beam contains a wide range of photon energies and the very soft components will be absorbed in the superficial layers of the patient and will not reach the film. An aluminium filter will absorb these soft rays thus reducing the skin dose to the patient and making little or no difference to the film dose.

No patient should be exposed unnecessarily to radiation and therefore it must be ascertained whether the relevant information can be obtained from films previously taken, possibly at another hospital, or by some completely different method. Fluoroscopy should not be used when the same information can be obtained by radiography as doses are invariably less for radiography.

In view of the importance of minimizing radiation to the foetus, no woman should be radiographed in the pelvic region during pregnancy unless this is absolutely necessary. It should be remembered that any woman of child-bearing age could be in the early stage of pregnancy, and to avoid this possibility radiographic examinations of the pelvis would be best undertaken during the first half of the menstrual cycle.

In considering the role of the radiographer in minimizing radiation to the patient the most important factor is good radiographic technique which will not only produce good radiographs, but also reduce to the minimum the irradiation of the patient, especially the gonads. In this, the following points are of importance:

(1) Always to position the patient accurately. Immobilizing devices should be used when necessary and practicable. If the exposure has to be repeated, the radiation to the patient is doubled.

(2) Always to use the smallest possible field sizes. If the edges of the beam show as a margin on the film one can be sure that an excessive field size was not used. This should, ideally, become the general practice. The use of a circular cone to cover a rectangular film exposes more of the patient than necessary (or otherwise wastes the corners of the film), so it is obviously preferable to have an adjustable rectangular aperture fitted with a light beam localizer which assists the accurate positioning of the beam.

(3) When possible to direct the beam away from the gonads, for example, when radiographing the upper limb with the patient in the sitting position.

(4) Gonad shields should be used where the gonads are likely to be in the primary beam, unless they interfere with the examination itself. Shields of 0·5 mm lead equivalent will reduce the gonad dose to about 5 per cent. of the unshielded dose, most of which is due to radiation scattered from the rest of the beam. A number of different devices for protecting the gonads have been designed in recent years (Ardran and Kemp, 1957; Abram, Wilkinson and Hodson, 1958; Whitehead and Griffiths, 1961) some of which are positioned on the patient and others attached to the cone or light beam diaphragm. Kendig (1960) has described a method of shielding the gonads of both mother and foetus in pelvimetry. Some of these devices are illustrated on page 127, Section 4.

(5) The fastest possible films and screens should be used which will give the required diagnostic information. The use of high speed films and screens tends to result in increased graininess in the radiograph, but where this does not interfere with the diagnosis, exposure to radiation is reduced and furthermore the shorter exposure time diminishes the effect of patient movement.

(6) The longest practicable focus–film distance should be used. For a given film dose the skin dose is less for a long than for a short focus–film distance. This is shown in the diagram which illustrates two situations: in the first, the focus–skin distance is 9 inches and the focus–film distance 18 inches; in the second, the distances are increased to 27 inches and 36 inches

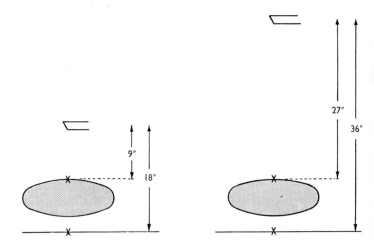

respectively. For the same tube exposure in the two examples the film dose in the second example will be a quarter, and the skin dose one-ninth of those in the first example. If, therefore, the tube exposure in the second example be four times that of the first, the film dose will be equal, but the skin dose will be reduced to four-ninths or less than half.

(7) The kilovoltage used should be neither too low nor too high.* Soft X-rays are readily absorbed by the body and therefore, to give the required film dose, a large dose must be given to the patient. On the other hand, if a very high kilovoltage is used, the penetrating power will be increased so much that the X-rays will tend to pass through the film as well as the patient. Also, scatter outside the beam is greater for high kilovoltage than for low kilovoltage radiation, so that if the gonads are out of the main beam they will receive a smaller dose at the appropriate lower kilovoltage. Thus, for minimum gonad

* As there is some confusion in the use of the terms "soft" and "hard" in describing radiation *versus* its photographic effect—high kilovoltage, therefore hard radiation, produces a flat effect in the radiograph; conversely, low kilovoltage, therefore soft radiation, produces a steep contrasty radiograph

doses the use of about 70 kv is recommended in the report "Radiological Hazards to Patients".

(8) A check on the alignment of the light and X-ray beams of all light beam localizers should be made periodically. This can easily be done with a large double-wrapped film. Using a field somewhat smaller than the film, small strips of metal should be laid along the four edges of the light beam to mark their positions on the film. An exposure sufficient to penetrate the metal and leave a clear outline of the X-ray field will show any discrepancy between the two fields. Correct alignment can make all the difference between the gonads being in or out of the beam, especially in chest radiography where the focus–film distance is considerable.

Estimation of skin dose from nomogram

Where an extensive radiological examination is contemplated it is advisable to keep a careful account of the skin dose from the beginning. A quick indication of skin dose received by the patient and how it varies with an added filter, kilovoltage and focus–skin distance can be obtained by referring to the nomogram on page 780. This has been constructed by measuring the output of a number of X-ray sets and taking the largest, a ward-mobile machine, as the "standard". The actual dose from other sets may be somewhat less but will not in general be less than half the value estimated from the nomogram, see Osborn (1955 and 1962). It is thus possible to get a reasonable estimate of skin dose.

To use the nomogram, a straight line is required, and this can conveniently be either a length of black thread stretched taut, or a fine black line ruled on celluloid. This line should be laid over the chart so as to cross the top and bottom scales at values corresponding to a specified exposure. The bottom horizontal scale represents kilovolts peak (kVp); the line should cross this scale at a position determined by the lower row of figures if *no* external filter is used, or by the upper row of figures if a 2 mm aluminium filter is used. (For undercouch work, the couch top may legitimately be regarded as a filter for the purpose of estimating radiation exposure, and this applies also to a vertical stand with the tube in the screening position). The top horizontal scale represents the focus–skin distance (FSD) *not* the focus–film distance (FFD) and it is scaled in centimetres as well as in inches for convenience.

When the line is correctly adjusted on the two outer scales, the point at which it crosses the middle horizontal scale should be observed, and the numerical value noted. This indicates the dose delivered in milliroentgens (mr) per milliampere-second (mAS), from which the total surface dose for any other value of milliampere-seconds can easily be calculated.

Example 1. A patient was radiographed at 90 kVp, 12 mAS, 2 mm aluminium filter at a focus–skin distance of 50 cm. From the nomogram is read the value of 38 mr per mAS, but the tube exposure was 12 mAS and therefore the dose was $38 \times 12 = 456$ mr. (N.B. With no added filter the dose would have been $95 \times 12 = 1140$ mr. This is two-and-a-half times the skin dose with 2 mm aluminium filter).

Example 2. A patient is screened at 85 kVp, 3 mA, 2 mm aluminium filter, at a focus–skin distance of 30 cm. How long is permitted for a maximum skin dose of 20 r (20,000 mr)? The nomogram value corresponding to the above conditions is 92 mr/mAS; hence for 20,000 mr we have $20{,}000/92 = 217.4$ mAS. At 3 mA, this would give an exposure time of 72.5 seconds.

Existing levels of genetic doses in Great Britain

In 1957 to 1958 a survey was made of genetic doses to the population of Great Britain, resulting from diagnostic and therapeutic radiology. A Committee was set up under the chairmanship of Lord Adrian and the results obtained are recorded in the Committee's Second Report "Radiological Hazards to Patients".

Table 2 on page 782 is taken from the report and gives the mean gonad doses received in different diagnostic examinations. It was calculated that doses from all diagnostic examinations in Great Britain are equivalent to an average gonad dose (ie genetic dose) of 14.1 mr per year to each person in the population. A similar calculation for genetic dose from radiotherapy gave a figure of 5.2 mr per year to each person.

Table 3 on page 782 shows the genetic doses per person from the different sources of radiation to which the population is exposed. These figures are derived from those in the Second Report of the Medical Research Council on radiation hazards (1960). The last column gives the genetic doses received in a generation of 30 years showing that this amounts to 0.08 rad above background plus 0.579 rad from medical exposure. This should be compared with the recommended maximum value of 5 rems above background plus the lowest practicable contribution from medical exposure. The first figure is obviously well below the acceptable level, but the contributions from medical exposure can be reduced considerably by the adoption of all possible protection measures.

A detailed analysis of the results obtained in the Adrian Committee survey has shown that the genetic dose from diagnostic radiology is as high as 14.1 mr to each person per year mainly because some hospitals do not take sufficient care to use low dose techniques. For example, it was found that in the chest examinations of the survey the ovaries of 51 per cent. of the adult females were in the X-ray beam as was also the scrotum of 10 per cent. of the adult males, for which there is no justification. It was shown that, if the techniques of the 10 per cent. of hospitals giving the largest doses were brought up to the average standard of all the others, the figure of 14.1 mr to each person per year would be reduced to about 10 mr. If all techniques were as satisfactory as that in the 25 per cent. of hospitals giving the lowest doses, then the genetic dose could be reduced to 2 mr to each person per year. With improvements also in techniques in the treatment of non-malignant disease by radiotherapy, it is estimated that the total genetic dose to each person per year from diagnostic and therapeutic radiology could be reduced from 19.3 mr to about 6 mr.

The importance of technique in reducing radiation hazards should not now need to be emphasized. Radiographers must surely realize that they are in control of a potentially hazardous machine and it is their duty to use it with the utmost care. Only then are they making their maximum contribution to the well-being of mankind by helping to diagnose disease in the present population with the minimum hazard to future generations.

779

NOMOGRAM FOR ESTIMATING THE SURFACE
RADIATION EXPOSURE TO THE PATIENT

FOCUS–SKIN DISTANCE

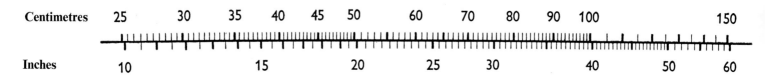

Centimetres   25   30   35   40   45   50   60   70   80   90   100   150

Inches   10   15   20   25   30   40   50   60

MILLIRÖNTGENS PER MILLIAMPERE-SECOND

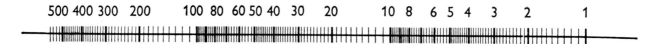

500 400 300 200   100 80 60 50 40 30   20   10 8 6 5 4   3   2   1

kVp

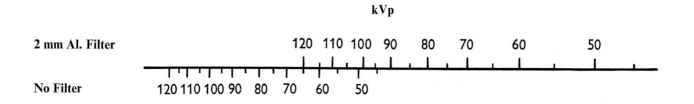

2 mm Al. Filter   120 110 100 90   80   70   60   50

No Filter   120 110 100 90 80   70   60   50

IMPORTANT· This nomogram is applicable only to half-wave and full-wave HT generators

Definitions of terms

(*Based on definitions in the Code of Practice for the Protection of Persons Exposed to Ionizing Radiations*).

Absorbed dose of any ionizing radiation: amount of energy imparted to matter by ionizing particles per unit mass of irradiated material at the place of interest. Expressed ideally in rads but for X and gamma rays of quantum energy up to 3 MeV, the roentgen (r) may be used.

Collimation. In radiology; the limiting of a beam of radiation to the required dimensions.

Cosmic rays. Ionizing rays entering the earth's atmosphere from unidentified extra-terrestrial space and resulting in the presence of photons, electrons, neutrons, protons, mesons, etc., by collision with atoms in the atmosphere.

Half-value layer (HVL). The thickness of a specified absorbing material which, when introduced into the path of an X-ray beam, reduced the dose-rate to half its original value.

Ionizing radiation. Electromagnetic radiation (X-ray or gamma-ray photons or quanta), or corpuscular radiation (alpha-particles, beta-particles, electrons, protons, neutrons, and heavy particles) capable of producing ions.

Lead equivalent. The thickness of lead affording the same protection under specified conditions of irradiation as the material in question. The lead equivalent of a substance, such as lead glass or lead rubber, which attenuates the radiation essentially by its lead content, is largely independent of the quality of the radiation. The lead equivalent of all other protective materials and also building material for protective walls (concrete, brick, etc.) and barium protective glass shows a dependence on the quality of the radiation.

Lead glass (protective glass). Glass, containing a high proportion of lead compounds, which absorbs radiation passing through it. Used as a transparent protective material.

Lead rubber. Rubber containing a high proportion of lead compounds. It is used as a flexible protective material.

Quantum. The smallest quantity of energy in the form of a bundle or packet of waves of electromagnetic radiation which can be associated with a given phenomenon. (Electromagnetic radiation sometimes appears to consist of waves and at other times of particles. Such particles may be regarded as bundles of waves.)

Quantum energy. Energy contained in a quantum of radiation and proportional to the frequency of the radiation waves. (The energy E of a quantum of radiation of frequency f if hf where h is Planck's constant.)

Rad. Unit of absorbed dose. It is 100 ergs per gramme. Millirad (mrad): 1/1,000 rad.

Radiation (as applied to X-rays):

1. Primary radiation: radiation coming directly from the target of the X-ray tube. Except for the useful beam, the bulk of this radiation is absorbed in the tube housing.

2. Secondary radiation: radiation, other than the primary radiation, emitted by any matter irradiated with X-rays. Often loosely called scattered radiation.

3. Scattered radiation: radiation which during passage through a substance has been deviated in direction. It may also have been modified by an increase in wavelength (Compton effect). It is one form of secondary radiation.

4. Stray radiation: radiation not serving any useful purpose. It includes secondary radiation and any radiation, other than the useful beam, coming from within the X-ray tube and tube housing (such as stem radiation). This is the radiation against which special protective measures have to be taken.

5. Useful beam: that part of the primary radiation which passes through the aperture, cone or other device for collimating the X-ray beam.

Relative Biological Effectiveness (RBE). Ratio of the dose (expressed in rads) of 200 to 250 kV X-rays to the dose (in rads) of any type of ionizing radiation which produces the same biological effect. Most of the clinical evidence on the effects of ionizing radiations has been obtained with 200 to 250 kV X-rays. Accordingly, this is used as the base line, being given a biological effectiveness of unity.

Rem (Rad-Equivalent-Man). Quantity of any ionizing radiation such that the energy imparted to a biological system per gramme of living matter by the ionizing particles present in the locus of interest, has the same biological effectiveness as 1 rad of 200 to 250 kV X-rays. Millirem (mrem): 1/1,000 rem.

Roentgen (r). Unit of dose of X and gamma rays, but not other ionizing radiation. Defined as below:

"The Roentgen shall be the quantity of X or gamma radiation such that the associated corpuscular emission per 0·001293 gramme of air produces, in air, ions carrying 1 electrostatic unit of quantity of electricity of either sign." (It becomes increasingly difficult to measure the dose in roentgens as the quantum energy of X or gamma radiation approaches very high values. The unit may, however, be used for most practical purposes for quantum energies up to 3 MeV.)

Milliroentgen (mr):	1/1,000 r.
Microroentgen (μr):	1/1,000,000 r.

X-ray tube housing. An enclosure which covers the tube and sometimes also other portions of the X-ray equipment (transformer) and which limits the major portion of radiation emitted from the tube to the useful beam.

TABLE 1

**SUMMARY OF RECOMMENDATIONS OF ICRP FOR MAXIMUM
PERMISSIBLE DOSES OF RADIATION, EXCLUDING MEDICAL EXPOSURE**

	Maximum Permissible Dose in rems			
	in 13 weeks	in 1 year	up to age N years	up to 30 years
A. Radiation Workers				
(i) Gonads, blood-forming organs, lens of the eye.	3	5	5 (N–18)	60
(ii) Skin and thyroid gland.	8	30		
(iii) Hands, forearms, feet, ankles.	20	75		
(iv) All other organs and tissues.	4	15		
B. Non-radiation Workers who work near or may occasionally enter areas where radiation is used				
(i) Gonads, blood-forming organs, lens of eye and all internal organs.		1·5	1·5 (N–18)	18
(ii) Skin and thyroid gland.		3		
C. Some members of the public, for example those living in the neighbourhood of radiation areas. (Including children and pregnant women)				
All tissues.		0·5	0·5N	15
D. Average gonad dose per head of population				5
E. Therefore all other members of the population (to maintain average of 5 rem)				less than 5

TABLE 2

MEAN GONAD DOSE PER EXAMINATION IN MILLIROENTGENS

Type of Examination	Male	Female	Foetus
1. Chest, heart, lung (excluding mass miniature radiography)	2·75	5·4	5·5
2. Barium meal	44	333	448
3. Abdomen	105	183	281
4. Abdomen obstetric	—	367	723
5. Intravenous Pyelography	765	585	843
6. Pelvimetry	—	745	885
7. Pelvis, lumbar spine, lumbo-sacral joint	370	392	536
8. Hip, upper femur	740	102	154

TABLE 3

APPROXIMATE GENETIC DOSES TO THE POPULATION OF GREAT BRITAIN IN 1957–1960

Source of Radiation	Genetic Dose per Person			
	in millirads per year		in rads per 30 years	
Natural Background		100		3
Medical Exposure:				
Diagnostic Radiology		14·1		0·423
Therapeutic Radiology		5·2		0·156
Total		19·3		0·579
Other Sources:				
Fall-out		1·2		0·035
Miscellaneous	Less than	1	Less than	0·03
Occupational exposure		0·5		0·015
Total	Less than	2·7	Less than	0·08

WORKING METRIC EQUIVALENTS OF DIMENSIONS AND QUANTITIES

SUPPLEMENT THREE

WORKING METRIC EQUIVALENTS OF DIMENSIONS AND QUANTITIES

LINEAR

Inches		Centimetres
$\frac{1}{8}$	=	0·32
$\frac{1}{4}$	=	0·64
$\frac{1}{2}$	=	1·3
$\frac{3}{4}$	=	1·9
1	=	2·5
$1\frac{1}{4}$	=	3·2
$1\frac{1}{2}$	=	3·8
$1\frac{3}{4}$	=	4·4
2	=	5·1
$2\frac{1}{4}$	=	5·7
$2\frac{1}{2}$	=	6·3
$2\frac{3}{4}$	=	7·0
3	=	7·6
$3\frac{1}{2}$	=	8·9
4	=	10
$4\frac{1}{2}$	=	12
5	=	13
$5\frac{1}{2}$	=	14
6	=	15
$6\frac{1}{2}$	=	17
7	=	18
$7\frac{1}{2}$	=	19
8	=	20
$8\frac{1}{2}$	=	22
9	=	23
$9\frac{1}{2}$	=	24
10	=	25
11	=	28
12 (1 foot)	=	30
13	=	33
14	=	36
15	=	38
16	=	41
17	=	42
18	=	46
19	=	48
20	=	51
22	=	56
24 (2 feet)	=	61
26	=	66

LINEAR

Inches		Centimetres
28	=	71
30	=	76
32	=	81
34	=	86
$35\frac{1}{2}$		90
36 (3 feet)	=	91
38	=	97
$39\frac{3}{8}$	=	100 (1 metre)

		Metres
40	=	1·02
42	=	1·07
44	=	1·12
46	=	1·17
48 (4 feet)	=	1·22
$49\frac{1}{2}$	=	1·25
50	=	1·27
54	=	1·37
56	=	1·42
59	=	1·50
60 (5 feet)	=	1·52
66	=	1·68
72 (6 feet)	=	1·83
79	=	2·0
84 (7 feet)	=	2·13
96 (8 feet)	=	2·44

Centimetres		Inches
1·0	=	0·4
2·0	=	0·8
2·5	=	1·0
3·0	=	1·2
4·0	=	1·6
5·0	=	2·0
6·0	=	2·4
7·0	=	2·8
8·0	=	3·2
9·0	=	3·6

To convert centimetres to inches multiply by 0·4
To convert inches to centimetres divide by 0·4

<table>
<tr><td colspan="3" align="center">

WEIGHT
</td></tr>
</table>

Pounds avoirdupois		Kilograms
1	=	0·4536
5	=	2·268
10	=	4·536
20	=	9·072
30	=	13·608
50	=	22·680
80	=	36·288
100	=	45·360
125	=	56·7
140	=	63·5
146	=	66·2
150	=	68·0
157	=	71·2
160	=	72·6
168	=	76·2
200	=	90·7

Kilograms		Pounds avoirdupois
1	=	2·2046 = 35·27 oz.
2	=	4·4092
3	=	6·6138
4	=	8·8184
5	=	11·0230
6	=	13·2276
7	=	15·4322
8	=	17·6368
9	=	19·8414
10	=	22·0460
15	=	33·069
20	=	44·092
25	=	55·115
30	=	66·138
35	=	77·161
40	=	88·184
45	=	99·207
50	=	110·230
55	=	121·253
60	=	132·276
65	=	143·299
70	=	154·322
75	=	165·345
80	=	176·368
85	=	187·391
90	=	198·414
95	=	209·437
100	=	220·460

FLUID

Millilitres		Ounces	Minims
1	=		16·9
2	=		33·8
3	=		50·7
4	=		67·6
5	=		84·5
6	=		101
7	=		118
8	=		138
9	=		152
10	=		169
20	=		338
30	=	1	27
40	=	1	196
50	=	1	365
60	=	2	54
70	=	2	223
80	=	2	391
90	=	3	80
100	=	3	249
200	=	7	19
300	=	10	268
400	=	14	37
500	=	17	287
600	=	21	56
700	=	24	305
800	=	28	75
900	=	31	324
1,000	=	35	94
(1 litre)			

35·2 ounces = 100 ml = 1 litre = 0·220 gal.
   1 gal. = 4·56 litres.

Drams		Fluid ounces		Millilitres
1	=	$\frac{1}{8}$	=	3·55
2	=	$\frac{1}{4}$	=	7·10
4	=	$\frac{1}{2}$	=	14·20
8	=	1	=	28·40
		2	=	57·00
		4	=	114·00
		8	=	228·00
		12	=	342·00
		16	=	456·00
			=	(1 USA pint)
		20	=	568·20
			=	(1 British pint)

TEMPERATURE CONVERSION CHART

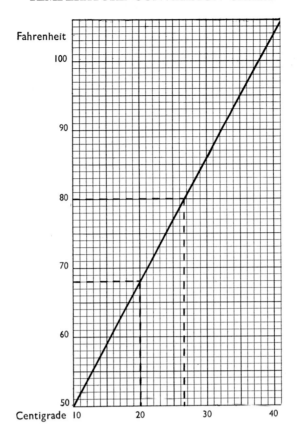

Ilford Rapid R film is available in the following centimetre and inch sizes:

cm		inches	
13 × 18	24 × 30	$4\frac{3}{4} \times 6\frac{1}{2}$	10 × 15
15 × 30	30 × 40	$6\frac{1}{2} \times 8\frac{1}{2}$	12 × 15
15 × 40	35·6 × 35·6	8 × 10	7 × 17
18 × 24	35·6 × 43·2	6 × 12	14 × 14
20 × 40		10 × 12	14 × 17

Roll film $\begin{cases} 30 \text{ cm} \times 15 \text{ metres} \\ 30 \text{ cm} \times 25 \text{ metres} \end{cases}$

INDEX

ABDOMINAL ANGIOGRAPHY

abdomino-peripheral angiography unit, (Bart's) 591
anaesthetic—general, local 592
cassette changers: manual, automatic to include limbs 572, 573, 591
exposure rate, exposure factors 592, 595
opaque media: quantity, catheterization, injection, interosseous, retrograde, translumbar 591, 592
  sensitivity test 580
  see also SUPPLEMENT 1 768
preliminary exposure 591
protection 574
AORTOGRAPHY
abdominal aorta and branches 590
vessels of lower limbs 590
PORTOPHLEBOGRAPHY, PORTOVENOGRAPHY
liver, spleen 595
PORTOSPLENOGRAPHY
direct injection—splenic vein 595
RENAL ANGIOGRAPHY
injection level, general, selective 593, 594, 595
kidneys, arteriogram, nephrogram 593, 594
TOMOGRAPHY 595
  see also ANGIOGRAPHY 572

ANGIOGRAPHY, GENERAL 572–574

automatic programme selector 572, 573
cassette and film changers:
  manual operation—longitudinal, transverse 572, 573
  mechanical operation 572, 573
  simultaneous biplane 572, 574
  skull table 576
exposure rate 572
methods: cine—35 mm 572
full size—cut film, roll film 572
miniature—roll film, 70 mm 574
opaque media, injection methods 572
  see also SUPPLEMENT 1
processing 574
protection 574, 576
  see also SUPPLEMENT 2 773

CARDIAC ANGIOGRAPHY

catherization 581, 584
conditions investigated: heart—congenital, rheumatic; lung tumours 580
exposure conditions 580–585
  films, grids, screens 572
film changers: large cut or roll film 572
            cine, 35 mm 586
            miniature, 70 mm 572
heart and great vessels 580
opaque media: allergic tendencies 580
            quantity—adult, child 580
            rate of injection 684
            sensitivity test 580
  see also SUPPLEMENT 1 768

CARDIAC ANGIOGRAPHY (*continued*)

positioning: simultaneous biplane—
            antero-posterior/lateral 582
            oblique/oblique 584
precautions 574
programme selector 573
simultaneous biplane technique 574

CEREBRAL ANGIOGRAPHY

anaesthetic 575
anatomical diagrams 575
arteriogram, phlebogram (venogram), sinogram 575
include 579
cassette changers—automatic, manual, Rapidex 572, 573, 576
exposure conditions, exposure rate 576, 577
immobilization 576
methods: direct—cut and roll film 572
        indirect—cine, 35 mm 572
                miniature, 70 mm 572
opaque media: injection—by incision 572
                    percutaneous 572, 575
            sensitivity test 575
  see also SUPPLEMENT 1 768
projections: antero-posterior, lateral, oblique, half-axial 578, 579
radiation exposure, filter 616, 618
  see also SUPPLEMENT 2
skull table 576
subtraction 588

CINERADIOGRAPHY

applications 758, 763–765
cine camera 760
cine speeds 760–763
cinefluorography 758, 760
exposure technique 762
film strips:
  angiocardiography 764
  bladder and urethra 765
  cerebral angiography 765
  oesophagus 765
  pyelogram 765
  stomach and duodenum 765
films used: 16 mm, 35 mm 758, 760
  frames per subject, frames per second 762
  fine-focus tube 760
  fluorescent screen 758, 761
  image intensifier 758
  intensification factor 758
  optics: lens, mirror 696
  processing and copying 763
  television: cameras 758, 760
            Orthicon 760
            monitoring 758, 760

DENTAL

anatomical features   470, 471, 473
cassette: collar   493
   flexible   495
cone, localizing, protective   472, 478
dentitions, deciduous, permanent   470–473
distortion—vertical, lateral   477
examination of mouth   472
exposure conditions, table   478, 479
film-holders, loaders   474
films: identification of   479
  types of   472
mouth: broad, narrow   475
   occlusal planes   476, 480, 486
positioning: vertical, horizontal   476, 477
processing, hangers, unit   479
request formula: adults, children   472, 473
units, output, timing, control   472
viewing   479

CHILDREN
presence of both dentitions   470, 473
request formula   472

CROWNS
caries dental film-holders, positioning   489

EDENTULOUS
film series   488
roots, buried   488

EXTRA-ORAL   470, 488, 492
edentulous   488
lower jaw   492, 493

INTRA-ORAL
lower jaw   484–487
upper jaw   480–483

OCCLUSAL PLANES   490
projections: lower jaw   491
    upper jaw   490

PANAGRAPHY (pan-oral)
enlargement, equipment   494, 495
flexible cassette   495
jaws, lower, upper   494, 496
tube in mouth, fine-focus   494, 495

RADIATION PROTECTION   478

ROTOGRAPHY (roto-tomography)
craniostat, equipment   496, 497
examples   498
facio-maxillary   497
positioning, movement   496, 497

TEETH
correct projection of   476, 477, 480–487
deciduous, permanent   470–473
position in jaw, alveolar (gum)   470, 471
unerupted   470, 498

FEMALE REPRODUCTIVE SYSTEM

GENERAL
anatomical features—ovaries, uterine tubes, uterus,
  vagina, vulva   682
BASIC positions   687–691
exposure conditions   684
genetic hazards   684
patient: care of, preparation of   683, 684
pelvis: types, public arch   683
range of examinations   683
sacral curve   683

GYNAECOGRAPHY
air insufflation, rate of injection   686
anaesthesia   686
exposure conditions, factors   712
positioning   686

FEMALE REPRODUCTION SYSTEM (continued)

premedication   686
rapid development   686

HYSTEROSALPINGOGRAPHY
anaesthetic   684
exposure factors   712
investigations for abortion, fibroids, sterility, tumours   684
opaque media, injection of   684, 685
positions: antero-posterior, oblique   684
premedication   684
uterine tubes, patency of   685
uterus, cervix of   682
see also PELVIMETRY   706, 710
see also PREGNANCY   687

FOREIGN BODIES

GENERAL
foreign bodies: non-opaque, of varying opacity,
  opaque   724, 740
opacified surgical swab   724
operative measures   734
stages in investigation   724
  (1) initial routine examination   724
  (2) anatomical location   724
  (3) localization of depth   724
war conditions   704, 705

INITIAL EXAMINATION
gas in tissues   724
position of surface wounds   724
routine projections: exploratory, of large area   724, 732, 733
soft tissue   724

ANATOMICAL LOCATION   724
positioning, general, localized   725–733
screening   725–733
soft tissue   733

ALIMENTARY TRACT
gastro-intestinal, barium meal   732
  children, clothing, opacities   732
  coin, swallowed, evacuation of   733
  ileocolic valve   713
  opaque bodies, small, diffusion of   732
  operative measures, screening   734
oesophagus, denture, needle   732, 733
  obstruction, opaque, non-opaque   732
  position: right anterior oblique   732
pharynx and upper oesophagus   732
  barium swallow, bolus   732
  fish bone, coin, gristle   732
  throat, abrasion of   732

HEAD
cranium, face—cheeks, jaw, lips, optic, canal, orbital cavity,
  tongue   726–727

LIMBS
positioning, screen examination   725

RESPIRATORY SYSTEM
bronchography   731
respiration, screen examination   730
tangential projections, tomography   730
tooth, inhaled   731

TRUNK
abdomen   729
clavicle   728
diaphragm   729
hip, metal rings over wound   729
pelvis   729
sacrum   729
scapula, shoulder   728
thorax: organs, ribs   729
vertebrae: cervical, lumbar   728

FOREIGN BODIES (*continued*)

LOCALIZATION OF DEPTH
basis, Mackenzie Davidson method   737
  general   719, 737
foreign bodies: number, opacity, size, type   724, 734
geometrical projection:
  flat, in three dimensions   737
  parallax   739
  triangulation   722, 723–725, 738
margin of error: general, for eye   737
marking skin surface:
  adjusting angle of approach   734
  metal markers on skin   734
  screening limitations, image intensifier   734
  sterile surgical needle   734
measurements:
  focus-table top, calculation   736
patient: compression avoided   734
  cassette and screen supported   734
  curved surfaces negotiated   734
  distance deducted, wound position indicated   734
preliminary experiments: for eye, general   736
processing: rapid development   735
tube shift: direction, centring, divided exposure   734, 735
          measurement, rule on couch   716, 717
METHODS:
  SCREEN AND FILM
    parallax
      localizer positioning, screening, tube shift   737, 739
    triangulation
      depth formula, table of calculations   737, 738
ORBITAL CAVITY
charts   745, 746, 748
cross-wires, use of   742
eye, diameter of   740
  mobility of, muscles of   741, 742
foreign body, confirmation of presence   740
immobilization of head   726, 730, 733
ocular fixation   741
positions: lateral   742
          occipito-mental   742

HIGH KILOVOLTAGE

Exposure time   714
Film Quality   714
focal spot size   714
Positive and Negative Contrast   714
Repetitive Exposure   714
Screen   714
Subject Contrast   714
Suitable Subjects   714

LACRIMAL SYSTEM

iodized oil, injection of   505
lacrimal apparatus: ducts, gland, sac   505
positions: lateral, occipito-mental   505
see also MACRORADIOGRAPHY   630–632

LYMPHANGIOGRAPHY

Anatomical features   601
  infection procedures   601, 602
  lower limb   601
  opaque media   601, 602
  upper limb

MACRORADIOGRAPHY

contrast and enlargement, kilovoltage control   621
definition   620, 626, 628
density control   621, 622
distance: focus-film, subject-film   620, 621
enlarged image, degree of   620, 622
film: screen, non-screen   621
immobilization   621
intensifying screens   620, 628, 668
localizing cone   621
Perspex: vertical support   628
         window in couch   621
regions: chest, lungs   628, 629
elbow, normal   624, 625, 638, 639
elbow, fracture—pinning screw   622
lacrimal system   630, 631
lower thigh, combined macro, contact   640, 641
public bone—ischium   632
temporal bones   626, 627
wrist, normal   623

MINIATURE RADIOGRAPHY

alignment   754
camera unit: horizontal, vertical, angled   751
cassettes: roll film, Rapidex   752
           cut film, Separator   752
control table, automatic sequence   751, 754
definition   686–688, 694
distance: focus-film   750
          focus-screen   750, 755
examinees: clothing, groups   750
           recalls   750
film: cut film, roll film   750
      dimensions, perforated, unperforated   688, 750, 753
      image size   753
      large film comparison   755
height adjustment: flexible cable system, lift   754
identification device   752
large films   750, 755, 756
mass examinations   750, 755
mirror optics: systems, field coverage, definition, resolution, speed relationship   751–752
Odelca camera unit   752
optics: lens, mirror, focusing   752
photo-timer   691
positioning: subject type   754
processing: roll film—daylight tank, frame   755
            cut film—frames, slotted carrier   755
projection: projector, screen   755
protection: lead, lead glass, scatter   752
record card   752
screen-film combination: blue, yellow-green   755
tube, diaphragm   752
viewing: magnification, projection   755

MULTIPLE RADIOGRAPHY

cassette, deepened   636
intensifying screens, two speeds arranged selectively in single cassette   634
DUPLICATION
example—lungs   636
SIMULTANEOUS CONTACT AND ENLARGEMENT
example—angiography of lower thigh   637, 638
WIDE-RANGE
examples—cervical region, bone and soft tissue; pregnancy, foetus and placenta; thoraco-lumbar vertebrae; bronchography, heart and lung densities   634, 635

III

MYELOGRAPHY

anatomical features   564, 565
cerebro-spinal fluid   564, 565
cisternal injection   567,
contrast media—air, opaque   565, 567, 568
image intensifier   565
injection—sub-occipital, lumbar   564
neural canal   565
spinal cord   564
   membranes—arachnoid, dura mater, pia mater   564
   spaces—extradural, subarachnoid, subdural   564
tilting couch: horizontal, erect, reverse   565–567
EXTRADURAL SPACE   564
INTERVERTEBRAL DISCS
calcification   569
opaque injection—discography   569
positioning   569
protrusion of disc   569
screen examination   569
SUBARACHNOID SPACE
air or oxygen, injection   564, 565
aspiration   568
exposures—general, localized, serial   567, 568
movements—longitudinal, rotational   566
obstruction—complete, partial   567

OPTIC FORAMINA

abnormalities   533
dry bone projections   531, 532
positioning: (1) general couch   532, 534
          (2) skull table   533

PANAGRAPHY

cassette, interior fluorescent coating, flexible,
   lead-backed   495
fast film   495
magnification   494
pan-oral panoramic survey of teeth   494
patient: anode stem—bite ridge, adjustable sterile cover;
   494, 495
positioning: lower jaw   495
         upper jaw   494, 495
radiation protection: anode stem lead covered,
   target area 2 mm aluminium filter   494
X-ray tube in mouth, fine-focus, low rating   494, 495

PELVIMETRY

angle of pelvic inclination   711
Caesarean operation   706
calculation of pelvic diameters by:
   geometrical correction scale   709
   mathematical formula   708
   perforated metal ruler   710
calipers   708
cephalometry, pelvicephalometer   600
distance: focus-film   707
        diameters to film   706
exposure conditions, table   712
foetal head diameters   711
grids, crossed   576
pelvic diameters: bi-ischial spinous, oblique, outlet,
   transverse, true conjugate   706
pelvimetry—backrest, chair, couch, vertical stand
   586, 587, 597, 598
positions: antero-posterior   579, 596–598, 706
        lateral erect   596, 706
        supero-inferior, inlet, outlet, 586, 587, 597

PELVIMETRY (*continued*)

pubic arch—subpubic arch   575, 586, 587
radiation protection, precautions   576
   foetal gonads   586
   see also SUPPLEMENT 2   776
see also FEMALE REPRODUCTIVE SYSTEM   682
see also PREGNANCY   687

PERIPHERAL ANGIOGRAPHY

ARTERIOGRAPHY
anaesthetic   596
cassette: changer   597, 598
     long—for one or three films   596, 597
collateral circulation—femoral block   599
exposure conditions: serial films   597
graduated wedge filter   597
injection: lower limb—single, both limbs   596, 597, 599
       upper limb—single   598
opaque media: rate of injection   596
scanography: movement, slit diaphragm   597
VENOGRAPHY
arterial graft   599
collateral circulation—incompetence, venal block   599, 600
couch tilted 15°, 65°   599
exposure: conditions, timing   596, 600
opaque media: injection—following incision,
   percutaneous, Polythene catheter   599, 600
   sensitivity test   599
positioning: antero-posterior   597, 599
       lateral   596, 599
Valsalva manoeuvre   599, 600
varicose veins, ulcers   599, 600
venous valves   599
see also ANGIOGRAPHY, GENERAL   572

PREGNANCY

ADVANCED
anencephalia   687
breech presentation   688, 689, 701
care of patient   684
compression, wide band   688, 689, 692
exposure conditions, table   712
filter—graduated, half-way, plastic lead   698, 699
hydramnios   687
hydrocephalus   687
investigations for—
   age of foetus   687, 703
   extension of limbs   701
   foetal abnormality   687
   foetal death   687, 701
   foetal maturity   687, 701
   foetus stillborn   703
   multiplicity   687, 702
   position of placenta   698–700
   presentation   687–697
placenta praevia   698–700
placental site   698–700
placentography   698, 700
positions: BASIC   683, 688, 689, 690, 691, 692
     antero-posterior   688, 693, 696, 708
     lateral, erect   692
       general   690, 708
        supine   691
     oblique   694
     postero-anterior   689, 693
     supero-inferior, inlet   695
        outlet   697

PREGNANCY (*continued*)

radiation protection, precautions 684
respiration 687, 689
Spalding's sign 701
vertex presentation 688, 689, 690
viewing illumination 698
see also FEMALE REPRODUCTIVE SYSTEM 682
see also PELVIMETRY 706
AMNIOGRAPHY
amniotic fluid 704
opaque media 704
EARLY PREGNANCY
exposure factors 712
location of foetus 687
postero-anterior 687
respiration 687, 689
FOETUS
stillborn 703
UROGRAPHY
cystography 704, 705
opaque media 704
pyelography 704

ROTOGRAPHY, ROTO-TOMOGRAPHY

curved cassette, adjustable, clamped to turntable 496, 497
curved objects examined 496
density wedges for uniformity 497
exposure conditions 497
exposure during 180° rotation, precautions, pituitary body 497
facio-maxillary investigation 497, 498
immobilization by modified craniostat 496, 497
patient/film rotation in opposite directions 496
specimen rotographs 498
condylar heads, mouth open 498
fracture, angle of mandible 498
showing both dentitions, fracture dislocation right condyle 498

SALIVARY GLANDS

anatomical features 500
calculi 500, 504
ducts: parotid 500
sublingual 312, 500
submandibular 500, 503, 504
iodized oil, injection of 500, 504
PAROTID
positions: antero-posterior 502
lateral-general, dental film 501
oblique 309, 501
profile 502
sialography 500–502
SUBLIGUAL
positions: inferio-superior 504
lateral 504
SUBMANDIBULAR (SUBMAXILLARY)
positions: infero-superior (1), (2) 503
lateral 504
sialograms 504

SELECTIVE FILTRATION

purpose of 719
use without grid 719
with grid 719

SOFT TISSUE

bone and soft tissue, hands 617
kilovoltage variation 610

SOFT TISSUE (*continued*)

limbs 612
multiple, wide-range 610
plastic bone replacement 616
SUMMARY OF CONDITIONS INCLUDED 611–618
ADENOIDS
operation, films exposed before, after 611
position: lateral 611
ANEURYSM 611
ARTHRITIS, RHEUMATOID 617
CALCIFICATION OF TENDONS 615
due to trauma 615
CALCIFIED ARTERIES
examples—foot, lower leg, pelvis 614
CYSTICERCOSIS 615
CYST 611
EMPHYSEMA
various causes 612
GAS GANGRENE 612
GOUT 617
HAEMATOMA 612
LIPOMA 613
LOSS OF TISSUE MASS 613
MAMMARY DUCTS, GLANDS (MAMMOGRAPHY) 604–609
carcinoma, female, male 605
exposure technique 608
fine-focus tube 608
industrial film 608
localizing cone, flattened 606
lead marker pellet 607

STEREOGRAPHY

films: exposure, marking, processing 676
focus-film distance 676
immobilization 676
localizing cone, use of 676
orthoscopic, pseudoscopic 678
steroscopic viewing, placing films correctly 676, 678
tube centring, tube shift 676, 678
STEREOMETRY
pelvic diameters 679
STEROSCOPE
binocular type 679
dual viewing 678, 679
precision 679
direct measuring 679
Wheatstone 677–679

STEREOTAXIS

cerebral localization, insertion of probe or needle for therapeutic injection 558
craniostat localizer 558, 559
methods—two described:
(1) air in ventricles 558
chiefly for Parkinson's disease 558
injection into thalamus 558
localizing instrument, external protractor, two-way adjustment 558
probe inserted, adjustable in three dimensions 559
projections: antero-posterior, lateral 418
(2) pre-selected objective, precision approach 559
burr holes in cranium 559
equipment:
arcuate instrument director, adjustable in three dimensions 558, 559
craniotsat fixed by four screws 559
double grids to check accuracy 559

V

STEREOTAXIS (*continued*)

    metal cap and ball apparatus for insertion of
      needle 559
    telescopic centring from 12 feet FFD 559
    opaque medium injected into frontal horn of
      lateral ventricle 559
    projections:
      antero-posterior, and confirmed with tube
        shift 559
      lateral 559
    therapeutic injection 559

SUBTRACTION

elimination of bone structures emphasizing opacified
  vessels 587
examples: abdominal 589
      cardiac 586–588
      cerebral 588
plain radiograph (control film) copied as positive
  transparency 587
positive copy superimposed on angiogram (contrast film)
  for transparency to produce subtraction copy 587
processing 587
technique 586–588
see ANGIOGRAPHY 572

TEMPORAL BONE

anatomical features 508, 509
angle board, use of 512, 515
equipment 510
film, definition, identification of 511
planes, lines and landmarks 510
technique 511
MASTOID—ANTRUM, PROCESS
positions: BASIC 512–518
      35° fronto-occipital 518
      lateral (1) head tilted 517
        (2) angle board 516
        (3) tube angled 517
      occipito-vertical 518
      profile (1) angle board 512
        (2) postero-anterior, oblique 514
PETROUS
auditory nerve tumour 519
auditory ossicles 508, 509, 520
equipment 522, 525
labyrinth—internal ear, cochlea, semicircular canals,
  vestibule 508, 509
macroradiography 528
positions: 35° fronto-occipital 527
      lateral 522, 525
      oblique: postero-anterior 523
        lateral 526
      submento-vertical 527
radiographs and tracing diagrams 520
skull table 525
tomography 529, 530
tympanic cavity—middle ear, incus, malleus, stapes
  508, 509
tympanic membrane 508, 509
see MACRORADIOGRAPHY 620
see TOMOGRAPHY 644

TOMOGRAPHY

GENERAL
apparatus 644, 646, 659
axis or fulcrum of movement 644, 645
charts—positioning and levels (approx.) 674–677

TOMOGRAPHY (*continued*)

confirmation of depth, of exposure angle 647, 648
depth scale 647
diffusion of unwanted shadows 644, 650, 652
estimation of number of layers 660
      spacings 660
exposure table, sequential method 662
film driving pin 645
focus-film distance 646, 647
linear, non-linear movement 652, 653, 654
localization—lungs 655, 656
movements, tube: circular, curvilinear, elliptical,
  hypocycloidal, rectilinear, sine wave, spiral 652, 653, 654
objective plane 644
operative angle—symmetrical, unsymmetrical 651
Polytome, tortuous movement 652, 654
principle of 654
respiration, same stage each level 665
section spacing, intervals 648, 660
tomographic switches 645
trisection 666
tube movement, angle 648, 661, 662, 663, 664
EXAMPLES
auditory ossicles 653, 654
chest—enlarged vessels 662
      foreign body 663
clavicle 656
dry bone skull—variable movements 652, 653, 654
larynx, vocal folds 651, 662
lungs—apices, lesion 659
mandible 664
petrous temporal 653, 654
skull 661
sterno-clavicular joints 662
temporo-mandibular joints 664
trachea—bifurcation, deviation 658
vertebrae—bone lesion. lumbar 663
      thoracic 663
AXIAL TRANSVERSE SECTIONS
alignment 673
equipment 673, 674
exposure conditions 673
focus-film distance 3 metres 673, 674
immobilization of patient 673
lung sections 673, 674
mandible 673
movement—film on turn table, patient on pedestal 673, 674
principle of 673
tube angle 30° 673, 674
SIMULTANEOUS MULTISECTION (MULTITOMOGRAPHY)
advantages—some reduction in radiation dosage, same
  phase of respiration, saves time 665
example, three layers: lung—antero-posterior, 667
fulcrum of movement levels shown, skull and step wedge
  665
intensifying screens, graduated speeds for even film
  density 665
magazine, five or more layers—films, intensifying
  screens, spacers, compression block 665
Polystyrene spacers 665
TRISECTION
deep cassette for three levels 666, 667
minimum spacings—middle ear 668
      auditory ossicles 668

VENTRICULOGRAPHY AND ENCEPHALOGRAPHY

anatomical features 538, 539
air injection: spinal canal, ventricles 540, 541

VENTRICULOGRAPHY AND ENCEPHALOGRAPHY
(*continued*)

apparatus: couch, skull table   542, 543
aqueduct of midbrain   538
autotomography   416, 417, 557
burr holes   414, 415, 538
cerebro-spinal fluid, air replacement   538, 540
child   555
comparative radiographs and
      tracing diagrams   545–554
encephalography   555
fourth ventricle   538, 541
interventricular foramen   538
lateral ventricles   538, 539
opaque injection   538, 556
planes, lines and landmarks   544
positions: (1) supine, fronto-occipital   545
    (2) supine, 30° fronto-occipital (half-axial)   546
    (3) supine, lateral   547
    (4) prone, occipito-frontal   548
    (5) prone, 30° occipito-frontal (reverse
    half-axial)   549
    (6) prone, lateral   550
    (7) lateral, right and left   551
    (8) supine, lateral, head lowered   552
    (9) erect, fronto-occipital   553
   (10) erect, lateral   554

skull table demonstrated   543
third ventricle   538, 539
AUTOTOMOGRAPHY
arcuate movement about axis 10°—spontaneous,
  controlled   557
third and fourth ventricles   557
ENCEPHALOGRAPHY   538, 555
encephalograms (child), eight positions   555
positions: occipito-frontal, lateral   555
posture for lumbar puncture   555
GAMMA RAY SCANNING
recording by thermo-electric marker,
     by photographic paper or X-ray film   561
scintillograms of cranium   561
selective concentration of radioactive material disclosing
  abnormal condition   561
OPAQUE INJECTION
biplane screening, television   556
controlled movement of head   556
lateral ventricle, passage to fourth ventricle   556
STEREOTAXIS   558
cerebral localization in three dimensions   558
localizer, craniostat; two methods   558, 559
therapeutic injection   558, 559
ULTRASOUND INVESTIGATION
recordings on oscilloscope   560
    by Polaroid camera   561
reflected ultrasound vibrations   561